The Excimer Manual

Ahmad,

It was a great pleasure for me to have you cooperate in the writing of this book as one of the coauthors. It has been a great 2 years working together with you on laser projects and I look forward to our future collaboration -

Best Regards,

[signature] MD

The Excimer Manual
A Clinician's Guide
to Excimer Laser Surgery

Jonathan H. Talamo, M.D.
Assistant Clinical Professor of Ophthalmology,
Harvard Medical School; Cornea Consultants; Medical Director,
The Laser Eye Center of Boston, Boston

Ronald R. Krueger, M.D., M.S.E.
Assistant Professor of Ophthalmology, Saint Louis University School
of Medicine; Cornea and Refractive Surgery, Anheuser-Busch Eye
Institute, St. Louis

Forewords by

Stephen Trokel, M.D.
Clinical Professor of Ophthalmology,
Columbia-Presbyterian Medical Center, New York

Theo Seiler, M.D., Ph.D.
Professor and Chairman, Department of Ophthalmology, Technical
University and University Eye Clinic, Dresden, Germany

Little, Brown and Company
Boston New York Toronto London

Library of Congress Cataloging-in-Publication Data

The excimer manual : a clinician's guide to excimer laser surgery
   [edited by] Jonathan H. Talamo, Ronald R. Krueger.
      p. cm.
   Includes bibliographical references and index.
   ISBN 0-316-83175-1
   1. Eye—Laser surgery. I. Talamo, Jonathan H. II. Krueger, Ronald R.
   [DNLM: 1. Keratectomy, Photorefractive, Excimer Laser—methods. 2. Cornea—surgery. 3. Refractive Errors—surgery.
WW 220 E96   1996]
RE86.E974   1996
617.7´19—dc20
DNLM/DLC
for Library of Congress   96-33145
                                                                   CIP

Printed in the United States of America

MV-NY

Editorial: Tammerly J. Booth, Joanne S. Toran
Production Editor: Marie A. Salter
Copyeditor: Joan Kocsis
Indexer: Alexandra Nickerson
Production Supervisor/Designer: Louis C. Bruno, Jr.
Cover Designer: Artillery Studios

To my loving wife, Andrea, and my daughters, Erica and Rachel, for their patience and support during this project; and

To my father, the late Richard C. Talamo, M.D., whose encouragement and example inspired me to strive for excellence in medicine

J.H.T.

To my father, the late Arthur M. Krueger, and my mother, Lucie Krueger, whose constant interest, support, and encouragement inspired me to pursue a career in medicine and to follow my research interests in excimer laser photoablation. Without their early influence and that of my mentor, Stephen Trokel, M.D., the groundwork for this book would not have been possible; and

To my niece, Kirsten Marie Krueger, who was conceived, born, and dedicated to Jesus Christ during the conception, writing, and publication of this book. It is my hope that this book will inspire her to pursue excellence and follow her dreams in life.

R.R.K.

Contents

Foreword

Excimer laser surgery has been in clinical development since 1985, when the first excimer clinical prototypes were built. The rate of its application to corneal surgery for refractive and therapeutic use accelerated with the successful treatment of the first pathological corneas reported in 1986 and the first successful photorefractive keratectomy (PRK) reported in 1988. In highly detailed and complex statistical studies designed to substantiate safety and efficacy for the United States Food and Drug Administration (FDA), thousands of patients were treated under rigorous and defined investigative protocols. The more flexible approach taken internationally fostered such rapid development of applications that excimer technology has displaced other refractive surgical procedures in most parts of the world. A number of ophthalmic surgeons now devote their practices full time to refractive surgery using the excimer laser. The recent approval by the FDA allows users in the United States access to this technology to a 7 diopter limit without treatment of associated astigmatism—finally this technology is available to ophthalmic surgeons in the United States.

This book, dedicated to the clinical, technical, and economic considerations of excimer laser corneal surgery, draws on the experiences of users in the United States and abroad. It is particularly timely as new users of this technology will want to know not only the approved labeling permitted by the FDA, but also the many innovative applications that have been devised by surgeons worldwide.

Practical experience is necessary to avoid and manage complications. This knowledge requires the kind of clinical exposure that can only be generated in an unregulated environment. The experience of many clinical investigators and laser users, both those working within the regulatory environment in the United States and international users working in an unregulated environment, have been brought together in this volume, which makes it a particularly useful clinical compendium.

Readers in the United States will find detailing of patient selection, surgical techniques, and management of complications of immediate interest and importance; however, they may be frustrated by the discussions of astigmatism, high myopia, and hyperopia—procedures not yet approved by the FDA for use in the United States. So-called nonapproved or "practice of medicine" applications of PRK—including laser in-situ keratomileusis (LASIK) and PRK following other surgical procedures, such as radial keratotomy (RK), corneal tranplantation, and cataract surgery—are presented with discussion of optimal techniques and the results obtained. This text is a rare source for this clinical information.

In one section of the book, the techniques and results of the LASIK procedure are presented in detail. LASIK is an exciting surgical application that creates the refractive change under a lamellar flap. This reduces postoperative pain, extends the stability of the refractive procedure to higher levels of myopia, and may produce a more stable refractive result.

Therapeutic uses of the excimer laser tend to be overshadowed by refractive applications. While the emphasis of this book is refractive surgery, the indications for therapeutic applications are well described, as are the different surgical techniques employed. Today, phototherapeutic keratectomy (PTK) plays an important role in corneal surgical practice, and knowing when and how to use the excimer laser in this context is essential.

Because the excimer laser is a new and evolving technology, the text describes this technology in detail and several chapters are devoted to the technical aspects of the different excimer laser systems. Both the scientific aspects and the variety of technical approaches to the problems of re-contouring the corneal surface are described. The Technical Considerations section is a valuable resource for specific information about individual excimer lasers that are commercially available for clinical use.

Cost and economic considerations are also addressed in detail by a group that has spent considerable time in the real world analyzing these factors using different refractive and excimer technologies. Discussion of informed consent and sample forms are also included for consideration by new users.

It is clear that the excimer laser has become an essential part of refractive and corneal surgery and now comprises a key element of ophthalmic practice. This book brings the ophthalmic surgeon into this emerging field and offers current information. *The Excimer Manual* is one of the first books to comprehensively cover all aspects of excimer corneal surgery; it is a practical resource that will greatly benefit the clinician using or considering use of this powerful new surgical technology.

Stephen Trokel, M.D.

erſt in ihrem Alter auf dieſe Kunſt begeben wollen: wie es zwar heut
zu Tage ihrer viel giebt/die dergleichen gethan.

Zum fünften ſo ſoll ein jeder Wund-Artzt und Barbierer/ der
die Augen und Schnitt-Artzney/ glücklich/ recht und mit Nutzen zu
treiben und zu practiciren begehret/ dieſelbige bey berühmten/ wol
erfahrnen und perfecten Oculiſten und Schnitt-Aertzten gelernet
und begriffen haben. Dann bey den jetzigen Wund-Aertzten und
Barbierern wird man dieſe Kunſt ſchwerlich recht lernen/ als wel-
che ſie ſelbſten wenigſten Theils recht verſtehen/ und heiſſet wol mit
ihnen/ wie der Poet Ovidius ſagt:

Quodcunque parum novit, nemo docere poteſt.

Fürs ſechſte iſt einem jeden Oculiſten und Schnitt-Artzt von-
nöthen/ daß er geſunde und friſche Augen/ und ein ſcharffes klares
und gutes Geſicht habe/ damit er ſeinem Patienten alle Gebrechen
und Mängel der Augen bald möge ſehen und eigentlich kennen/ wor-
zu dann ein gutes und ſcharffes Geſicht nothwendig erfordert wird.

Zum ſiebenden ſoll ein Oculiſt und Schnitt-Artzt nicht lahme
etwan gar zu grobe und ungeſchickte/ ſondern fein gerade/ ſubtile
und geſunde Arme/ Hände und Finger haben/ auch damit hurtig
und geſchwind/ und gleich Lincks und Rechts ſeyn/ damit er beyde
Hände zugleich miteinander führen und brauchen können möge/ welches dann ſonderlich im Staarn-würcken und Staarn-ſtechen hoch
vonnöthen iſt/ da ſonſten diejenige/ die nicht Lincks ſeyn/ den Staa-
ren von hinterwärts würcken müſſen/ welches aber gantz wider die
Natur iſt/ und gar nicht fein ſtehet/ auch denen Patienten öffters ſo
viel ſchadet/ daß ſie dadurch ehender blind als ſehend gemacht wer-
den. Damit ſich nun ein Oculiſt deſto leichter darzu gewähnen mö-
ge/ als wird es nicht undienlich für ihn hierzu ſeyn/ wann er ſich
etwan für die lange Weile auf künſtlichen Inſtrumenten/ als Harf-
fen/ Lauten und dergleichen zu Zeiten exerciren und üben wird.

Achtens/ dieweil ein Oculiſt und Schnitt Artzt viel ſubtile
Inſtrumenta ſo von Gold/ Silber und Eiſen müſſen gemacht wer-
den/ bedarff und brauchen muß/ als iſt ihme ſehr nöthig/ daß er des
mahlens und reiſſens erfahren ſey/ alldieweilen es nicht wol moglich/

daß

Excerpt from *Augendienst* by Georg Bartisch.

Foreword

One of the landmarks in modern ophthalmology dates back to 1583—*Augendienst*, a book written by the Dresden ophthalmologist Georg Bartisch. Early on, Bartisch describes the twelve conditions he believes an ophthalmologist must fulfill in order to be successful. Among others, he demands that an ophthalmologist be educated by famous, experienced, and "perfect oculists." In addition, he complains that there are many doctors in the field who do not understand what they are doing.

Although written in 1583, Bartisch's comments are still relevant today. If we consider the current state of refractive laser surgery in light of Bartisch's recommendations, we realize that, as surgeons, we should be educated by teachers who are experienced and who understand the basic principles of laser photoablation, techniques, and wound healing and its modulation—the editors of this book are such teachers.

Dr. Jonathan Talamo is a refractive surgeon with many years experience who has extensive PRK expertise as a result of his active cooperation with Mexican refractive surgery centers (Monterrey, Mexico) and University Eye Clinics in Europe (Dresden, Germany). Dr. Ronald Krueger has worked with the excimer laser both experimentally and clinically since 1984, long before he became a doctor of medicine. His outstanding contributions to the field are well recognized and demonstrate his continual interest. I had the opportunity to regard both Dr. Talamo and Dr. Krueger's expertise during their fellowships in Dresden and Berlin, and I remember many exciting discussions where we learned from each other.

Because the field of laser corneal surgery is rapidly evolving, one potential problem with any book on this subject would be the book's currency. However, because most of the authors who contributed to this text are involved in the research and development of new techniques, this book offers a recent review.

Refractive surgery has evolved into a significant economic factor in ophthalmic practice and will probably surpass cataract surgery in frequency within 10 years. As a consequence, ophthalmologists will experience a pressure to get involved from optometrists, commercial laser centers, and their patients. Although primarily written for ophthalmologists, this book provides useful information and insight to any individual working in the field of refractive surgery.

The editors have carefully selected a distinguished group of authors to share their knowledge and experience with the reader to the patient's benefit. Obviously, this book cannot and does not hope to teach skill; however, it may provide new insight into the different techniques of photorefractive keratectomy, and thus may help the surgeon discover a unique, personal approach.

Theo Seiler, M.D., Ph.D.

Preface

During the past 3 to 5 years, refractive surgery in general and excimer laser surgery in particular have become subjects of intense scrutiny among both the ophthalmic community and the general public. As a result, the rapidly increasing body of knowledge in this area is rather intimidating to the ophthalmologist or optometrist seeking to enter this burgeoning area of ophthalmic practice. The volume of literature on this subject is ever-expanding, and to date there are very few single source documents to which one can turn for both introductory and practical reference information.

With these facts in mind, we have endeavored to create a practical, well-illustrated, and user-friendly book emphasizing both basic principles of patient management and recent (often yet-unpublished) developments in excimer laser surgical techniques and management of postoperative complications. Each of the contributing authors was selected for his or her particular expertise in the field of photorefractive and phototherapeutic excimer laser surgery and laser in-situ keratomileusis.

Although it is impossible to compile a textbook with complete up-to-date clinical results and references in such a rapidly expanding field, we nevertheless hope that *The Excimer Manual* will be consulted to solve frequently encountered problems related to the evaluation, treatment, and postoperative management of patients undergoing photorefractive and phototherapeutic corneal surgery. As an aid to those surgeons just beginning to perform PRK, we have included samples of essential forms in Appendix B.

In addition to coverage of patient management–related issues, the book includes a section devoted entirely to describing and illustrating the unique features of the excimer and solid-state laser systems currently available for photorefractive corneal surgery. Whenever possible, a summary of clinical results for each system is also provided. A "master table" has been included in Appendix A for quick reference and comparisons between laser systems for the prospective user or buyer.

The last chapter of the book deals with the economic aspects of photorefractive surgery. The decision to devote one's time and energy to the practice of refractive surgery can be costly, both in terms of time and capital equipment expeditures. The issues of laser equipment purchases and practice marketing are discussed in detail so that individual practitioners may make careful, informed decisions as to how they will participate.

Finally, this book would not have been possible without the tremendous effort expended by our contributors and the editorial staff at Little, Brown. We are greatly indebted to them for their enormous contributions to this book.

J.H.T.
R.R.K.

Contributing Authors

Juan Carlos Abad, M.D.
Clinical Fellow, Cornea Service, Harvard Medical School and Massachusetts Eye and Ear Infirmary, Boston

Ahmad Abu-Shumays
Director of Photorefractive Systems, Coherent Medical Group, Palo Alto, California

Maria Clara Arbelaez, M.D.
Director of Refractive Surgery, Clinica de Oftalmologia de Cali, Colombia, South America

Penny Asbell, M.D.
Professor of Ophthalmology, Mount Sinai School of Medicine of the City University of New York; Director of Cornea Service, Mount Sinai Medical Center, New York

Kerry K. Assil, M.D.
Director of The Sinskey Eye Institute, Santa Monica, California

Dimitri T. Azar, M.D.
Associate Professor of Ophthalmology, Harvard Medical School; Director, Cornea Service, Massachusetts Eye and Ear Infirmary, Boston

Craig F. Beyer, D.O.
LaserSight Technologies, St. Petersburg, Florida

Stephen M. Blinn
Chief Operating Officer, Sight Resource Corporation, Burlington, Massachusetts

Nils Bonde-Henriksen
Corporate Communications Manager, Sight Resource Corporation, Burlington, Massachusetts

Shu-Wen Chang, M.D.
Lecturer in Ophthalmology, National Taiwan University, Taipei, Taiwan, Republic of China; Fellow in Ophthalmology, The Wilmer Eye Institute, Johns Hopkins University School of Medicine, Baltimore

Arturo S. Chayet, M.D.
Director of Refractive Surgery, Codet Eye Institute, Tijuana, Baja California, Mexico

Daniel S. Durrie, M.D.
Clinical Associate Professor of Ophthalmology, University of Kansas Medical Center; Director of Refractive Surgery, Hunkeler Eye Centers, Kansas City, Missouri

Robert E. Fenzl, M.D.
The Gills Eye Center, Tarpan Springs, Florida

Werner N. Förster, M.D.
Priv-Doz., University Eye Hospital, Munster, Germany

Andrew Garfinkle, M.D., Ph.D.
Assistant Professor of Ophthalmology, McGill University, Montreal, Quebec, Canada

Uwe Genth
Chief Research Scientist, Department of Ophthalmology, Technical University, Dresden, Germany

Marco C. Helena, M.D.
Clinical Fellow in Refractive Surgery, Eye Institute, The Cleveland Clinic Foundation, Cleveland

Kristian Hohla, M.S.C.
Vice President, Chiron Vision, Chiron Technolas GmbH, Dornach, Germany

Sandeep Jain, M.D.
Resident in Ophthalmology, The Harkness Eye Institute, Columbia-Presbyterian Hospital, New York

Paul M. Karpecki, O.D.
Director of Cornea and Refractive Surgery Studies, Indiana University School of Medicine, Bloomington, Indiana

Ernest W. Kornmehl, M.D.
Clinical Instructor in Ophthalmology, Harvard Medical School, Boston

Ronald R. Krueger, M.D., M.S.E.
Assistant Professor of Ophthalmology, Saint Louis University School of Medicine; Cornea and Refractive Surgery, Anheuser-Busch Eye Institute, St. Louis

Shui T. Lai, Ph.D.
President and Founder, Novatec Laser Systems, Inc., Carlsbad, California

Jeffery J. Machat, M.D.
Medical Director, TLC, The Laser Center, Inc., Toronto, Ontario, Canada

Robert J. S. Mack, M.D.
Assistant Professor of Ophthalmology, Rush Medical College of Rush University; Ophthalmologist, Rush Presbyterian-St. Luke's Medical Center, Chicago

Jonathan I. Macy, M.D.
Assistant Clinical Professor of Ophthalmology, University of California, Los Angeles, School of Medicine, Los Angeles

Shareef Mahdavi
Director of Marketing, VISX, Inc., Santa Clara, California

Marguerite McDonald, M.D.
Clinical Professor of Ophthalmology, Tulane University School of Medicine; Chairman, Refractive Surgery Center of the South; Eye, Ear, Nose, and Throat Hospital, New Orleans

Peter J. McDonnell, M.D.
Professor of Ophthalmology, University of Southern California School of Medicine; Director of Refractive Surgery, Doheny Eye Institute, Los Angeles

Martin P. Nevitt, M.D.
Medical Monitor, LaserSight, Orlando, Florida

Ioannis Pallikaris, M.D.
Professor of Ophthalmology, University of Crete Medical School; Director of Ophthalmology Clinic, University Hospital of Heraklion, Heraklion, Crete, Greece

Paul M. Pender, M.D.
Director of Refractive Surgery, Optima Health Eye Center, Manchester, New Hampshire

Peter A. Rapoza, M.D.
Clinical Assistant Professor of Ophthalmology, Harvard Medical School; Cornea Consultants, Boston

Michael A. Romansky, J.D.
Partner, Health Law Department, McDermott, Will and Emery, Washington, D.C.

Alex Sacharoff
Director of Product Development, Summit Technology, Inc., Waltham, Massachusetts

Richard Saver, J.D.
McDermott, Will and Emery, Washington, D.C.

R. Ray Sayano, Ph.D.
Vice President and General Manager, Nidek Technology, Inc., Pasedena, California

David J. Schanzlin, M.D.
Professor of Ophthalmology and Director of Keratorefractive Surgery, Shiley Eye Center, University of California, San Diego, School of Medicine, San Diego

Eckhard Schroder, Ph.D.
Director of Product Management and Applications, Aesculap-Meditec, Jena, Germany

Theo Seiler, M.D., Ph.D.
Professor and Chairman, Department of Ophthalmology, Technical University and University Eye Clinic, Dresden, Germany

Berthold Seitz, M.D.
Research Fellow in Ophthalmology, Doheny Eye Institute, University of Southern California, Los Angeles; Oberarzt, Department of Ophthalmology, Eye Hospital, University of Erlangen-Nurnberg, Erlangen, Germany

Neal A. Sher, M.D.
Associate Clinical Professor of Ophthalmology, University of Minnesota Medical School; Attending Surgeon in Ophthalmology, Phillips Eye Institute, Minneapolis

Dimitrios Siganos, M.D.
Professor of Ophthalmology, University of Crete Medical School, and Consultant in Cornea and Refractive Surgery, Vardinoyannion Eye Institute of Crete; Head of Ophthalmology Clinic, University Hospital of Crete, and Registrar in Ophthalmology, Heraklion University Hospital, Heraklion, Crete, Greece

Walter J. Stark, M.D.
Professor of Ophthalmology, Johns Hopkins University School of Medicine; Director of Cornea Service, The Wilmer Eye Institute, Baltimore

Gerhard Stenger
Herbert Schwind GmbH and Company, Kleinostheim, Germany

Casimir A. Swinger, M.D.
Assistant Clinical Professor of Ophthalmology, Mount Sinai School of Medicine of the City University of New York, New York

Jonathan H. Talamo, M.D.
Assistant Clinical Professor of Ophthalmology, Harvard Medical School; Cornea Consultants; Medical Director, The Laser Eye Center of Boston, Boston

Audrey R. Talley, M.D.
Medical Director and Director of Corneal and Refractive Surgery, TLC Northwest Laser Center, Seattle

Suhas W. Tuli, M.D.
The Wilmer Eye Institute, Johns Hopkins University School of Medicine, Baltimore

Larry C. Van Horn
Autonomous Technologies Corporation, Orlando, Florida

Jesus Vidaurri-Leal, M.D.
Professor of Surgery, Escuela de Medicina I.A. Santos; Chairman, Eye Department, Hospital San Jose, Monterrey N.L., Mexico

Excimer Laser Landmarks

1973 Charles Brau and James Ewing, encouraged by Donald Setser, start work on using rare halides to produce laser action.

1975 Stuart Searles produces the first excimer laser action by bombarding a medium of xenon-bromide with an electron beam gun.

1976 Argon fluoride (ArF) is found to lase, releasing 193 nm photons of laser light.

1979 The first commercial system is made by Tachisto.

1980 Excimer laser designs improve in reliability and output energy, making them suitable for general laboratory use.

1981 The United States Air Force School of Aerospace Medicine first investigates the use of these new lasers on the eye. ArF laser light shows an immediate but temporary indentation of the corneal epithelium, which takes on the shape of the beam. IBM researcher R. Srinivasan patents *photoetching* using the excimer laser and describes the mechanism of action as *photoablative decomposition* (later referred to as *photoablation*).

1983 Stephen Trokel first experiments on the cornea with excimer photoablation and publishes the first article describing its surgical potential. Separate patents on photorefractive keratectomy (PRK) are filed by Stephen Trokel and Francis L'Esperance.

1985 Theo Seiler of Germany performs the first excimer laser phototherapeutic keratectomy (PTK) in a sighted eye. Laser companies such as VISX (Santa Clara, CA) and Summit Technologies (Waltham, MA) begin to emerge.

1987 Francis L'Esperance performs the first PRK in the United States on a blind eye, as the first U.S. Food and Drug Administration (FDA) trial begins.

1988 Marguerite McDonald is the first to achieve a successful refractive result with PRK in a normally sighted myope.

1994   The FDA Ophthalmic Device Panel recommends that the FDA approve the Summit and VISX excimer lasers for PTK and the Summit laser for PRK, with conditions.

1995   The FDA issues premarket approval of the Summit and VISX lasers for PTK and the Summit laser for PRK. The FDA Ophthalmic Device Panel recommends the FDA approve the VISX laser for PRK.

1996   The FDA issues premarket approval of the VISX laser for PRK.

Excimer Laser Glossary

Ablation rate Amount of tissue removed per laser pulse; also known as *ablation depth*.

ALK Automated lamellar keratoplasty.

Argon fluoride (ArF) The rare earth–halogen gas mixture that is excited to stimulate emission of 193-nm excimer laser light.

CVK Computerized videokeratography; this is another name for *corneal topography*. The corneal surface power is recorded on a point-by-point basis on a two-dimensional multicolored map.

Excimer Short for *excited dimer*, which describes the combination of two rare gas atoms. Present-day excimer lasers use the combination of two different elements, a rare gas and a halide, which form an *excited molecular complex*.

Fluence A misnomer because it refers to energy per unit volume instead of energy per unit area. Better terms would be *energy density* or *irradiance*, but "fluence" has become popular.

Haze The increased scattering of light in the anterior corneal stroma secondary to the wound-healing process after a corneal reprofiling procedure.

Lamellar Resection of parallel sides; devoid of refractive power.

LASIK Laser in-situ keratomileusis. Corneal reprofiling procedure in which the excimer laser is applied to the corneal stroma after a lamellar flap of epithelium and anterior stroma are removed temporarily with a microkeratome.

Lenticular Corneal resection of nonparallel sides. It has either positive, negative, or astigmatic power.

Overcorrection The obtained refractive error is of opposite sign or axis to the patient's initial refraction.

PARK (PRKa) Photoastigmatic refractive keratectomy; surface corneal reprofiling procedure using an excimer laser to correct for astigmatism.

Photoablation Newly described mechanism of laser-tissue interaction; shortened from *photoablative decomposition*, described by Srvinivasan in 1983.

PRK Phtorefractive keratectomy; surface corneal reprofiling procedure using an excimer laser.

Pseudomembrane An electron-dense condensation less than 100 nm thick that borders the excimer ablated surface. It has membrane-like properties because it maintains the integrity of a severed cell, is a barrier to water transport, and serves as a template for smooth and easy re-epithelialization.

PTK Phototherapeutic keratectomy; surface corneal reprofiling procedure using an excimer laser to correct for a therapeutic corneal abnormality.

Regression The loss of the initially obtained refractive correction, or *regression*, toward the patient's original refractive error. Regression generally occurs 3 months or longer after surgery. (If regression occurs sooner, often it results from primary undercorrection.)

Repetition rate The frequency of the laser firing rate; expressed in hertz (Hz).

Reprofile To change the curvature of the cornea and hence its refractive power.

Scanning laser A type of laser delivery system in which the ablating spot or slit "scans" or travels across the corneal surface as it reshapes the surface.

Solid-state laser A laser system that generates ultraviolet light from non-gaseous components; it is not an excimer laser.

Steep central islands Areas of central corneal steepening noted by corneal topography following excimer laser PRK. Typically, their diameter ranges from 1–3 mm and their power from 1–3 diopters.

Undercorrection The obtained refractive error is of the same sign or axis as the patient's original refraction and falls short of the target refraction; generally observed within 3 months of surgery. Also referred to as *primary undercorrection*.

I Clinical Considerations

1 Basic Science and Principles

Juan Carlos Abad and Ronald R. Krueger

Laser Physics

How the Excimer Laser Works

The excimer gas laser is a high-energy ultraviolet (UV) laser that has been used with increasing frequency in corneal surgery. First developed in 1975, the excimer laser is used industrially to etch a variety of materials. Taboada [1] reported in 1981 on the corneal epithelial damage from an excimer laser, but it was not until 1983 that Trokel et al. [2] reported that UV light at 193 nm ablated corneal tissue at a predictable rate and, more important, that it produced minimal damage to the surrounding structures [3, 4]. Basic and clinical research on laser corneal surgery in general and excimer lasers in particular has undergone explosive growth since that time, making laser refractive surgery the fastest changing field in ophthalmology today.

Excimer stands for "excited dimer," a term first used by photochemists in 1960 to describe an energized molecule with two identical components. The gas mixture in most excimer lasers is composed of two different molecules instead of one, so the term *excimer* is a misnomer, but its usage is so widespread that it has persisted.

At the heart of the excimer laser is a cavity containing a mixture of a rare gas (i.e., argon, xenon, or krypton) and a halogen (i.e., fluoride, chloride, or bromide) (Fig. 1-1). This gas mixture is pre-ionized by a set of electrodes before a high-voltage current (about 30,000 electron volts [eV]) is applied, with the consequent formation of highly unstable rare gas-halide molecules, which rapidly dissociate, emitting UV light whose wavelength is determined by the particular gas mixture (Table 1-1).

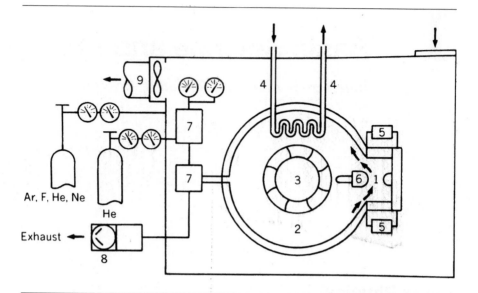

Fig. 1-1. A cross section of a typical excimer cavity shows the internal structural elements of the cylindrically shaped excimer laser in a plane oriented perpendicular to the laser beam path. Water or nitrogen cooling (4) may be necessary to maintain a sustained high output. The laser gas is circulated into the laser channel by the fan (3). The exciting energy is an electrical discharge across the electrodes (6), which creates the ArF-excite molecule. Mirrors that bound the cavity create the laser action. (From SL Trokel. History and mechanism of action of excimer laser corneal surgery. In JJ Salz, PJ McDonnell, MB McDonald [eds]. *Corneal Laser Surgery*. St. Louis: Mosby–Year Book, 1995. P 1.)

To maintain the purity of this mixture, two mechanisms have been employed: (1) frequent replacement with fresh gases, which presents the problem of disposal of the used mixture, and (2) cleansing of the cavity with a nitrogen (cryogenic) device that precipitates contaminants. Both approaches were used in first-generation lasers, but, with improvements in laser construction, contaminant-free cavities are being developed that allow repeated use of a single mixture for longer periods.

Recently, other solid-state UV laser sources have attempted to replace excimer lasers by eliminating the need for using expensive space-occupying gases. The 1064-nm emission of an infrared neodymium:yttrium-aluminum-garnet (Nd:YAG) laser can be modified by nonlinear optics to yield a UV wavelength of 213 nm [5]. Similarly, a neodymium:yttrium-lithium-fluoride (Nd:YLF) laser at 1053 nm can be frequency-quintupled to a wavelength of 211 nm. Although nondisclosed, the Novatec Lightblade laser (Carlsbad, CA) is rumored to use this latter optical setup [6]. However, others believe it uses a frequency-quadrupled titanium:sapphire laser to achieve a wavelength output of 208 nm [6].

Table 1-1. Excimer laser wavelength according to the gas mixture

Gas mixture	Wavelength (nm)
Fluorine (F_2)	155
Argon fluoride (ArF)	193
Krypton chloride (KrCl)	222
Krypton fluoride (KrF)	248
Xenon chloride (XeCl)	308
Nitrogen (N_2)	337
Xenon fluoride (XeFl)	351

Modes of Laser Application

When the excimer laser was introduced to ophthalmology, it was considered a much more accurate scalpel than the diamond blades then available for incisional keratotomy [7]; however, it was soon apparent that the unique characteristics of excimer laser–cornea interaction made it possible to actually reprofile the anterior surface of the cornea [8–11]. This technique, now known as *photorefractive keratectomy* (PRK), allows tissue removal from the anterior surface of the cornea to compensate for the patient's refractive error.

Another way of changing the curvature of the anterior surface of the cornea (and hence the refractive status of the eye) is to apply the laser directly to the corneal stroma after lifting a hinged disc of epithelium and anterior stroma with the microkeratome in a modification of the keratomileusis in-situ procedure [12–14] (Fig. 1-2). Once the laser ablation is done, the disc is repositioned and held in place by the action of the endothelial pump. Usually, no sutures are

Fig. 1-2. Schematic representation of laser in-situ keratomileusis (LASIK). **A.** The microkeratome and the creation of the corneal flap. **B.** The laser irradiation of the corneal stroma underlying the flap. (From IG Pallikaris et al. Laser in situ keratomileusis. *Lasers Surg Med* 10 : 463–468, 1990.)

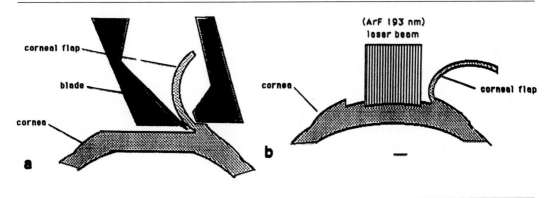

needed. This procedure has been named *laser in-situ keratomileusis* (LASIK); other terms include *excimer keratomileusis* (Excimer-KM) or *"flap-and-zap."*

Biophysics of Corneal Photoablation

Comparison with Other Lasers

Wavelengths from different parts of the electromagnetic spectrum can interact with a variety of ocular tissues, such as the cornea. The following is a brief description of how the other types of lasers used in ophthalmology compare with the excimer laser.

Visible Light Lasers

Wavelengths from 400 nm (violet) and 760 nm (red) comprise the visible part of the electromagnetic spectrum. "Colored" lasers (e.g., argon, krypton, diode) require the absorption of the light energy by tissue pigment (melanin, hemoglobin), which raises the temperature of the pigment in a process known as *photocoagulation* [15, 16].

Infrared Lasers

Infrared wavelengths range from slightly beyond 760 nm (near infrared) to 100,000 nm (far infrared). The near-infrared Nd:YAG laser is used to deliver high amounts of energy to a small area for a short period of time with resultant optical breakdown and "plasma" formation. Nd:YAG lasers are commonly used to perform capsulotomy and iridotomy [17]. The picosecond Nd:YLF laser is being employed to perform intrastromal corneal ablations [18–20]. Mid-infrared lasers, such as the holmium:YAG laser, are used to heat corneal tissue, inducing shrinkage of the stromal collagen fibers to modify the shape of the cornea [21]. Holmium:YAG energy can be delivered by direct contact or a slit-lamp delivery system. Far-infrared lasers, such as the carbon dioxide (CO_2) [22, 23] and erbium:YAG [24], are highly absorbed by water, producing an effect called *photovaporization*, which may have potential for keratorefractive surgery.

Ultraviolet Lasers

Electromagnetic wavelengths in the 100–400 nm range are called ultraviolet. They are divided into UVA (320–400 nm), UVB (290–320 nm), and UVC (100–290 nm). The smaller the wavelength, the greater the energy per photon. The UV wavelengths farther from the visible light band are known as *far-UV*. It is in this latter category of UV lasers that the excimer laser is found.

Mechanism of Photoablation

Theory of Interaction

The far-UV photons emitted by excimer or solid-state UV lasers are of sufficient energy to break intramolecular bonds. This bond-breaking minimizes heating of the tissue and thermal damage to surrounding structures. When the concentration of photons or energy density of laser light exceeds a critical value, the broken bonds no longer recombine, and the material decomposes ablatively, hence the name *ablative photodecomposition* or *photoablation* [25–27]. The driving forces for this ejection of molecular fragments are twofold: First, there is a large increase in the volume of tissue in the decomposed state compared with the polymer chains it replaced. Second, the excess energy of the photons produce kinetic energy to eject this decomposed tissue from the surgical plane. Figure 1-3 demonstrates the process of ablative photodecomposition. Photons are absorbed into the tissue sample, leading to the bond-breaking phenomenon and subsequent ablation. The precision of this type of tissue removal is far superior to that of both photovaporization with a CO_2 laser and photodisruption with a Nd:YAG laser, as shown by the ablation polymethylmethacrylate plastic in Figure 1-4.

Wavelength Dependence

Krueger et al. [28] studied four excimer-generated UV wavelengths in terms of their interaction with corneal tissue by changing the type of gas mixture in the laser cavity: argon-fluoride (193 nm), krypton-fluoride (248 nm), xenon-chloride (308 nm), and xenon-fluoride (351 nm). The smoothness and precision of the 193-nm wavelength can be seen in Figure 1-5, compared with the increased thermal damage to adjacent tissue seen with the longer wavelengths. Based on this and other studies, argon-fluoride (ArF) is the more common gas mixture used in clinical excimer lasers today.

Ablation Threshold

The irradiance, or energy density, is a measure of the amount of laser light energy per unit area projected onto the target tissue. This has often been incorrectly termed *fluence,* which actually is a measure of energy per unit volume. *Irradiance* is a function of the output energy and beam diameter of the laser and describes the density of photons striking the cornea with each laser pulse.

At low irradiance levels, the cornea remains grossly unaffected by the laser energy. As irradiance of the laser exposure progressively

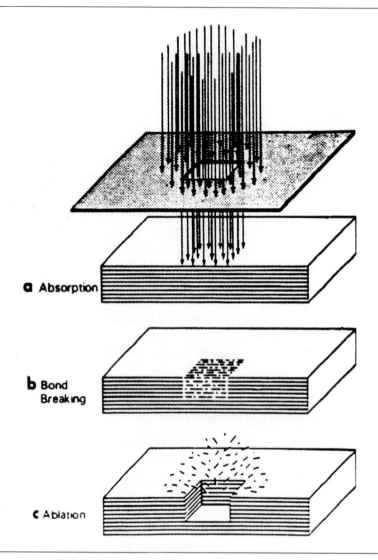

Fig. 1-3. Pictorial demonstration of ablative photodecomposition. **A.** The laser photons are first absorbed, leading to bond-breaking **(B)**. **C.** The subsequent ablation occurs as the fragments assume a larger volume and are ejected from the surface. (From R Srinivasan et al. Kinetics of the ablative photodecomposition of organic polymers in the far ultraviolet (193 nm). *J Vac Sci Technol* B1 : 923–926, 1983.)

increases, a faint clouding of the exposed corneal tissue occurs before the onset of clearly perceptible ablation [28]. Some have suggested that a transition threshold zone exists. The threshold for ablation at 193 nm is 50 mJ/cm^2, is independent of the pulse frequency (which speaks for a nonthermal mechanism of ablation), and is the lowest among the excimer laser wavelengths that have been tested (Fig. 1-6).

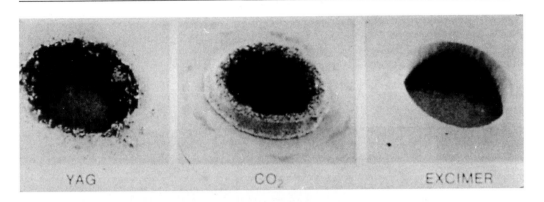

Fig. 1-4. Comparison of the differences in polymer ablation using a CO_2 laser, Nd:YAG laser, and ArF excimer laser. The excimer ablation shows a much smoother border. (From RR Krueger et al. The effects of excimer laser photoablation on the cornea. In JJ Salz, PJ McDonnell, MB McDonald [eds.]. *Corneal Laser Surgery*. St. Louis: Mosby–Year Book, 1995, P 11.)

Ablation Depth (Ablation Rate)

As energy density increases above threshold, each pulse of laser light removes a constant amount of corneal tissue proportional to the amount of energy striking the cornea (as shown in Fig. 1-6). This amount varies depending on the wavelength. In bovine eyes, at 193 nm the tissue removed varies from 0.13 microns at 150 mJ/cm² to 0.45 microns at 200 mJ/cm² and tends to plateau thereafter. This is in contrast to the ablation depth at 249 nm, which may be as high as 6.25 microns per pulse and follows a steep sigmoidal pattern as irradiance is increased or decreased. The small ablation depth at 193 nm and its relative independence of the irradiance allow for a more precise tissue ablation using this wavelength.

Krueger and Trokel [29] postulated in 1985 that the most efficient energy density for ablation with the 193-nm wavelength was 200 mJ/cm², the inflection point of the irradiance-ablation depth curve. This irradiance requires the least amount of total energy to remove a given amount of tissue, leaving less expenditure of energy for interactions other than ablation. In 1987, Puliafito et al. [30] repeated the ablation rate studies, demonstrating reproducible curves; however, they concluded that 400–600 mJ/cm² would be the best energy density of ablation because it represented an area in the curve with minimum variation (minimum slope). Van Saarloos and Constable [31] repeated this work in 1990 and concluded that the ablation efficiency was greater over a range of 150–400 mJ/cm² rather than just a single value. In the same year, Seiler and colleagues [32] went

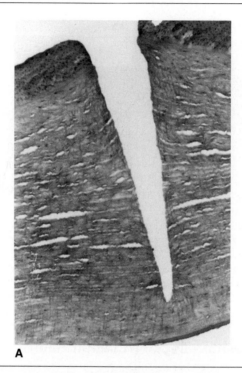

A

Fig. 1-5. Comparison of histologic views of linear excisions using different excimer wavelengths (×24). **A.** ArF excimer laser at 193 nm. Note the smooth ablation edge without apparent adjacent tissue damage.

a step further and determined the ablation rate for epithelium, Bowman's layer, and the stroma in human eyes, rather than in the bovine eyes studied previously. They showed that at 205 mJ/cm^2, the ablation rate was lower in Bowman's layer (0.38 microns/pulse) than in stroma (0.55 microns/pulse) or the epithelium (0.68 microns/pulse).

With all these factors to consider, clinical studies began using an empiric value for ablation depth, which was then altered by trial and error to compensate for the healing response. Using 160–180 mJ/cm^2, an ablation rate between 0.21 and 0.27 microns per pulse (VISX laser; Santa Clara, CA) and 0.26 microns per pulse (Summit laser; Waltham, MA) was estimated when human trials began. Seiler et al. [33] used Scheimpflug photography of the cornea before and after PRK, confirming the previous values. Extra care should be taken during photo-therapeutic keratectomy (PTK) because the ablation rate of corneal scars can differ from that of stromal tissue and may be highly variable [34].

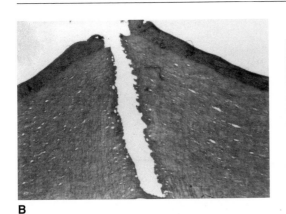
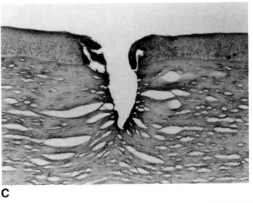

B   C

Fig. 1-5 (continued). **B.** KrF excimer laser at 248 nm. Note the jagged excision edge with cavitation vacuoles and small 10-micrometer zone of thermal damage. **C.** XeCl excimer laser at 308 nm. Note the zone of adjacent thermal damage with localized tissue shrinkage. (From RR Krueger et al. Interaction of ultraviolet laser light with the cornea. *Invest Ophthalmol Vis Sci* 26 : 1455–1464, 1985)

Pulse Frequency (Hz)

Most excimer lasers work at a frequency of 6–10 Hz (pulses per second). There is a trend toward faster repetition rates in order to decrease the total lasing time to redeem the effects of variables, such as stromal hydration and patient fixation. A limiting factor, however, is excess thermal damage if the laser frequency is faster than the thermal relaxation time of the adjacent tissues. Bende et al. [35], using rabbit eyes, determined that for an irradiance of 300 mJ/cm^2, the repetition rate should not exceed 63 Hz. With an irradiance of 150 mJ/cm^2, the upper limit increases to 82 Hz.

Consequences of Photoablation

Shock Waves

The impact of the excimer laser energy on the cornea produces an acoustic shock wave, creating an audible snap. The shock wave has been photographed in the air above the eye [36] (Fig. 1-7A) and recorded posteriorly underneath the cornea using piezoelectric transducers. In each case, the velocity of the leading edge of the shock wave is a function of the material through which it propagates. In air, shock wave velocity is 3–4 km/sec; in helium, 6 km/sec; and passing through the cornea it travels at the speed of sound (1.6 km/sec). The laser-induced shock wave has been shown to generate a pressure of up to 100 atm, resulting in mechanical stress to the cornea. This may

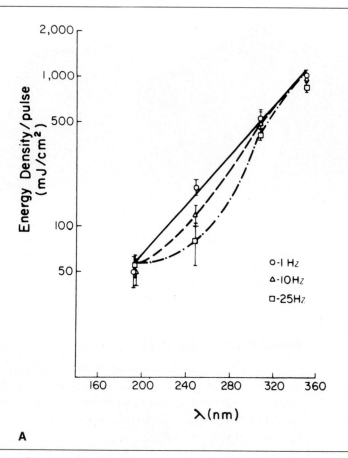

A

Fig. 1-6. **A.** Threshold for ultraviolet laser corneal ablation, as tested for the four major wavelengths produced by the excimer laser. There is a semilogarithmic relationship with increasing wavelength at 1 Hz. The decreasing threshold with increasing repetition rate at 248 nm implies a thermal component.

lead to structural damage to adjacent collagen layers or cellular alterations in keratocytes or endothelial cells, or both.

Gaseous and Particulate Ejection

In 1987, Puliafito and colleagues [37] used high-speed photography to investigate excimer laser ablation and found that a plume of particulate material was ejected from the cornea on a time scale ranging from 500 nanoseconds to 150 microseconds. Figure 1-7B shows the ablation plume at 193 nm, which resembles a mushroom cloud of smoke similar to that seen after an atomic bomb explosion. The individual particles were too small to resolve optically but traveled at velocities on the order of several hundred meters per second. Using mass spectroscopy, the majority of ejected material was of smaller

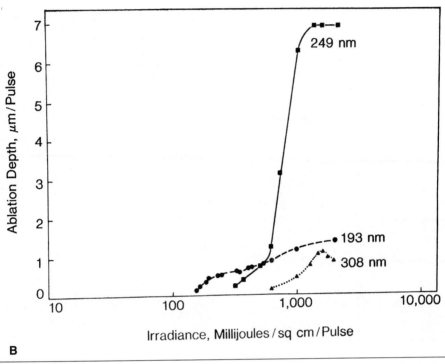

B

Fig. 1-6 (continued). **B.** Corneal ablation depth as a function of pulse radiance for three wavelengths produced by the excimer laser. Note the flatness of the 193 nm curve compared with the others, allowing a more controlled ablation of the tissue. (From RR Krueger et al. Interaction of ultraviolet laser light with the cornea. *Invest Ophthalmol Vis Sci* 26:1455–1464, 1985; RR Krueger et al. Quantitation of corneal ablation by ultraviolet laser light. *Arch Ophthalmol* 103:1741–1742. Copyright 1985, American Medical Association.)

molecular weight, consistent with free radicals and other simple carbons and hydrocarbons.

Surface Waves

The high-velocity particles and gases of the ejection plume are released as the potential energy of the molecular bonds is converted to kinetic energy. The recoil of the ejection plume results in a surface wave emanating from the point of laser impact [38]. This surface wave has an initial amplitude as high as 150–400 microns, and it propagates along the surface at several meters per second. The surface wave can significantly displace corneal tissue, which could result in damage or tearing of the layers of the cornea, but these effects have yet to be observed histopathologically.

Both the shock wave and the later surface wave may result in the production of surface fluid from within the cornea, possibly leading to

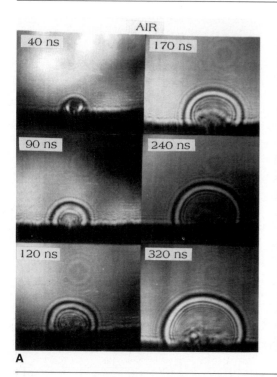 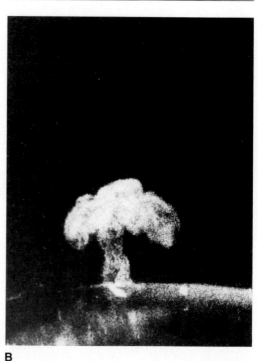

Fig. 1-7. Mechanical effects of the excimer laser ablation. **A.** Shock wave in air followed by **(B)** an ejection plume. (**A** From RR Krueger et al. Photography of shock waves during excimer laser ablation of the cornea. Effect of helium gas on propagation velocity. *Cornea* 12:330–334, 1993; **B** From Puliafito CA et al. High-speed photography of excimer laser ablation of the cornea. *Arch Ophthalmol* 105: 1255–1259. Copyright 1987, American Medical Association.)

attenuation of corneal ablation centrally and topographic steep central island formation.

Pseudomembrane Formation

The formation of a pseudomembrane in association with excimer laser photoablation was first described in 1985, when Marshall and colleagues [39] noted that some epithelial cells adjacent to the ablated area had a pale-staining cytoplasm. On closer examination, these pale-staining cells had no cell membrane along the border adjacent to the ablated area and had actually been cleaved by the photoablation process (Fig. 1-8). The severed edge was bounded by an electron-dense condensation of less than 100-nm thickness that seemed to maintain the integrity of the cell, hence the term *pseudomembrane*. Along the ablation edge, individual collagen fibers cleaved by the laser seem to converge and are pinched together as if the ends have been sealed [40]. The greater the energy density, the greater the thickness

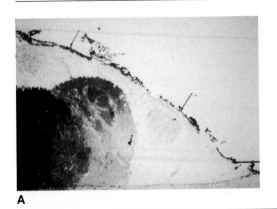 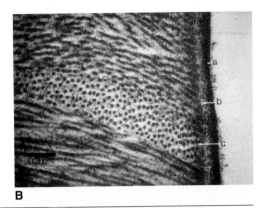

A   B

Fig. 1-8. Pseudomembrane formation. **A.** Pale-staining epithelial cell cleaved by the excimer laser and maintained by an electron-dense condensation with membranelike properties. **B.** High-power electron micrograph of a pseudomembrane showing an outer dense-staining region (a), middle light-staining region (b), and an inner region (c), where the fine structure of collagen is partially preserved. (From J Marshall et al. An ultrastructural study of corneal incisions induced by an excimer laser at 193 nm. *Ophthalmology* 92 : 749–758, 1985; CA Puliafito et al. Excimer laser ablation of cornea and lens: Experimental studies. *Ophthalmology* 92 : 741–748, 1985.)

of the pseudomembrane. Although the cause of the pseudomembrane is unknown, some believe that it is caused from uncoupled organic double bonds created during photoablation, and others contend that it might be related to a thermal effect. Corneal dehydration seems to have a detrimental effect on the pseudomembrane, whereas hydration at physiologic levels keeps it thin and uniform. Perhaps the water in the cornea helps to dissipate any heat generated during the procedure. This suggests a possible thermal mechanism for pseudomembrane formation, but even if this is so there is no damage seen beyond it.

The membranelike properties of pseudomembranes appear to have a beneficial effect: Their smooth, uniform surfaces may act as a template for re-epithelialization during healing and may serve as a barrier to water transport, thus limiting significant corneal swelling after PRK, as compared to conventional lamellar keratectomy.

Controllable Variables in Photoablation

Surface Smoothness

The smoothness of the anterior corneal surface after lamellar keratectomy seems to correlate with the degree of haze and scarring that develops. The excimer laser allows for a more precise reprofiling of the anterior corneal surface [41] (Fig. 1-9).

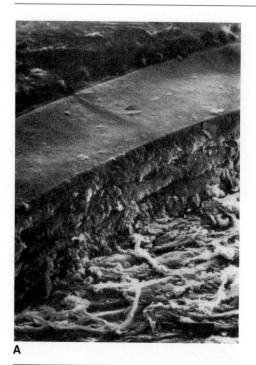
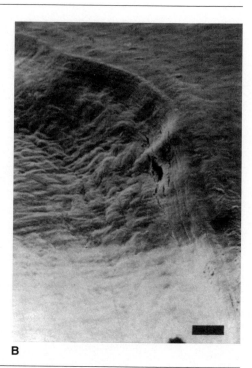

A   B

Fig. 1-9. Scanning electron micrographs of manual (**A**) and 193-nm excimer laser (**B**) keratectomies. Notice the smoothness and improved regularity of the floor of the surgical site with the excimer ablation. (From MG Kerr-Muir et al. Ultrastructural comparison of conventional surgical and argon fluoride excimer laser keratectomy. *Am J Ophthalmol* 103 : 448–453, 1987.)

One of the most important factors in surface smoothness and uniformity is homogeneity of the laser beam. The excimer laser beam profile as it exits the laser cavity is rectangular and has a gaussian distribution along its short axis. Additionally, there are often energy spikes of higher intensity ("hot spots"), which could lead to focal areas of greater ablation. The beam energy must be redistributed into a homogeneous pattern before exiting the clinical laser system. If the beam profile is not homogeneous, then corneal ablation will not be uniform but will mimic the spatial intensity of the laser beam [42].

Corneal Hydration

One of the most important environmental factors during excimer laser ablation is tissue hydration. After removal of the corneal epithelium, the corneal stroma can swell while the light of the operating microscope promotes superficial dehydration. As previously mentioned, the ablation rate of the excimer depends strongly on the level of tissue hydration [43, 44] with deeper ablations occurring when the tissue is dehydrated.

What seems more important during excimer surgery is to maintain a constant level of tissue hydration, mimicking physiologic conditions as much as possible. This helps to achieve a uniform ablation rate and fosters the development of a smooth pseudomembrane. To achieve this, the time elapsed from the removal of the corneal epithelium to the application of laser energy should be minimized, and no additional fluid should be applied to the corneal surface. The deeper the ablation, the closer it is to the aqueous humor and the wetter the corneal stroma will be, thereby decreasing the ablation depth per pulse. One manufacturer (VISX) varies the predicted ablation depth (rate) per pulse according to the depth of the ablation. When performing LASIK, because the ablation starts in the mid-stroma, the ablation rate might be lower than after PRK. Central surface fluid accumulation can lead to a nonuniform ablation rate and result in topographic central islands [45]. More recent software in some laser systems takes this into account and delivers additional pulses to the central cornea.

In early clinical studies with the nitrogen gas blower, tissue dehydration resulted in good predictability of the ablation rate, but increased reticular corneal haze was noted. An animal study was then performed that examined the effects of the nitrogen gas blower and demonstrated a greater surface roughening and greater corneal haze when the nitrogen gas blower was used [46]. As a result of this finding, the clinical use of the nitrogen gas blower was abandoned. Since that time, further clinical studies have demonstrated a significant decrease in corneal haze and a more predictable refractive outcome. Another animal study compared the effects of blowing both dry and humidified gas over the corneal surface during PRK [47]. The results showed that corneas ablated using humidified gases were smooth and equivalent to those ablated under ambient conditions, whereas those ablated using a dry gas blower again showed surface irregularity. When using an ablatable mask or a slit mask, gas blowing must be used because the ablation by-products deposit on the undersurface of the mask and interfere with passage of the laser light. In this case, humidified gas blowing would probably be best.

Ablation Depth and Diameter

The correction of myopia using the excimer laser is based on a graded removal of tissue resulting in a decreased corneal radius of curvature. The ablation process is analogous to the removal of a biologic contact lens from the central corneal surface (PRK) [9], as shown in Figure 1-10. Here the thickness of this biologic contact lens (t_0) depends on the diameter of tissue removal (S), as well as the desired amount of myopic correction (D), and can be expressed by the following equation:

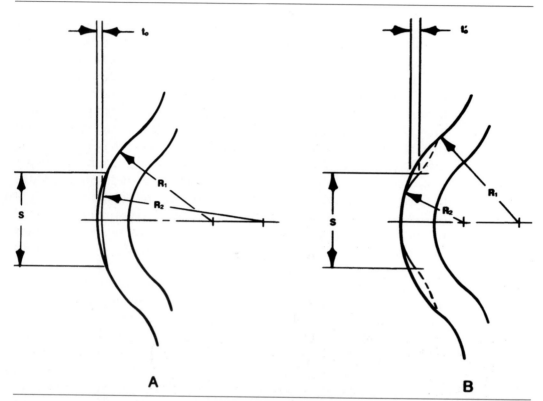

Fig. 1-10. Anterior corneal reprofiling for the correction of myopia **(A)** and hyperopia **(B)**. S is the diameter of the optical zone, t_o is the depth of the ablation, and R_1 and R_2 are the initial and final radii of curvature. (From CR Munnerlyn et al. Photorefractive keratectomy: A technique for laser refractive surgery. *J Cat Refract Surg* 14:48, 1988. © *Journal of Cataract and Refractive Surgery.*)

$$t_o = \frac{-S^2 D}{8(n-1)} \quad or \quad \frac{-S^2 D}{3}$$

Thus, for a given amount of myopic correction, the depth of ablation increases in proportion to the square of the ablation diameter. When performing LASIK, similar principles apply, but in this case the lenticule is resected from the mid-corneal stroma.

Although the maximum depth of tissue removal for a given dioptric correction can be minimized by reducing the diameter of the ablation zone, optical zones less than or equal to the pupil diameter can result in significant glare and halos due to light refraction through peripheral unablated cornea. This can have disturbing consequences, especially in younger people, who have a greater pupillary diameter in both dim and bright light.

It is clear that a sufficiently large ablation zone diameter is required for asymptomatic excimer PRK. Most reports suggest that 6 mm is sufficient to reduce postoperative glare in the vast majority of cases, whereas ablation zone diameters of 5.0 and 5.5 mm are associated with 37% and 5.5%, respectively, of patients reporting significant glare [48].

For higher myopic corrections, a compromise has been achieved with the multizone ablation technique, in which part of the ablation is done at a large diameter to minimize glare and the rest of the ablation is performed at progressively smaller diameters to minimize depth. Earlier experience with keratomileusis showed that at least 300 microns of undisturbed corneal stroma should be left if progressive ectasia of the cornea is to be avoided. This is important for doing LASIK in high myopes, in which case either a multizone program can be used or the thickness of the superficial flap can be reduced.

For hyperopic corrections, the excimer is used to excavate a groove in the periphery to steepen the central part of the cornea. The fact that there is an abrupt transition in the shape of the cornea requires increased optical zones up to 8 mm to blend the groove with the peripheral cornea, thereby inducing less haze and regression.

Biologic Response to Corneal Photoablation

Postoperative Pain

One of the major concerns associated with excimer PRK is that of postoperative pain. During early investigational trials in the United States and elsewhere, severe postoperative pain was a significant complication. Neurophysiologic studies of corneal nerves in rabbits have demonstrated an exaggerated neural response to stimulation with return to baseline more slowly after PRK than after manual keratectomy wounds [49]. Severe pain was experienced by the majority of patients in the first 12–36 hours following excimer laser PRK, and they required large doses of strong analgesics for relief. As with any large corneal abrasion, the use of a bandage contact lens promotes epithelial healing and permits an earlier return to work.

Experimental data in rabbits show a dramatic increase in the level of prostaglandin E_2 after PRK. This level decreases more after the administration of diclofenac sodium than fluorometholone [50]. Subsequent clinical studies comparing the degree of pain and discomfort of patients undergoing bilateral PRK with one eye treated with a contact lens, cycloplegics, and fluorometholone 0.1%, and the other eye treated with the same regimen plus diclofenac sodium 0.1%, reveal markedly less pain in the diclofenac-treated eye [51, 52]. Case reports from Canada suggest that sterile stromal infiltrates may occur in as many as 1 out of 250 PRK-treated eyes when the eyes are treated with nonsteroidal anti-inflammatory drugs (NSAIDs) alone, highlighting the importance of using NSAIDs in combination with the steroids to counteract the migration of polymorphonuclear neutrophil leukocytes (PMNs) induced by NSAIDs [53].

Recent work by Verma et al. [54] suggested the use of topical anesthetics for the first 24 hours after PRK; they demonstrated a dramatic reduction in the amount of pain and no impairment of the re-epithelialization process.

After LASIK, there is mild pain associated with the shock wave and the surgical trauma, but the absence of an epithelial defect seems to speed recovery from the surgery.

Because the laser removes the subepithelial nerve plexus, PRK is associated with a transient decrease in corneal sensitivity for approximately 3 months [55]. This does not seem to be associated with re-epithelialization problems. There is less corneal anesthesia after LASIK than after PRK [56].

Epithelial Wound Healing

Following PRK, the corneal epithelium covers the denuded stroma in 3–5 days, and this initial epithelial thickness consists of three to five layers. For up to 6 months following the ablation, the epithelium thickens primarily at the deepest part of the ablation site, thus attenuating the reprofiling effect of the excimer laser [57–61] (Fig. 1-11).

Fig. 1-11. Light micrograph of the interface between corneal epithelium and stroma in an area of excimer laser ablation 6 months after exposure. Note the increase of the number of epithelial cell layers at the edge of the ablation. (From J Marshall et al. Long-term healing of the central cornea after photorefractive keratectomy using an excimer laser. *Ophthalmology* 95 : 1411–1421, 1988.)

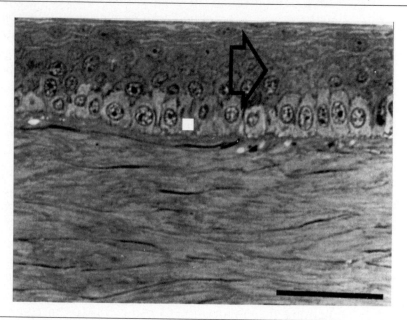

At present, we are unsure of the stimulus for epithelial hyperplasia. One theory suggests that tear film thickness is responsible. Others have suggested that it is related to the abrupt change in shape of the ablated area, with smaller (< 5 mm), single-zone ablation stimulating a greater hyperplastic response. The clinical implication of epithelial hyperplasia is thought to be early regression of the refractive effect.

One of the initial concerns following PRK was the possibility of recurrent epithelial erosions caused by abnormalities of epithelial adhesion to bare stroma. Several studies of the epithelial cells have documented normal anchoring complexes as evidenced by the presence of type VII collagen (anchoring fibrils), β_4-integrin (epithelial hemidesmosomes) and type IV collagen (basement membrane) [62]. In fact, the excimer laser is an excellent treatment for recalcitrant recurrent corneal erosions, promoting the adhesion of the epithelial cells to Bowman's or corneal stroma [63].

During LASIK, the epithelial layer is left undisturbed centrally, leaving only a linear circular defect where the microkeratome enters the stroma. Although rare, one complication of this technique is the ingrowth of the epithelium across the stromal interface. Most of the time it is self-limited and innocuous. If symptoms occur, the stromal cap can be lifted and the undersurface cleaned of epithelium.

Stromal Wound Healing

Destruction of the acellular Bowman's layer has previously been associated with permanent corneal scarring in the area of its removal. The reason for this is unknown but might be related to the activation of the stromal keratocytes by the discontinuity in the stroma plus the influence of PMNs or cytokines in the tear film, which gain access to the stroma via the denuded epithelium or by cell-to-cell interaction of the keratocytes with the epithelial cells as they migrate to cover the epithelial defect. As mentioned previously, the smoothness of the ablation with the excimer laser plays an important role in minimizing scarring after PRK.

Acute morphologic studies after PRK demonstrate the presence of a thin pseudomembrane over the abated surface and vacuolization of the keratocytes of the anterior collagen layers of the stroma. Within the first 24 hours, stromal wound healing begins, as inflammatory cells (PMNs) invade the corneal stroma from the tear film. Within the first 3 days, both the anterior stromal keratocytes and PMNs disappear [64, 65]. The marked decrease in keratocytes also can be seen following de-epithelialization without stromal ablation, and repopulation occurs over a 2-week period. Following excimer laser PRK, the keratocytes not only repopulate but also increase in density, being seen in more than three times their normal number by the third postoperative week. The increased number of activated keratocytes deposit new

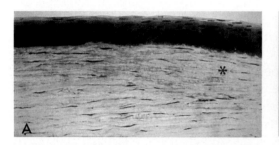 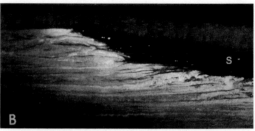

Fig. 1-12. Histologic view of corneal remodeling 3 months following excimer laser keratectomy. **A.** Note the new collagen fibers with an altered orientation suggestive of scar tissue (*). **B.** Fluorescent microscopy demonstrates unlabeled connective tissue scar (*S*) in contrast with the native collagen, as labeled with dichlorotriazinyl aminofluorescein (DTAF) dye. (From SJ Tuft et al. Corneal repair following keratectomy: A comparison between conventional surgery and laser photoablation. *Invest Ophthalmol Vis Sci* 30 : 1769–1777, 1989.)

collagen and proteoglycans, which are responsible for the high level of light scatter, resulting in corneal haze [66, 67] (Fig. 1-12). This haze can be seen as early as 1 week following treatment, and it peaks at 1 month in the rabbit [68], at 3 months in the nonhuman primate [69–71], and at 3–6 months in the human [72]. In the latter, haze tends to disappear by 12–18 months in almost all cases [73]. The degree of haze does seem to correlate with the late regressive refractive changes after PRK (3–18 months) [74].

The stromal changes after LASIK have been studied less extensively. Tuft et al. [67] reported less collagen deposition after intrastromal (mechanical) keratectomy compared with anterior (mechanical and excimer) keratectomies [7]. Another study revealed decreased metalloprotease (a collagenase involved in wound repair) levels after LASIK compared to PRK [75]. Clinical studies seem to support such findings, as the incidence of significant haze is dramatically lower after LASIK than after PRK [76–78].

Wound Healing Modulation

Because a mild to moderate amount of epithelial hyperplasia and haze is expected after PRK, most excimer lasers overcorrect patients initially and allow the healing response to bring the patient's refraction back toward the target value.

According to Durrie et al. [79], there seems to be three types of healing response following PRK. Type I is what is considered the "normal" healing response, with mild haze and refractive regression occurring in the vast majority of patients. Type II results in clear corneas and refractive overcorrection. Type III results in intense haze or refractive regression, or both.

The presence of activated fibroblasts has been demonstrated after excimer PRK, and it is known that corticosteroids inhibit fibroblast proliferation [80], so it is logical to treat corneas with topical steroids following excimer photoablation. Early experimental studies have demonstrated the effectiveness of topical steroids in reducing corneal haze [81], and retrospective clinical experience has verified this finding. In a prospective double-blind trial to determine the efficacy of topical steroids in reducing stromal haze, however, topical steroid use was shown to have no statistically significant effect on anterior stromal haze in comparison to placebo control [82, 83]. It was recommended that topical steroids not be used after PRK, but others suggest that there exists a high-risk subgroup in which the absence or discontinuation of topical steroids will lead to significant haze formation. Furthermore, in cases of refractive regression, steroids can reverse both haze and regression by an as yet unknown mechanism [84–86].

The potential for side effects from topical steroids, such as glaucoma and cataract, has spurred continued research regarding the efficacy of other pharmacologic modulators in reducing corneal haze. These have included antifibrotic agents, such as mitomycin [81], interferon-alfa-2b [87], pirenzepine (a muscarinic antagonist) [88]; protease inhibitors, such as aprotinin (plasmin inhibitor) [89, 90]; minoxidil; antibodies against tissue growth factor–beta, sodium hyaluronate [91]; NSAIDs [92]; pentoxifylline [93]; and even cooling the cornea during photoablation to reduce the production of heat-shock proteins [94].

Excimer Laser Safety

Laser Beam Safety

Far-UV–induced Fluorescence

When far-UV laser light strikes the cornea, a broad-spectrum band of UV light of longer wavelengths is created. Several investigators have studied the luminance associated with excimer laser corneal ablation and have shown the spectral pattern of fluorescence to cover a broad range of wavelengths from as low as 260 to more than 500 nm [95]. The peak wavelength for laser-induced fluorescence of human epithelium is 460 nm (in the blue region of the visible electromagnetic spectrum), whereas that for human corneal stroma is 310–320 nm (UVB). This color change of the excimer-induced fluorescence has been used to monitor the removal of epithelium [96].

Photokeratitis is a known side effect of UVA and UVB light exposure [97]. Krueger et al. [98] studied the effects of 193-nm UV light in rabbit cornea and found minimal damage to the surrounding tissues because of the short penetration of excimer radiation. The possible effect that the excimer-induced fluorescence might have was deemed minimal.

Such longer-wavelength UV light may pass through the cornea, affecting intraocular structures. Knowing that these UVA and UVB wavelengths are transmitted by the cornea and absorbed partially by the lens, the possibility of cataract formation remains a concern [99, 100], although this has not been born out in clinical trials.

Mutagenesis

Because UV light can result in mutations of DNA, some concern over the potential mutagenesis of 193-nm excimer laser radiation has been raised. A number of experimental studies have been performed to address this issue, and each one has shown that 193-nm radiation does not result in cytotoxic damage to DNA and mutagenicity [101, 102]. One way of measuring mutagenic damage to DNA is by monitoring the amount of unscheduled DNA synthesis. This was tested at the edge of ablated human skin and rabbit cornea, suggesting no replacement of damaged DNA with 193-nm radiation but significant replacement when the tissue was irradiated with a germicidal lamp at 254 nm or with 248-nm excimer laser [103]. The reasons proposed for this lack of damage to DNA at 193 nm are absorption of that wavelength by protein surrounding the nucleus (a protein shield), lack of cytotoxicity of DNA photoproducts produced by 193-nm light, DNA damage that can be readily repaired by the cells, or such lethal damage that potential mutagenic repair processes are not possible. Gebhardt et al. [104] irradiated mouse corneas and implanted subcutaneously those keratocytes in syngeneic recipients that showed no evidence of tumor growth after many months. Although one might think that the secondary UV fluorescence could lead to DNA damage, this level of exposure is 10,000 times lower than the minimum average annual exposure to solar UVB radiation.

Endothelial Damage

A major concern about operating on normal, healthy corneas for refractive purposes has been the potential for endothelial cell damage, especially considering the history of late-onset corneal edema following radial keratotomies performed in Japan. Acute morphologic studies of primate and human endothelium have failed to demonstrate endothelial changes, unless the excimer laser beam approaches Descemet's membrane [105, 106]. Clinically significant endothelial cell loss after excimer laser PRK has not been recorded [107, 108]. In fact, endothelial morphology seems to improve after PRK in contact lens wearers, perhaps reflecting its elimination. There was also concern about endothelial integrity when performing LASIK because the ablation was started in the mid-stroma, rendering it closer to the endothelial layer [109]. This possible mode of endothelial damage is currently being evaluated in clinical trials.

Laser System Safety and Reliability

Gases

All commercially available excimer lasers employ an ArF mix, with the exception of the Novatec system, which is a far-UV solid-state laser, not an excimer laser. The gas mix should be replaced after a certain number of treatments, and with newer models this period has been extended up to 1 year. Replacement is handled by the distributing company, and it is one factor that contributes to the high maintenance costs of this equipment [110]. The distributing company handles gas replacement because of the toxic nature of the fluorine within the ArF mixture. The safety rating of fluorine is one part per million, which means that once you can smell its odor, it has exceeded its safety rating [110].

The other gas that has to be changed periodically is nitrogen, which has several uses: (1) as a coolant, (2) as a particle precipitator in the main gas chamber, and (3) to purge the optical components in order to increase mirror lifetime and reduce transmission losses. Using nitrogen gas to blow the corneal surface during ablation has been abandoned. Because ablated particles are ejected in the direction of the next oncoming laser pulse, it was suggested that they might interfere with the uniformity of the energy profile. One manufacturer (VISX) designed a nitrogen blower to eliminate the gaseous and particulate debris, but an increased amount of haze and scarring was noted, possibly due to roughening of the corneal surface [46].

Calibration

Use of the excimer laser differs from that of other ophthalmic lasers in that there is no modification of the laser energy based on any clinical indication of tissue response. When we perform retinal photocoagulation, for example, we adjust the power or the spot size according to the amount of whitening of the retina or choroid. When we perform excimer surgery, there is no endpoint that will make us change the laser energy being delivered; therefore, preoperative calibration is one of the more important steps in this type of refractive surgery [111].

The beam diameter must possess a homogeneous distribution of energy and a constant fluence from pulse to pulse, making optical performance and its verification extremely important. Several methods of beam calibration have been employed. The VISX laser is calibrated by doing a myopic ablation on a polymethylmethacrylate (PMMA) block, and the machine is reprogrammed based on the myopic ablation reading. The Summit laser is optionally checked by doing a 90% gelatin film ablation, but there is no reprogramming involved. The Chiron-Technolas laser (Irvine, CA) is reprogrammed after counting the number of pulses needed to perforate a special foil. The Coherent-Schwind (Kleinostheim, Germany) laser utilizes a gelatin film for calibration, and reprogramming is done based on the number of pulses for 10–90% perforation of the film. The LaserSight laser uses a patented device, called Ex-Calibur, which allows for preoperative calibrations using commercially available corneal topography systems.

Eye Tracking

The proper centration of the laser procedure is a major concern in excimer refractive surgery. Ablation decentration leads to under-corrections, glare, and irregular astigmatism, with decreased best-corrected visual acuity [112]. Another concern is the effect of the fixation microsaccades by the patient, but those seem to have a blending effect on the ablation steps, although excessive oscillations may decrease the achieved correction.

A fixating suction ring was proposed initially for PRK, but this was soon abandoned. The procedure is typically performed under topical anesthesia without akinesis, and it is the surgeon's most important task to coach the patient to fixate properly in the coaxial fixation light. When performing LASIK, the surgeon can either use the suction ring to hold and center the patient's eye or rely on the patient's fixation.

The VISX and Summit lasers do not use an eye tracking device. Other lasers employ a passive eye tracking system, in which a video camera "locks" the pupil and automatically stops the firing of the laser if the eye moves outside the preset range. The Autonomous [113], Chiron Technolas, and Novatec lasers each use active eye tracking devices that adjust the laser beam position with respect to the globe during surgery.

Delivery Systems

There are two ways of delivering the laser energy to the cornea. The first one uses a broad laser beam and a variable spot size centered on the visual axis to correct the different refractive errors. The second strategy uses a scanning laser slit or spot that travels across the cornea, shaping it according to the refractive correction desired. Because the second strategy uses a laser beam of smaller energy, the manufacturers claim that it induces less tissue reaction than the other lasers. This has yet to be proved in clinical trials.

Regardless of the method employed, a uniform "top hat" energy configuration is needed to avoid hot and cold spots that will alter the predicted ablation pattern. After the UV laser beam exits the laser cavity, several methods of beam reshaping have been used to achieve a uniform beam profile. These include, in addition to a series of lenses and mirrors, a rotating dove prism, a rotating [114] or scanning slit beam, and a prismatic integrator.

Once a uniform beam shape has been obtained, various strategies are used to project the desired laser pattern correction onto the cornea. They include an opening or closing iris diaphragm [115], opening parallel blades, a scanning mirror, zoom optics, or even a mask held against the cornea. The exceptions are the laser systems that already have a scanning laser beam, in which case this is applied directly onto the cornea. All the commercial lasers employ quartz optics, which are not affected by the high-energy UV light [116].

For myopic ablations, almost all the lasers use spots of varying size centered around the visual axis. The most common pattern shaper used is an expanding mechanical iris. The Meditec laser (Heroldsberg, Germany) uses a contracting iris diaphragm. The greater the number of steps as the iris opens, the greater the surface smoothness and subsequent successful healing. When performing PRK using the iris diaphragm system, the VISX laser initially used a contracting iris diaphragm but later changed to an expanding aperture because of discontinuities in the pseudomembrane with the former method [117]. Even with an expanding aperture system, stepped edges sometimes can be seen acutely after excimer PRK. These steps can be attenuated by defocusing the image of the aperture [42]. Whether this leads to any benefit in the optical or refractive outcome is unknown. The Schwind laser uses a telescopic zoom to progressively change the diameter of the ablation. An ablatable mask has also been used to create myopic ablations.

For hyperopic ablations, there are two strategies. One involves the use of a scanning laser that creates a groove in the periphery of the cornea that is shaped like a doughnut, steepening the central part. The other involves a special rotating diaphragm with two opposing holes that preferentially ablates the periphery of the cornea.

For astigmatic ablations, separating parallel blades or a scanning spot are used. Current technology usually corrects the refractive error by *flattening* the steep meridian, in cases of both myopic and hyperopic astigmatism. There is always some degree of flattening of the flat meridian as well. This might not be important in cases of compound myopic astigmatism, but it is relevant in cases of simple myopic astigmatism and hyperopic astigmatism. Early studies are under way using the Aesculap-Meditec and the Coherent-Schwind laser to perform selective *steepening* of each meridian in cases of compound hyperopic astigmatism.

For presbyopic ablations, most of the work has been done by increasing the power of the central 2–3 mm of the cornea. It can be done combined with other refractive corrections, or more rarely as the sole refractive procedure. In cases of hyperopic ablations, the multifocality of the cornea might help with unaided near vision. There are still many problems to be solved with this technique, such as ghosting, decreased contrast sensitivity, and decreased best corrected distance visual acuity.

All of these unique delivery system features are designed to deliver a safe and efficacious pattern of energy for the correction of refractive error. The differences among excimer laser systems and in the type of refractive error corrected are in part responsible for the detailed investigational studies and restrictions imposed by the FDA. Understanding the many features and differences in energy delivery, calibration, tracking, and maintenance are important in understanding how the excimer laser works and how to keep it safe. Consequently, greater detail regarding the technical features of each individual laser system are covered in the Technical Considerations section of the book. More specific information regarding surgical technique and features for correcting myopia, astigmatism, hyperopia, and presbyopia are reviewed in Chapter 4.

References

1. Taboada JM, Kessel GW, Reed RD. Response of the corneal epithelium to KrF excimer laser pulses. *Health Phys* 40:677, 1981.
2. Trokel SL, Srinivasan R, Braren B. Excimer laser surgery of the cornea. *Am J Ophthalmol* 96:710, 1983.
3. Seiler T, Wollensak J. In vivo experiments with the excimer laser— Technical parameters and healing processes. *Ophthalmologica* 192: 65–70, 1986.
4. Srinivasan R, Sutcliffe E. Dynamics of the ultraviolet laser ablation of corneal tissue. *Am J Ophthalmol* 103:470–471, 1987.
5. Ren Q, et al. Ultraviolet solid-state laser (213 nm) photorefractive keratectomy: In vivo study. *Ophthalmology* 101:883–889, 1994.
6. Swinger CA, Lai ST. Solid-state photoablative decomposition—the Novatec laser. In JJ Salz, PJ McDonnell, MB McDonald (eds.). *Corneal Laser Surgery.* St. Louis: Mosby–Year Book, 1995, P 261.
7. Marshall J, et al. An ultrastructural study of corneal incisions induced by an excimer laser at 193 nm. *Ophthalmology* 92:749–758, 1985.

8. Marshall J, et al. Photoablative reprofiling of the cornea using an excimer laser. Photorefractive keratectomy. *Lasers Ophthalmol* 1:21, 1986.

9. Munnerlyn CR, Koons SJ, Marshall J. Photorefractive keratectomy: A technique for laser refractive surgery. *J Cataract Refract Surg* 14:46–52, 1988.

10. Trokel S. Evolution of excimer laser corneal surgery. *J Cataract Refract Surg* 15:373–383, 1989.

11. Taylor DM, et al. Human excimer laser lamellar keratectomy: A clinical study. *Ophthalmology* 96:654–664, 1989.

12. Barraquer JI. Queratoplastia refractiva. *Estudios Inform Oftal Inst Barraquer* 10:2–10, 1949.

13. Ruiz LA, Rowsey JJ. In situ keratomileusis. *Invest Ophthalmol Vis Sci* 29(Suppl.):392, 1988.

14. Pallikaris IG, et al. Laser in situ keratomileusis. *Lasers Surg Med* 10:463–468, 1990.

15. Cherry PM, et al. Argon laser treatment of corneal neovascularization. *Ann Ophthalmol* 5:911–920, 1973.

16. Sugar J, Jampol LM: Photocoagulation therapy of a pigmented retrocorneal plaque. *Ophthalmic Surg* 13:562–563, 1982.

17. Aron Rosa D, et al. Use of a neodymium YAG laser to open the posterior capsule after lens implant surgery: A preliminary report. *J Am Intraocul Implant Soc* 6:352–354, 1980.

18. Stern D, et al. Corneal ablation by nanosecond, picosecond and femtosecond lasers at 532 and 625 nm. *Arch Ophthalmol* 107:587–592, 1989.

19. Del Pero RA, et al. Intrastromal YAG laser refractive surgery in the cat model with the Phoenix laser knife. *Invest Ophthalmol Vis Sci* 36(Suppl.):S578, 1995.

20. Speaker MG, et al. Results of a safety study of myopic intrastromal photorefractive keratectomy (IPRK) with the Nd:YLF picosecond laser in blind human eyes. *Invest Ophthalmol Vis Sci* 36(Suppl.):S985, 1995.

21. Seiler T, Matallana M, Bende T: Laser thermokeratoplasty by means of a pulsed holmium:YAG laser for hyperopic correction. *Refract Corneal Surg* 6:355–359, 1990.

22. Fine BS, et al. Preliminary observations on ocular effects of high-power, continuous CO_2 laser irradiation. *Am J Ophthalmol* 64:209–222, 1967.

23. Peyman GA, et al. Modification of rabbit corneal curvature with the use of carbon dioxide laser burns. *Ophthalmic Surg* 11:325–329, 1980.

24. Bende T, Kriegerowski M, Seiler T. Photoablation in different ocular tissues performed with an Er:YAG laser. *Lasers Light Ophthalmol* 2: 263–269, 1989.

25. Srinivasan R. Kinetics of the ablative photodecomposition of organic polymers in the far ultraviolet (193 nm). *J Vac Sci Technol B* 1:923–926, 1983.

26. Keyes T, Clarke RH, Isner JM. Theory of photoablation and its implications for laser phototherapy, *J Phys Chem* 89:4194–4196, 1985.

27. Krauss JM, Puliafito CA, Steinert RF. Laser interactions with the cornea. *Surv Ophthalmol* 31:37–53, 1986.
28. Krueger RR, Trokel SL, Schubert HD: Interaction of ultraviolet laser light with the cornea. *Invest Ophthalmol Vis Sci* 26:1455–1464, 1985.
29. Krueger RR, Trokel SL. Quantitation of corneal ablation by ultraviolet laser light. *Arch Ophthalmol* 103:1741–1742, 1985.
30. Puliafito CA, Wong K, Steinert RF. Quantitative and ultrastructural studies of excimer laser ablation of the cornea at 193 and 248 nanometers. *Lasers Surg Med* 7:155–159, 1987.
31. Van Saarloos PP, Constable IJ: Bovine corneal ablation by ultraviolet laser light. *Arch Ophthalmol* 103:1741–1742, 1985.
32. Seiler T, et al. Ablation rate of human corneal epithelium and Bowman's layer with the excimer laser (193 nm). *Refract Corneal Surg* 6:99–102, 1990.
33. Seiler T, Hubscher J, Genth U. Corneal curvature change immediately after PRK as detected by Scheimplug photography. *Invest Ophthalmol Vis Sci* 34(Suppl.):S703, 1993.
34. McDonnell JM, Garbus JJ, McDonnell PJ. Unsuccessful excimer laser phototherapeutic keratectomy: Clinicopathologic correlation. *Arch Ophthalmol* 110:977–979, 1992.
35. Bende T, Seiler T, Wollensak J. Side effects in excimer corneal surgery: Corneal thermal gradients. *Graefes Arch Exp Ophthalmol* 226:277, 1988.
36. Krueger RR, et al. Photography of shock waves during excimer laser ablation of the cornea: Effect of helium gas on propagation velocity. *Cornea* 12:330–334, 1993.
37. Puliafito CA, et al. High-speed photography of excimer laser ablation of the cornea. *Arch Ophthalmol* 105:1255–1259, 1987.
38. Bor Z, et al. Plume emission, shock wave, and surface wave formation during excimer laser ablation of the cornea. *Refract Corneal Surg* 9(Suppl.):S111-S114, 1993.
39. Marshall J, et al. A comparative study of corneal incisions induced by diamond and steel knives and two ultraviolet radiations from an excimer laser. *Br J Ophthalmol* 70:482–501, 1986.
40. Puliafito CA, et al. Excimer laser ablation of the cornea and lens: Experimental studies. *Ophthalmology* 92:741–748, 1985.
41. Kerr-Muir MG, et al. Ultrastructural comparison of conventional surgical and argon fluoride excimer laser keratectomy. *Am J Ophthalmol* 103:448–453, 1987.
42. Krueger RR, et al. Diffractive smoothing of excimer laser ablation using a defocused beam. *J Refract Corneal Surg* 10:20–26, 1994.
43. Dougherty PJ, Wellish KL, Maloney RK. Excimer laser ablation rate and corneal hydration. *Am J Ophthalmol* 118:169–176, 1994.
44. Filatov V, et al. The effect of tissue hydration on the corneal surface smoothness following excimer photorefractive keratectomy in rabbits. *Invest Ophthalmol Vis Sci* 36(Suppl.):S707, 1995.
45. Krueger RR, Saedy NF, McDonnell PJ. Clinical analysis of steep central islands after excimer laser photorefractive keratectomy. *Arch Ophthalmol* 114:377–381, 1996.

46. Campos M, et al. Corneal wound healing after excimer laser ablation: Effects of nitrogen gas blower. *Ophthalmology* 99:893–897, 1992.
47. Krueger RR, et al. Corneal surface morphology following excimer laser ablation with humidified gases. *Arch Ophthalmol* 111:1131–1137, 1993.
48. DelloRusso J. Night glare and excimer laser ablation diameter. *J Cat Refract Surg* 19:565, 1993.
49. Beuerman RW, et al. Neurophysiological evaluation of corneal nerves in rabbits following excimer photorefractive keratectomy. *Invest Ophthalmol Vis Sci* 34:704, 1993.
50. Phillips AF, et al. Arachidonic acid metabolites after excimer laser corneal surgery. *Arch Ophthalmol* 111:1273–1278, 1993.
51. Eiferman RA, Hoffman RS, Sher NA. Topical diclofenac reduces pain following photorefractive keratectomy. *Arch Ophthalmol* 111:1022, 1993.
52. Sher NA, et al. Topical diclofenac in the treatment of ocular pain after excimer photorefractive keratectomy. *Refract Corneal Surg* 9:425, 1993.
53. Sher NA, et al. Role of topical corticosteroids and nonsteroidal anti-inflammatory drugs in the etiology of stromal infiltrates after excimer photorefractive keratectomy. *J Refract Corneal Surg* 10:587–588, 1994.
54. Verma S, Corbett MC, Marshall J. A prospective, randomized, double-masked trial to evaluate the role of topical anesthetics in controlling pain after photorefractive keratectomy. *Ophthalmology* 102:1918–1924, 1995.
55. Campos M, Garbus J, McDonnell PJ. Corneal sensitivity after photorefractive keratectomy. *Am J Ophthalmol* 114:51–54, 1992.
56. Delargyris EN, et al. Comparison of postoperative corneal sensation following photorefractive keratectomy and laser in-situ keratomileusis. *Invest Ophthalmol Vis Sci* 37(Suppl.):S58, 1996.
57. Gibson IK, Cintron C, Binder PS. Corneal epithelial and stromal reactions to excimer laser photorefractive keratectomy. *Arch Ophthalmol* 108:1539–1541, 1990.
58. Amano S, Shimizu D, Tsubota K. Corneal epithelial changes after excimer laser photorefractive keratectomy. *Am J Ophthalmol* 115:441–443, 1993.
59. Amano S, Shimizu K, Tsubota K. Specular microscopic evaluation of the corneal epithelium after excimer laser photorefractive keratectomy. *Am J Ophthalmol* 117:381–384, 1994.
60. Lohmann C, Marshall J. The importance of the corneal epithelium in excimer laser photorefractive keratectomy: A histopathological study in rabbits. *Invest Ophthalmol Vis Sci* 36(Suppl.):S708, 1995.
61. Epstein D, et al. Epithelial hyperplasia causes the initial myopic shift after excimer photorefractive keratectomy. *Invest Ophthalmol Vis Sci* 36(Suppl.):S704, 1995.
62. Fountain R, et al. Reassembly of corneal epithelial adhesion structures following human excimer laser keratectomy. *Arch Ophthalmol* 112:967–972, 1994.
63. Dausch D, et al. Phototherapeutic keratectomy in recurrent corneal epithelial erosion. *Refract Corneal Surg* 9:419–424, 1993.

64. Aron-Rosa DS, et al. Corneal wound healing after excimer laser keratotomy in a human eye. *Am J Ophthalmol* 103:454–464, 1987.

65. Hanna KD, et al. Corneal stromal wound healing in rabbits after 193-nm excimer laser surface ablation. *Arch Ophthalmol* 107:895, 1989.

66. Marshall J, et al. Long-term healing of the central cornea after photorefractive keratectomy using an excimer laser. *Ophthalmology* 95: 1411–1421, 1988.

67. Tuft SJ, Zabel RW, Marshall J. Corneal repair following keratectomy: A comparison between conventional surgery and laser photoablation. *Invest Ophthalmol Vis Sci* 30:1769–1777, 1989.

68. Goodman G, et al. Corneal healing following laser refractive keratectomy. *Arch Ophthalmol* 107:1799–1803, 1989.

69. Fantes F, et al. Wound healing after excimer laser keratomileusis (photorefractive keratectomy) in monkeys. *Arch Ophthalmol* 108:665–675, 1990.

70. Hanna K, et al. Corneal wound healing in monkeys 18 months after excimer laser photorefractive keratectomy. *Refract Corneal Surg* 6:340–345, 1990.

71. Malley D, et al. Immunofluorescence study of corneal wound healing after excimer laser anterior keratectomy in the monkey eye. *Arch Ophthalmol* 108:1316–1322, 1990.

72. Binder PS. What we have learned about corneal wound healing from refractive surgery. *J Refract Corneal Surg* 5:98–120, 1989.

73. Lohman C, et al. Haze in photorefractive keratectomy: Its origins and consequences. *Lasers Light Ophthalmol* 4:15–34, 1991.

74. Lohmann CP, et al. Corneal haze after excimer laser refractive surgery: Objective measurements and functional implications. *Eur J Ophthalmol* 1:173–180, 1991.

75. Pluznik DT, et al. Matrix metalloproteinase expression and corneal haze measurement after excimer keratomileusis in situ. *Invest Ophthalmol Vis Sci* 36(Suppl.): S29, 1995.

76. Buratto L, Ferrari M, Rama P. Excimer laser intrastromal keratomileusis. *Am J Ophthalmol* 113:291–295, 1992.

77. Pallikaris IG, Siganos DS. Excimer laser in situ keratomileusis and photorefractive keratectomy for correction of high myopia. *J Refract Surg* 11(Suppl.):498–510, 1995.

78. Kremer FB, Dufek M. Excimer laser in situ keratomileusis. *J Refract Surg* 11(Suppl.):244–247, 1995.

79. Durrie DS, Lesher MP, Cavanaugh TB. Classification of variable clinical response after photorefractive keratectomy for myopia. *J Refract Surg* 11:341–347, 1995.

80. Aquavella J, Gasset A, Dohlman C. Corticosteroids in corneal wound healing. *Am J Ophthalmol* 58:621–626, 1964.

81. Talamo J, et al. Modulation of corneal wound healing after excimer laser keratomileusis using topical mitomycin C and steroids. *Arch Ophthalmol* 109:1141–1146, 1991.

82. Gartry D, et al. The effect of topical corticosteroids on refractive outcome and corneal haze after photorefractive keratectomy. *Arch Ophthalmol* 110 : 944–952, 1992.

83. Gartry DS, Kerr-Muir MG, Marshall J. The effect of topical cortico-steroids on refraction and corneal haze following excimer laser treatment of myopia: An update. A prospective, randomized, double-masked study. *Eye* 7:584–590, 1993.

84. Brancato R, et al. Corticosteroids vs diclofenac in the treatment of delayed regression after myopic photorefractive keratectomy. *J Refract Corneal Surg* 9:376–379, 1993.

85. Fitzsimmons TD, Fagerholm P, Tengroth B. Steroid treatment of myopic regression: Acute refractive and topographic changes in excimer pho-torefractive keratectomy patients. *Cornea* 12:358, 1993.

86. Marques EF, Leite EB, Cunha-Vaz JG. Corticosteroids for reversal of myopic regression after photorefractive keratectomy. *J Refract Surg* 11(Suppl.):302–307, 1995.

87. Morlet N, et al. Effect of topical interferon-alpha 2b on corneal haze after excimer laser photorefractive keratectomy in rabbits. *Refract Corneal Surg* 9:443–451, 1993.

88. Lam D, et al. Modulation of corneal wound healing after excimer laser keratoplasty with muscarinic and histamine receptor antagonists. *Invest Ophthalmol Vis Sci* 34(Suppl.):S705, 1993.

89. Lohmann CP, Marshall J. Plasmin- and plasminogen-activator inhibitors after excimer laser photorefractive keratectomy: New concept in pre-vention of postoperative myopic regression and haze. *J Refract Corneal Surg* 9:300–302, 1993.

90. O'Brart D, et al. The effects of topical corticosteroids and plasmin inhibi-tors on refractive outcome, haze and visual perfomance after photore-fractive keratectomy. *Ophthalmology* 101:1565–1574, 1994.

91. Algawi K, et al. Randomized clinical trial of topical sodium hyaluronate after excimer laser photorefractive keratectomy. *J Refract Surg* 11:42, 1995.

92. Nassaralla BA, et al. Effect of diclofenac on corneal haze after photo-refractive keratectomy in rabbits. *Ophthalmology* 102:469–474, 1995.

93. Abad JC, et al. Evaluation of pentoxifylline in the prevention of haze after photorefractive keratectomy (PRK) in the rabbit. *Invest Ophthalmol Vis Sci* 37(Suppl.):S58, 1996.

94. Tsubota K, Toda I, Itoh S. Reduction of subepithelial haze after photo-refractive keratectomy by cooling the cornea (letter). *Am J Ophthalmol* 115:820–821, 1993.

95. Tuft S, et al. Characterization of the fluorescence spectra produced by excimer laser irradiation of the cornea. *Invest Ophthalmol Vis Sci* 31:1512–1518, 1990.

96. Gimbel HV, et al. Comparison of laser and manual removal of corneal epithelium for photorefractive keratectomy. *J Refract Surg* 11:36–41, 1995.

97. Sliney D, et al. Photokeratitis from 193 nm argon-fluoride laser radia-tion. *Photochem Photobiol* 53:739–744, 1991.

98. Krueger RR, Sliney D, Trokel S. Photokeratitis from subablative 193 nm excimer laser radiation. *Refract Corneal Surg* 8:274–279, 1992.

99. Muller-Stolzenburg NW, et al. UV exposure of the lens during 193 nm excimer laser corneal surgery. *Arch Ophthalmol* 108:915–916, 1990.

100. Ediger MM. Excimer-laser induced fluorescence of rabbit cornea: Radiometric measurement through the cornea. *Lasers Surg Med* 11:93–98, 1991.

101. Trentacoste J, et al. Mutagenic potential of a 193-nm excimer laser on fibroblasts in tissue culture. *Invest Ophthalmol Vis Sci* 94:125, 1987.

102. Nuss RC, Puliafito CA, Dehm E. Unscheduled DNA synthesis following excimer laser ablation of the cornea in vivo. *Invest Ophthalmol Vis Sci* 28:287–294, 1987.

103. Seiler T, et al. Side effects in excimer corneal surgery: DNA damage as a result of 193 nm excimer laser radiation. *Graefe's Arch Clin Exp Ophthalmol* 226:273–276, 1988.

104. Gebhardt B, Salmeron B, McDonald M. Effect of excimer laser on energy growth potential of corneal keratocytes. *Cornea* 9:210–250, 1990.

105. Asano Y, Mizuno K. The effect of ultraviolet irradiation on the corneal endothelium. *Acta Soc Ophthalmol Jpn* 92:578–583, 1988.

106. Binder P, et al. Endothelial cell loss associated with excimer laser. *Ophthalmology* 97:107, 1993.

107. Carones F, et al. The corneal endothelium after myopia excimer photo-refractive keratectomy. *Arch Ophthalmol* 112:920–924, 1994.

108. Stulting RD, Thompson KP, Lynn MJ. (Summit PRK Endothelial Cell Investigator Group). The effect of excimer laser photorefractive keratectomy (PRK) on the human corneal endothelium. *Invest Ophthalmol Vis Sci* 36(Suppl.):S1062, 1995.

109. Cano DB, et al. Endothelial changes with mid-stromal excimer laser ablations in human and porcine eyes. *Invest Ophthalmol Vis Sci* 36(Suppl.):S710, 1995.

110. Sliney D. Safety of ophthalmic excimer lasers with an emphasis on compressed gases. *Refract Corneal Surg* 7:308–314, 1991.

111. Krueger RR. Excimer laser: A step-up in complexity and responsibility for the ophthalmic laser surgeon? *J Refractive Surg* 10:83–86, 1994.

112. Sachs H, et al. Centration of excimer laser photorefractive keratectomy for myopia relative to the pupil with and without the use of an active eye tracking system. *Invest Ophthalmol Vis Sci* 36(Suppl.):S190, 1995.

113. McDonald M, et al. First clinical evaluation of autonomous technologies, scanning and tracking excimer laser: A primate study. *Invest Ophthalmol Vis Sci* 36(Suppl.):S710, 1995.

114. Hanna K, et al. A rotating slit delivery system for excimer laser refractive keratoplasty. *Am J Ophthalmol* 103:474, 1987.

115. Sinbawy A, McDonnell PJ, Moreira H. Surface ultrastructure after excimer laser ablation: Expanding vs contracting apertures. *Arch Ophthalmol* 109:1531–1533, 1991.

116. Foster W, Beck R, Busse H. Design and development of a new 193-nanometer excimer laser surgical system. *Refract Corneal Surg* 9:293–299, 1993.

117. Campos M, et al. Corneal wound healing after excimer laser ablation in rabbits: Expanding versus contracting apertures. *Refract Corneal Surg* 8:378–381, 1992.

2 Patient Selection and Evaluation

Audrey R. Talley, Kerry K. Assil, and David J. Schanzlin

The most important aspect of any keratorefractive practice is proper patient selection and evaluation. This pertains not only to medical and surgical criteria but also to patient expectations. Even if a patient meets the medical and surgical requirements for keratorefractive surgery, unrealistic patient expectations can render a patient ineligible for surgery. In this chapter, we address the evaluation of the keratorefractive patient, including history taking, clinical examination, preoperative testing, and the informed consent procedure.

History

As with any other ophthalmologic surgical evaluation, a complete patient history should be obtained and include medical and ocular history, family history, a list of medications, refractive stability, history of contact lens use, and relevant social and occupational history. Table 2-1 lists absolute and relative medical contraindications to radial keratotomy (RK), photorefractive keratectomy (PRK), and laser in-situ keratomileusis (LASIK).

Medical and Ocular History

Collagen vascular diseases, including rheumatoid arthritis and Sjögren's disease, affect corneal wound healing and are therefore contraindicated in RK and PRK. LASIK has been safely and successfully performed in selected patients with rheumatoid arthritis [1] and therefore is relatively rather than absolutely contraindicated in this disease. The potential for corneal melting and perforation due to stromal lysis induced by the inflammatory response following PRK

Table 2-1. Absolute and relative contraindications to keratorefractive surgery

	RK		PRK		LASIK	
	Absolute	Relative	Absolute	Relative	Absolute	Relative
Age < 18 years	X		X		X	
Refractive instability	X		X		X	
Rheumatoid arthritis	X		X			X
Collagen vascular disease	X		X			X
Scleritis	X		X		X	
Severe ocular surface disorders (ocular cicatricial pemphigoid, alkali burns)	X		X		X	
Moderately dry eyes		X		X		X
Neurotrophic corneal disease	X		X		X	
Diabetes mellitus		X		X		X
AIDS, other immunosuppression	X		X		X	
Herpes simplex virus		X		X		X
Blepharitis, rosacea		X		X		X
Keratoconus	X		X		X	
Glaucoma		X		X	X	
Pregnancy	X		X		X	
Cataracts	X		X		X	

RK = radial keratotomy; PRK = photorefractive keratectomy; LASIK = laser in-situ keratomileusis.

make this a poor choice for patients with this disease. Similarly, a history of scleritis disqualifies patients from all keratorefractive procedures. Patients with a history of inflammatory bowel disease, such as Crohn's disease or ulcerative colitis, or Wegener's granulomatosis also have the potential for corneal melting and are poor candidates for keratorefractive surgery.

Ocular surface abnormalities resulting from Sjögren's disease, alkali burns, or ocular cicatricial pemphigoid are absolute contraindications to keratorefractive surgery. Moderate to severe dry eye syndromes resulting in surface abnormalities are relative contraindications to keratorefractive surgery. Punctal occlusion and tear replacement therapy are often necessary to stabilize the patient's ocular surface prior to surgery. Patients with a history of immunosuppression from AIDS or chronic active hepatitis and those who are pharmacologically immunosuppressed from systemic corticosteroids or other cytotoxic agents are also poor candidates for keratorefractive surgery.

A history of neurotrophic corneal ulcers, herpes zoster ophthalmicus, or nonhealing epithelial defects makes these patients ineligible for keratorefractive surgery due to the delay in epithelial wound healing. Similarly, diabetes mellitus is a relative contraindication to keratorefractive surgery, due to concerns about delayed wound healing and abnormal immune responses. Certainly, any diabetic patient with a documented history of delayed corneal epithelial healing or a history of proliferative diabetic retinopathy (indicating more severe or advanced disease) would not be a good candidate for any keratorefractive procedure.

A history of herpes simplex (HSV) keratitis presents another relative contraindication to keratorefractive surgery. PRK and phototherapeutic keratectomy (PTK) performed on patients with a history of HSV have resulted in cases of reactivation of latent virus [2]. Patients without a history of stromal disease who have been free from HSV keratitis for at least 1 year may still be good surgical candidates. Oral acyclovir given in the perioperative period may also be beneficial in preventing recurrence of the disease [3].

Blepharitis, ocular rosacea, and meibomitis can also be relative contraindications to keratorefractive surgery. These conditions need to be adequately treated preoperatively with lid hygiene and, in some cases, with oral tetracycline or doxycycline. Aggressive medical treatment of these disorders must also continue postoperatively to minimize the chances of abnormal corneal wound healing.

Keratoconus, as viewed by these authors, is an absolute contraindication to keratorefractive surgery. This progressive corneal ectasia can cause wide variations and fluctuations in pre- and postoperative refractions. There have been some anecdotal cases of keratoconus treated with PRK, but no long-term data are available [4].

A history of glaucoma is a relative contraindication to RK and PRK and an absolute contraindication to LASIK. The postoperative steroid regimen in PRK may lead to poor control of intraocular pressure due to a steroid response. The increased intraocular pressure that occurs during the LASIK procedure with the placement of the suction ring can further damage an optic nerve that is already compromised or damaged from glaucoma.

Atopic disease is a relative contraindication for keratorefractive procedures. Atopic individuals with severe lid abnormalities, cataracts, keratoconus, or severe eye rubbing behavior are ineligible for surgery. Eye rubbing can lead to an increased incidence of infection, a delay in wound healing, and instability of postoperative refraction. Antihistamines and behavioral modification may be beneficial in preventing and treating ocular itching.

Cataracts are an absolute contraindication to keratorefractive surgery. The patient's refractive status can be corrected by intraocular lens implantation at the time of cataract surgery.

Pregnancy is another contraindication to keratorefractive surgery due to the changes in corneal curvature and refraction that can occur during this time. Keratorefractive procedures should be delayed until stability of refraction is documented in the postpartum period or thereafter.

Family History

Family history should include a history of corneal dystrophies, keratoconus, glaucoma, retinal detachment, retinal dystrophies, optic nerve abnormalities, diabetes mellitus, collagen vascular disease, early cardiovascular disease, and any other hereditary diseases. This information should be an adjunct to the information already obtained from the patient's medical and ocular history.

Medications

A complete list of systemic and ophthalmic medications should be obtained. Although the majority of keratorefractive candidates are young, healthy myopes on few medications, this part of the history should not be omitted. A list of medications can provide clues to the existence of diseases that may have been overlooked or forgotten by patients during the medical and ocular history.

Antihistamines, decongestants, and some antidepressants can exacerbate dry eye problems, immunosuppressants can delay wound healing, and oral contraceptive pills can cause changes in corneal curvature and refraction. Amiodarone and acutane (Isotretinoin) are also contraindicated in patients undergoing PRK or PTK. Although the benefits of these and other medications may clearly outweigh the risks of discontinuance, it is important to be aware of the potential effects of these and other drugs when planning the surgical procedure.

Refractive Stability

Refractive stability is imperative for obtaining the desired keratorefractive surgical results. Patients younger than 18 and those who have had a 0.50 or greater diopter change in sphere or cylinder per year over the preceeding 2 years are not eligible for surgery.

Contact Lens History

Candidates for keratorefractive surgery should discontinue soft contact lens wear 2 weeks prior to surgical evaluation. Rigid gas-permeable (RGP) lens wearers must discontinue lenses for a minimum of 3 weeks prior to surgical evaluation. Manifest and cycloplegic refractions along with corneal topography should be used to monitor and confirm stabilization of the corneal curvature and of refraction before the surgery can be planned. The existence of corneal warpage due to contact lens wear (usually RGP) is a contraindication to keratorefractive surgery until the condition has stabilized. It may take months or years for some corneas to recover from warpage secondary to contact lens wear [5].

Social and Occupational History

Evaluating the patient's vocational and recreational refractive needs is important for optimal surgical planning. Patients of presbyopic age may benefit from monovision, whereas younger patients (< 35–40 years of age) are usually not tolerant of this approach.

Patients involved in boxing or other contact sports where blunt head trauma is likely are better suited for PRK or LASIK and clearly should not be considered good RK candidates.

Patients who are pilots, law enforcement agents, or who have other careers that have strict visual acuity requirements are encouraged to check with their employers before undergoing keratorefractive surgery. Some airlines and military branches do not recognize refractive surgery as a valid means of visual correction.

Clinical Examination

A complete ophthalmologic examination must be performed, including measurements of ocular dominance and motility, pupillary examination, retinoscopy, manifest and cycloplegic refractions, external examination, slit-lamp examination, measurement of intraocular pressure, and dilated funduscopic examination.

Ocular Dominance and Motility

Ocular dominance may be established by patient history or by testing distance fixation. The examiner can ask the patient about his or her preferred viewing eye when looking through the lens of a camera. If the patient is unsure, the examiner can employ standard tests of distance fixation. One simple method is to have the patient line up an outstretched thumb or finger with a distant object. By alternating right and left eye closure, the fixating eye, and therefore the dominant eye, can be established.

Many surgeons prefer to operate on the nondominant eye first because visual fluctuations, glare, and halos will be less problematic for the patient if the dominant eye is still functioning normally in the early postoperative period. This also allows the surgeon to assess the effects of wound healing and under or overcorrections in the nondominant eye, which may provide important information for planning the surgery on the dominant eye.

Motility testing should include evaluation of ductions, versions, and measurement of any tropias or phorias. Any motility abnormality that could result in diplopia should be fully evaluated before keratorefractive surgery. Any history or finding on examination that suggests amblyopia should also be carefully documented.

Pupillary Examination

Pupillary examination should include the measurement of pupillary size, shape, and direct and concentric light responses. Pupil size and shape are especially important when planning the optical zone size for RK or photoablative procedures. Any abnormalities noted with the pupillary light response deserve further evaluation.

Retinoscopy and Manifest and Cycloplegic Refractions

Retinoscopy and manifest and cycloplegic refractions are imperative for assessing refractive stability. Any significant discrepancies among these measurements require further evaluation for the presence of overaccommodation, latent hyperopia, progressive myopia or astigmatism, corneal warpage syndromes, and other corneal, lenticular, or retinal pathology. Refractions should also be compared with the patient's current spectacle correction and with corneal topography. It is also important to record the patient's uncorrected and best corrected visual acuities. As stated previously, refractive stability must be documented before any keratorefractive procedure can be performed.

External Examination

External examination should focus on the lids, lashes, and lacrimal apparati. Any lid abnormalities, such as lagophthalmos, entropion, ectropion, trichiasis, blepharitis, chalazia, or other lid lesions should be treated before planning surgery. Lagophthalmos, ectropion, entropion, and trichiasis can cause problems with corneal exposure and ocular surface instability. Blepharitis, canaliculitis, and dacryocystitis can predispose patients to infection in the perioperative period. Chalazia and other lid lesions can cause astigmatism and corneal warpage syndromes. Obviously, any indication of accompanying systemic medical disease warrants further evaluation.

Slit-Lamp Examination

Slit-lamp examination should include a thorough examination of all anterior segment structures with special attention focused on the conjunctiva, cornea, and lens. Further evaluation of any lid abnormalities noted on external examination should also be included.

Examination of the conjunctiva should detect any scarring from previous trauma, surgery, inflammatory disease, or infection and any conjunctival lesions. The presence of conjunctival pathology can potentially interfere with proper lid closure and create corneal dellen and other ocular surface abnormalities.

The cornea should be examined for evidence of any epithelial, stromal, or endothelial pathology. The tear film should be observed and tear break-up times recorded. If a decreased tear film or tear break-up time is noted, further evaluation, including Schirmer testing, is indicated. Epithelial dystrophies (including anterior basement membrane disease) do not present a contraindication to keratorefractive procedures. PTK and PRK have been successfully used in the treatment of recurrent corneal erosions [6] and therefore may play a therapeutic role in such cases. Other ocular surface disorders need more complete evaluation and treatment, as has been previously discussed. Corneal sensitivity should be tested, and if decreased, a search for potential causes of neurotrophic corneal disease should be undertaken.

The corneal stroma should be examined for thickness and clarity. An increase in corneal thickness should prompt the examiner to evaluate endothelial cell function. Corneal thinning may be due to keratoconus; pellucid degeneration; previous infection with loss of stroma; inflammatory disease, such as immune corneal melts; or trauma. A decrease in corneal clarity may result from stromal dystrophies or scarring from trauma or infection. Stromal opacity with neovascularization may indicate previous herpetic infection or other chronic ocular surface inflammatory processes.

The corneal endothelium should be evaluated for the presence of guttae. Any evidence of increased corneal thickness associated with endothelial dystrophy or dysfunction can cause instability of refraction.

Examination of anterior chamber depth should be recorded and any pupillary or iris abnormalities of size or shape should be noted. The presence of iris atrophy may indicate previous herpes zoster infection, trauma, anterior segment dysgenesis syndromes, or glaucoma.

The lens should be examined for any evidence of cataract formation. With the exception of very small, visually insignificant congenital cataracts, lens opacities represent an absolute contraindication to keratorefractive surgery.

Measurement of Intraocular Pressure

Intraocular pressure should be measured using applanation tonometry. If increased intraocular pressure is found, the patient should have an evaluation for glaucoma. If the patient is known to have glaucoma, better intraocular pressure control should be attained before proceeding with keratorefractive surgery. Patients with ocular hypertension who plan to have RK or PRK should be aware of the risk of steroid response in the postoperative period that may necessitate treatment with glaucoma medications. LASIK is an absolute contraindication in patients with ocular hypertension or glaucoma.

Funduscopic Examination

A dilated funduscopic examination should be performed using indirect ophthalmoscopy and slit-lamp biomicroscopy. Any evidence of macular or other retinal pathology that could affect visual acuity should be noted. Macular edema or proliferative diabetic retinopathy are contraindications to keratorefractive procedures.

Optic nerve pathology, such as increased cup to disc ratios, optic pits, or nerve head drusen, should be further evaluated with visual field testing. Any significant optic nerve or retinal pathology may indicate a relative or absolute contraindication to keratorefractive surgery.

Peripheral retinal pathology, such as lattice degeneration, atrophic holes, and white appearance without pressure, should be carefully documented. Such abnormalities are common in myopic individuals, and retinal consultation should be obtained where appropriate prior to refractive surgery.

Preoperative Testing

Preoperative testing should include corneal topography, a demonstration of the expected refractive outcome, and screening pachymetry.

Corneal Topography

Corneal topography is now considered an integral component of preoperative evaluation of the keratorefractive patient. The advent of corneal topography has obviated the need for manual keratometry. Corneal topography can be used to detect regular and irregular astigmatism, corneal warpage from contact lens wear or compressive lid lesions, clinical and preclinical or forme fruste keratoconus, pellucid marginal degeneration, and the postoperative refractive effects of keratorefractive surgery. Corneal topography is also helpful in determining refractive stability when used as an adjunct to manifest and cycloplegic refractions.

At the present time, placido-disc–based computerized video keratography (CVK) is the technique most commonly used to assess corneal curvature prior to refractive surgery. As such, we will devote our efforts here to defining and illustrating commonly encountered normal and abnormal CVK patterns. Newer technologies with a potentially greater range of technical capabilities are under development (e.g., rasterstereography, interferometry, holography, scanning slit technology) but have yet to find widespread application in clinical practice.

The normal cornea is asymmetrically aspheric, with 90% of the refractive power at the anterior surface. There is a changing radius of curvature in the normal cornea, with the steepest area centrally, and a gradual flattening peripherally. According to the Bogan and Waring system of classification of normal corneal topography using CVK [7], 23% of corneas have a round classification, 21% are oval, 18% have a symmetric bowtie shape, 32% have an asymmetric bowtie shape, and 7% are irregular. The following corneal topographic maps (Figs. 2-1 through 2-5) demonstrate the Bogan and Waring classification system. Although not illustrated here, it is important when inspecting any CVK map to carefully study the accompanying dioptric power scale to better determine the clinical significance of the color-coded changes observed.

In cases of corneal warpage from contact lenses, CVK shows irregular astigmatism that is greatest centrally, without a set pattern. This

Fig. 2-1. Round CVK pattern. (From Bogan et al. Classification of normal corneal topography based on computer-assisted videokeratography. *Arch Ophthalmol* 108:945–949. Copyright 1990, American Medical Association.)

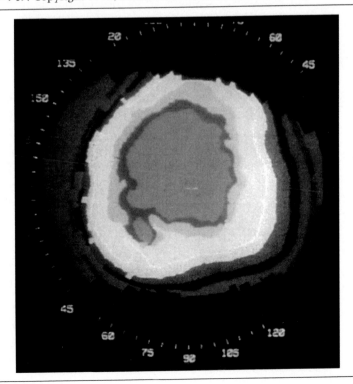

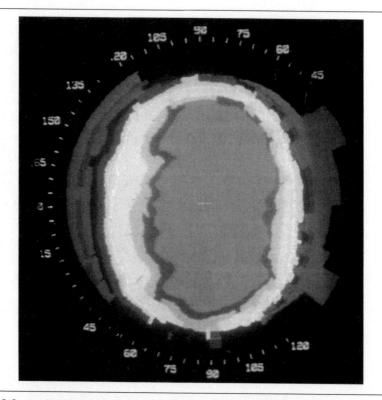

Fig. 2-2. Oval CVK pattern. (From Bogan et al. Classification of normal corneal topography based on computer-assisted videokeratography. *Arch Ophthalmol* 108:945–949. Copyright 1990, American Medical Association.)

may be accompanied clinically by an unstable refraction, decreased visual acuity, spectacle blur, or decreased contrast sensitivity. The following corneal topographic map shows corneal warpage in an RGP lens patient. As previously stated, keratorefractive procedures should not be performed on patients with corneal warpage until refractive and topographic stability have been achieved (Plates 1 and 2).

CVK maps in both clinical and preclinical (forme fruste) keratoconus demonstrate conelike or asymmetric bowtie-like steepening, usually inferiorly, although the entire cornea may be involved. The following corneal topographic maps illustrate examples of clinical (Plate 3) and preclinical or forme fruste keratoconus (Plate 4). Clinical and forme fruste keratoconus are contraindications to keratorefractive surgery.

In pellucid marginal degeneration, corneal topography demonstrates inferior steepening with against-the-rule astigmatism. Pellucid marginal degeneration is a contraindication to keratorefractive surgery. Stromal thinning extending to the limbus in the zone of topographic steepening is sometimes evident with careful slit-lamp

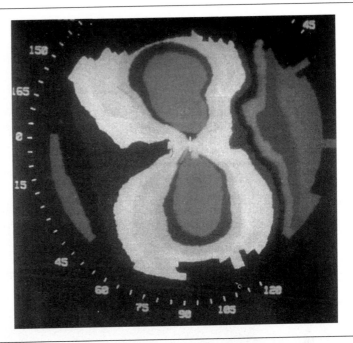

Fig. 2-3. Symmetric bowtie-shaped CVK pattern. (From Bogan et al. Classification of normal corneal topography based on computer-assisted videokeratography. *Arch Ophthalmol* 108:945–949. Copyright 1990, American Medical Association.)

biomicroscopy. Terrien's marginal degeneration can also show a similar CVK pattern but usually manifests itself by a superficial vascular pannus with intrastromal lipid deposition.

In the postoperative keratorefractive surgical patient, corneal topography can be used to assist in assessing the refractive outcome and in planning enhancement procedures. After succesful RK, PRK, or LASIK procedures in the myope, there should be a uniform region of central corneal flattening (Plate 5). One topographic complication of PRK is the formation of central islands. These are regions of central elevation in the treatment zone that may cause clinically significant irregular astigmatism (Figure 2-6). Although many of these central islands resolve with time, enhancement procedures may be indicated in some patients. Illustrations of other abnormal topographic patterns after PRK and LASIK can be found in Chapters 5, 8, and 9.

Demonstration of the Expected Refractive Outcome

Demonstration of the expected refractive outcome can be beneficial in some patients by helping to provide them with realistic expectations from their planned keratorefractive procedure. This may be accomplished by having them look through a phoropter or trial frame

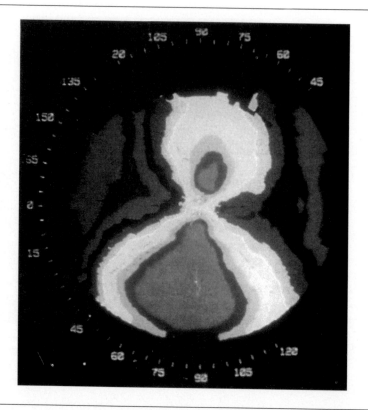

Fig. 2-4. Asymmetric bowtie-shaped CVK pattern. (From Bogan et al. Classification of normal corneal topography based on computer-assisted videokeratography. *Arch Ophthalmol* 108:945–949. Copyright 1990, American Medical Association.)

with a refraction that enables them to see the 20/40 or 20/30 line clearly but shows slightly defocused 20/25 and 20/20 lines. The patient is then allowed to compare this refraction with his or her current or best corrected visual acuity. The examiner should explain that a realistic goal of keratorefractive surgery is for uncorrected visual acuity at the level of legal driving vision (20/40 or 20/30). Although many patients achieve better postoperative vision, their uncorrected postoperative visual acuity may not be as sharp and clear as their preoperative best corrected visual acuity. In a similar fashion, the examiner may use trial frames to demonstrate monovision and a presbyopia. These demonstrations are useful tools in obtaining informed consent and in attempting to clarify the patient's expectations.

Pachymetry

Although pachymetry is an invaluable tool in the measurement of corneal thickness during the RK procedure and in planning PTK or

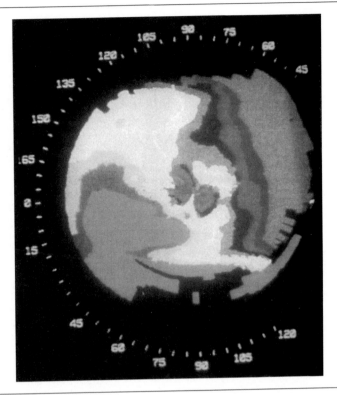

Fig. 2-5. Irregularly shaped CVK pattern. (From Bogan et al. Classification of normal corneal topography based on computer-assisted videokeratography. *Arch Ophthalmol* 108:945–949. Copyright 1990, American Medical Association.)

LASIK procedures, it has limited value as a general screening tool for all keratorefractive procedures. If there is evidence of an increase or decrease in corneal thickness during the clinical examination, as in cases of endothelial dystrophy or stromal loss, then pachymetry is certainly warranted. Pachymetry also may be useful in planning enhancement procedures following PRK and LASIK. No one would fault the cautious keratorefractive surgeon for obtaining this test on all patients, but it should not be used as a substitute for a thorough clinical corneal examination.

Contrast Sensitivity

Contrast sensitivity may be measured using the standard early treatment diabetic retinopathy study (ETDRS) contrast sensitivity visual charts. This test, although initially required by the Food and Drug Administration (FDA) in the United States PRK trials, has yet to prove valuable as a general screening tool in the evaluation of keratorefractive patients.

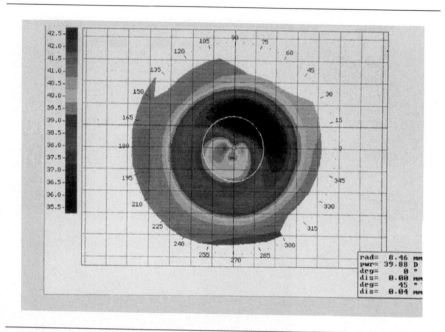

Fig. 2-6. Postoperative photorefractive keratectomy showing the formation of a central island.

Informed Consent

Informed consent should include apprising the patient of both surgical and nonsurgical refractive options; the risks, benefits, side effects, and expected outcome of the procedure; and a discussion of enhancement procedures. The patient who meets medical and surgical criteria for a keratorefractive procedure but who has unrealistic expectations is not a good candidate for keratorefractive surgery.

The patient must be required to read and sign an informed consent document and should discuss the planned procedure with the kera-torefractive surgeon before doing so. In general, it is wise to have the patient read and sign the informed consent document prior to dilation or at a later date. A portion of this document may be in the form of a true/false "quiz," which serves to further educate the patient about the planned procedure. There should be ample opportunity during the surgeon-patient discussion for the patient to ask questions. In addi-tion, it is useful for the patient to attend educational seminars and to read brochures and watch videotapes that contain informational material about refractive surgery. An example of informed consent for laser vision correction is included in Appendix B.

Refractive Options

The patient should be informed about surgical and nonsurgical refractive options, including glasses, contact lenses, RK, PRK, and LASIK. The selection of the appropriate keratorefractive surgical procedure is discussed in detail in Chapter 3.

The patient should also be made aware that refractive surgery usually does not eliminate the need for additional reading correction once the patient has entered the presbyopic age group. For the patient nearing or of presbyopic age, the concept of monovision should also be discussed.

Risks

Risks of all keratorefractive procedures include the risk of infection, overcorrection, undercorrection, regression, loss of best corrected visual acuity, scarring, night glare, and blindness. Rupture of incisions leading to a permanent decrease in best corrected visual acuity has been reported after severe trauma in patients that have had RK [8], but this is a very rare ocurrence. There have not been any cases of blindness reported to date in the peer-reviewed literature after PRK or LASIK. Blindness remains a theoretical risk of any ophthalmologic surgical procedure and therefore should be discussed.

An additional risk of RK is the structural weakening of the cornea. For this reason, RK is not recommended for individuals who are involved in contact sports and others who are likely to sustain blunt trauma. Other risks specific to RK include the risk of micro- and macroperforation during the procedure. These complications are usually easily treated with patching and occasionally by suturing of the cornea. Progressive hyperopia is another documented risk of RK. As the incidence and magnitude of long-term hyperopic shift appears to increase in direct proportion to incision length and number [9], modern techniques tend to limit optical zone size and incision number more strictly than in the past. This issue is discussed in greater detail in Chapter 3.

Haze formation is an additional risk of PRK and LASIK. Clinically significant haze has been reported, mostly in high myopes that have undergone PRK [10, 11]. This haze may lead to a loss of best corrected visual acuity. As a result, PRK is not recommended for patients who are known to be keloid formers. The use of the microkeratome in the LASIK procedure adds the additional theoretical risk of perforation of the anterior chamber with suction engaged, potentially resulting in loss of the eye. Although this has occurred during automated lamellar keratoplasty (ALK) procedures, it has not been reported, to date, with LASIK.

Side Effects

The most common side effects of all keratorefractive procedures are postoperative discomfort or pain, glare, and the starburst or halo symptoms. Postoperative pain has been minimized in all keratorefractive procedures and especially in PRK with the use of topical nonsteroidal anti-inflammatory drops, such as sodium diclofenac [12]. PRK patients are often fitted during the acute postoperative period with a bandage contact lens. Most patients describe only mild discomfort, increased light sensitivity, and a "scratchy" feeling in the eye after keratorefractive surgery. Almost all keratorefractive patients describe halos or a starburst effect when looking at bright lights in the early postoperative period. This effect usually, but not always, diminishes with time.

Patients undergoing PRK may have a delay in visual recovery lasting from a few days (when epithelial healing is complete) up to several months after surgery. This is in distinct contrast to individuals undergoing RK, ALK, or LASIK, where visual recovery is often quite rapid.

Expected Outcome

Patients need to be aware that the goal of any keratorefractive procedure is to make them less dependent on glasses or contact lenses, but it seldom completely eliminates the need for nonsurgical refractive correction. As was previously discussed, patients should be informed about presbyopia and the need for reading correction. Demonstration of expected refractive outcomes, as described in the preoperative testing section of this chapter, can be useful in helping the patients achieve realistic expectations of the planned keratorefractive procedure.

Need for Further Surgery

The concept of the enhancement procedure and the need for further surgery to achieve the desired visual outcome should also be discussed with every patient. Enhancement rates vary with each surgeon but are generally in the range of 25% for RK procedures, 2–10% for PRK procedures, and 10–25% for LASIK procedures. The informed consent process for an enhancement procedure should not differ significantly from the original keratorefractive procedure.

Conclusions

The evaluation of the keratorefractive surgical candidate includes recording a thorough history, performing a complete clinical ophthalmologic examination, utilizing appropriate preoperative tests, and obtaining informed consent for the surgical procedure. At the completion of the process, the surgeon should be certain that the patient has realistic expectations of the planned keratorefractive surgery. Surgeons must remember that not every patient who meets the medical and surgical criteria for keratorefractive procedures is a good surgical candidate. Unrealistic expectations can lead to both disgruntled patients and unhappy surgeons.

References

1. Machat JJ. Personal communication. October, 1995.
2. Fagerholm P, Ohman L, Orndahl M. Phototherapeutic keratectomy in herpes simplex keratitis. Clinical results in 20 patients. *Acta Ophthalmol* 72:457–460, 1994.
3. Barney NP, Foster CS. A prospective randomized trial of oral acyclovir after penetrating keratoplasty for herpes simplex keratitis. *Cornea* 13:232–236, 1994.
4. Mortensen J, Ohstrom A. Excimer laser photorefractive keratectomy for the treatment of keratoconus. *Refract Corneal Surg* 10:368–372, 1994.
5. Wilson SE, Klyce SD. Screening for corneal topographic abnormalities before refractive surgery. *Ophthalmol* 101:147–152, 1994.
6. Talley AR, et al. Phototherapeutic keratectomy for the treatment of recurrent corneal erosion syndrome. Proceedings of the 42nd Annual Symposium on Medical Cornea. *Corneal Refract Surg* New Orleans Acad of Ophthalmol Proceed 10:121–126, 1994.
7. Bogan SJ, et al. Classification of normal corneal topography based on computer-assisted videokeratography. *Arch Ophthalmol* 108:945–949, 1990.
8. McDermott ML, et al. Corneoscleral rupture ten years after radial keratotomy. *Am J Ophthalmol* 110:575–576, 1990.
9. Waring GO, McDonnell PJ, Lynn MJ. Results of the Prospective Evaluation of Radial Keratotomy Study (PERK) 10 years after surgery. *Arch Ophthalmol* 112:1298–1308, 1994.
10. Sher NA, et al. Excimer laser photorefractive keratectomy in high myopia: A multicenter study. *Arch Ophthalmol* 110:935–943, 1992.
11. Menezo J, et al. Excimer laser photorefractive keratectomy for high myopia. *J Cataract Refract Surg* 21:393–396, 1995.
12. Sher NA, et al. Topical diclofenac in the treatment of ocular pain after excimer photorefractive keratectomy. *J Refract Corneal Surg* 9:425–436, 1993.

3 Selecting the Right Surgical Procedure: Clinical Results and Other Considerations

Paul M. Pender, Paul M. Karpecki, and Daniel S. Durrie

Some surgeons wishing to offer keratorefractive surgical options might ask for a simple answer to the question, "Which procedure is right for a given patient?" Here we will discuss the reasoning behind our qualified answer: The "right" keratorefractive procedure is the one most likely to result in a satisfactory outcome for both the patient and surgeon and the one least likely to cause problems.

We accept the premise that recommendations made in this text based on recent results may well be out of date in a relatively short time, given the pace of development [1–29]. We also believe that there is value in providing an overview of the literature and clinical results of keratorefractive procedures. We distinguish between generally accepted procedures and merely promising ones. What follows are guidelines for procedure selection from among commonly used procedures based on reports and clinical experience.

We assume that many readers have taken a course in radial keratotomy (RK) and photorefractive keratectomy (PRK) as well as attended conferences featuring refractive surgery topics. Our goal is not to revisit all the information derived from such sources but to distill the essentials and to offer our perspective on the subject for those about to begin performing refractive surgery in earnest. Surgeons preparing to begin a practice in keratorefractive procedures may have some feel for the incidence and severity of complications, but they may not have had personal experience in the management of complications. The procedures discussed in this chapter are characterized by a performance envelope, within which a low complication rate is observed. Consideration of the "maximum performance" for a given procedure is helpful in procedure selection. We are all aware of the temptations to stretch the performance envelope for a given procedure; that is not our goal. Here we develop the concept of the

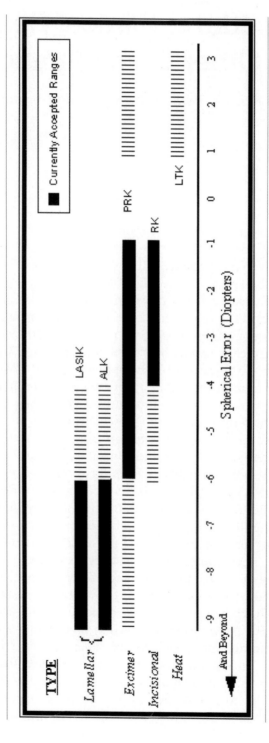

Fig. 3-1. Flow chart for procedure selection by range of refractive error.

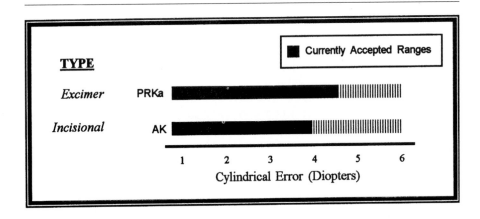

Fig. 3-2. Flow chart for procedure selection by range of cylindrical error.

performance envelope to meet the previously stated goals of a satisfied patient with the lowest risk for problems.

Our overview of clinical results of common procedures is further qualified by other considerations, such as patient age, systemic condition, lifestyle, occupation, and history of prior procedures. We cover the issues of surgical planning with regard to timing between eyes and staging of procedures, if indicated by the degree of ametropia. Finally, flow charts (Figs. 3-1, 3-2) are offered for suggested procedure selection according to the degree and type of ametropia.

Myopia

Radial Keratotomy

Surgery performed to reduce or eliminate myopia has evolved a great deal since Fyodorov popularized RK in the mid-1970s. Fyodorov's early concepts and experience challenged our thinking about operating on the so-called "normal eye" of the patient with myopia. At first, the technique was recommended for a very wide range of myopia. Enthusiastic supporters of Fyodorov seemed satisfied that the procedure worked well, even in high myopia. The amount of myopia that could be corrected seemed limited only by the surgeon's imagination and the number of radial incisions the cornea could tolerate. We now realize that the trade-off of a less stable cornea is not worth the price of attempting correction of high myopia with RK [6]. When no other alternative was practically available, it seemed reasonable to attempt such correction, whereas today that is not the case.

RK has been the most widely practiced keratorefractive technique to date. The 10-year results of the Prospective Evaluation of Radial Keratotomy (PERK) study [2] show that RK is a relatively safe and effective treatment for myopia of low to moderate degree (< −6 D). However, progressive corneal flattening is more severe as the attempted correction increases. The PERK study showed that 43% of eyes experienced a hyperopic shift of 1 D or more over the decade following surgery. More than one-third of all eyes were overcorrected by more than 0.50 D. The mean hyperopic shift in years 2 through 10 was 0.06 D per year. An important related finding was that hyperopic shift was reduced in eyes that had lower preoperative refractive errors. Patients who underwent RK with a 3-mm central optical zone (for treatment of high myopia) experienced about 0.50 D more hyperopic shift on average than those with a central optical zone of 3.5 mm (moderate myopia treatment) or 4 mm (low myopia treatment). The finding of greater hyperopic shift in higher myopes was confirmed by Werblin and Stafford using the Casebeer nomograms for age-dependent treatment of myopia by RK [13].

Although newer techniques will become more popular, we believe that RK will continue to occupy a niche in the armamentarium of refractive surgeons [6, 14]. Over the next 5 years, the primary uses of RK will be for low myopia and for enhancements of other keratorefractive procedures. As PRK becomes more established, it is likely that the vast majority of myopia surgical candidates will undergo PRK rather than RK.

Excimer Photorefractive Keratectomy

The Phase III Food and Drug Administration (FDA) studies of PRK for myopia between −1.5 and −6 D show greater predictability for patients receiving PRK than those receiving RK over the same myopia range when compared to results from the PERK study (Table 3-1) [15, 16]. With higher degrees of myopia, however, PRK may regress in the absence of appropriate medical intervention [17, 18]. Additionally, safety of PRK for eyes with myopia greater than −6 D remains an issue for additional study: Seiler and colleagues have reported that visually significant corneal haze and scarring developed in 7% of treatments above −6 D [15], but in less than 1% of eyes treated for under −6 D.

Does this mean that it is inadvisable to treat beyond −6 to −8 D of myopia with PRK? Preliminary international experience with surface PRK suggests that modifications in postoperative medications and surgical technique permit treatments of greater than −6 D of myopia. Multiple optical zones may provide higher corrections without uniformly deeper ablations. Multipass techniques to blend the edges of

Table 3-1. Clinical results for low myopia at 1 year: RK and PRK[a]

	PERK [12]	Werblin [13]	Verity [14]	Summit[b]	VISX[b]
UCVA ≥ 20/40	81%	99%	95%	98%	93.8%
UCVA ≥ 20/20	47%	45%	NR	80%	60%
Actual SE vs intended					
± 1 D	64%	NR	92%	85%	87%
± 0.5 D	36%	NR	NR	51%	48%
Loss of BCVA ≥ 2 lines	0.7%	NR	0.3%	1.2%	0.3%
Enhancement rate	NR	48%	27%	NA	NA

PERK = Prospective Evaluation of Radial Keratotomy study; UCVA = uncorrected visual acuity; SE = spherical equivalent; BCVA = best spectable-corrected visual acuity; NR = not reported; NA = not applicable.
[a]Summit (Waltham, MA) and VISX (Santa Clara, CA) data for 6-mm ablations up to −6 D; PERK to −8.75 D; Werblin to −8.87 D; Verity to −9.50 D.
[b]Source: Food and Drug Administration Panel Presentations October 19, 1994 (Summit) and October 20, 1995 (VISX), Gaithersburg, MD.

the treatment zones are intended to reduce the likelihood of regression and scarring. Although excimer laser investigators in the United States may feel constrained by the protocol restrictions imposed by the FDA, most realize the importance of application of standardized techniques for data collection and trend analysis. As we look at other techniques for treating high myopia (defined here as > −6 D) we will return to the issue of safety and the risk-benefit ratio of PRK compared to other modes of treatment.

Radial Keratotomy vs. Photorefractive Keratectomy

Both RK and PRK are equally safe in the range of low to moderate myopia with respect to preservation of best corrected visual acuity (BCVA). Comparable results are found in the PERK study and in the FDA's PRK Phase III study for preservation of best corrected acuity in the treatment of spherical myopia in the range of −1 to −6 D (see Table 3-1). Prior to the discontinuation of nitrogen blowing across the cornea in the VISX series (Santa Clara, CA) of PRK for low myopia (phase II-A), higher rates of BCVA loss were observed. It is likely that intraoperative drying of the stromal surface created abnormalities that resulted in irregular astigmatism postoperatively. Recent reports by both Summit and VISX investigators indicate that FDA criteria for safety and efficacy are met by PRK for low to moderate myopia (Table 3-2). These criteria are useful to keep in mind when evaluating clinical results following RK or other procedures as well.

The two most important factors favoring PRK over RK for low myopia are PRK's decreased need for enhancements and greater long-term stability of refractive correction. Although RK as it is cur-

Table 3-2. FDA Safety and efficacy criteria for photorefractive keratectomy

Less than 5% of eyes lose 2 or more lines of BCVA
Less than 1% of eyes lose 3 or more lines of BCVA
For eyes that started with 20/20 or better visual acuity, no more than 1% would become worse than 20/25 BCVA, and no more than 0.2% would become worse than 20/40 BCVA
20/25 or better UCVA in 75% of eyes with cycloplegic refraction between −1.00 D and +0.50 D

BCVA = best corrected visual acuity; UCVA = uncorrected visual acuity.
Source: The Scientific Advisory Panel, Ophthalmic Devices Division, Gaithersburg, MD, October 21, 1994.

rently practiced allows the prudent surgeon and the informed patient the ability to titrate the correction required with additional surgery, PRK may yield a higher percentage of desired corrections with a single treatment. Recent reports of RK employing Russian technique (centripetal), American technique (centrifugal), or a technique combining both methods (combined, Genesis, Duotrak) still show additional surgery required in one-fourth to one-third of eyes [13, 14]. As market pressures force surgeons to be more economical in their global surgical encounters, the cost to the surgeon's time for additional enhancements may become prohibitive.

With respect to stability of correction, PRK will probably prove more stable than RK over time. Attempts to modify RK technique to avoid problems with progessive flattening of the cornea by shortening the length of incisions ("mini-RK") may offer some hope of greater stability for 4-incision procedures with large optical zones [6]. For most patients with low to moderate myopia, however, PRK will likely prove more stable than RK.

As surgeons who perform both RK and PRK are aware, there are distinct benefits and drawbacks to each technique that may make one preferable to another for a given patient. Although PRK offers greater long-term refractive stability and less risk of subsequent ocular rupture from blunt trauma, the early postoperative pain can be severe and the visual recovery prolonged in a substantial minority of patients. For patients with low myopia (≤ −3 D) who lead an extremely active lifestyle or have a visually demanding occupation, the inconvenience of prolonged healing following PRK may be too great. Additionally, further studies may quite possibly demonstrate that large optical zone, 4-incision mini-RK is as safe, effective, and stable for *low* myopia as PRK and can be provided at lower cost as well.

Laser In-Situ Keratomileusis

There is a general perception of reduced risk for late regression and scarring from lamellar corneal surgery compared to surface ablation.

Laser in-situ keratomileusis (LASIK) and automated lamellar kerato-plasty (ALK) have been advocated in the treatment of high myopia [19–22]. It appears that the second, or refractive, cut in the stromal bed during ALK may be more accurately performed with an excimer laser. Early reports in the literature give LASIK the edge over ALK for safety and efficacy, particularly if the excimer ablation is performed in the stromal bed rather than on the back of the corneal flap or cap. Results at the present time are still very preliminary, however, and the promise of LASIK in the stromal bed awaits further confirmation in the peer-reviewed literature (Table 3-3). Problems with decentration, irregular astigmatism, and undercorrection and overcorrection may be reduced when the laser, rather than the mechanical micro-keratome, completes the refractive cut. There is also a general belief among some surgeons performing lamellar corneal surgery that LASIK appears to cause less trauma to the cornea than does PRK for high myopia. Additional prospective clinical studies will better define the reasons for the perceived advantage of lamellar techniques in treating high myopia, as well as the long-term safety, efficacy, predictability, and stability of this procedure.

Recent meetings of the International Society of Refractive Surgery (ISRS) and the American Society of Cataract and Refractive Surgery (ASCRS) [1] provided an opportunity to poll participants on their approaches to the treatment of high myopia, as shown in Table 3-4.

One-fourth of the respondents chose not to treat high myopia surgically. Because more needs to be learned about lamellar surgical procedures, it appears that any recommendation for treatment of high myopia must be based on impression rather than hard fact. In another poll, although only 14% of ISRS members had performed LASIK, 89% of these respondents considered it the treatment of choice for high myopia.

It may be prudent for the refractive surgeon to develop his or her own procedure nomograms to serve as a guide for procedure selection according to the degree of myopia being treated. One such approach might include the following procedures for the degrees of myopia specified:

RK	−1 to −4 D
PRK	−1 to −6 D
ALK or LASIK	−6 D and above

Although the presenters at the 1994 ISRS meeting set the upper limit of RK at −3 to −4 D, the majority of the audience set the RK ceiling at −5 to −6 D. The presenters felt that the risk of progressive hyperopia increased as the degree of intended correction increased. Based on the

Table 3-3. Clinical results of laser in-situ keratomileusis

Author	# Eyes	Range	Follow-up	UCVA > 20/40	SE within 1 D	BCVA loss > 2 lines	Complications	Comment
Pallikaris [21]	20	Up to −26 D	1 yr	NA	67%	0%	Interface haze	Partially sighted eyes Meditec laser (Heroldsberg, Germany)
Ruiz[a]	119	Up to −7.5 D	6 mo	94.8%	NA	0%	None listed	PRK vs. LASIK Summit laser (Waltham, MA)
Salah[b]	59	Mean −9.36	3 mo	76%	73%	10%	Epithelial ingrowth	Summit laser
Fiander[c]	124	Up to −27 D	3 mo	81%	70%	0%	Cap off in 10% Overcorrection	Summit laser
Bas[d]	97	Mean −10.75	3 mo	50%	47%	13.4%	Decentration Epithelial cysts Incomplete flap Irregular astigmatism	Summit laser
Salah [22]	88	Up to −20 D	3–8 mo	71%	73%	3.6%	Irregular astigmatism Macular degeneration	Summit laser

UCVA = uncorrected visual acuity; SE = spherical equivalent; BCVA = best corrected visual acuity; NA = not applicable.
[a]L Ruiz, SG Slade, SA Updegraff. Excimer Myopic Keratomileusis: Bogota Experience. In JJ Salz (ed), *Corneal Laser Surgery*. St. Louis: Mosby–Year Book, 1995. Pp. 195.
[b]T Salah, GO Waring, A El-Magrahby. Excimer Laser Keratomileusis (part I). In JJ Salz (ed), *Corneal Laser Surgery*. St Louis: Mosby–Year Book, 1995. Pp. 187–194.
[c]DC Fiander, F Tayfair. Excimer laser in situ keratomileusis in 124 myopic eyes. *J Refract Surg* 11 : S234–238, 1995.
[d]AM Bas, R Onnis. Excimer laser in situ keratomileusis for myopia. *J Refract Surg* 11 : S229–233, 1995.

Table 3-4. International Society of Refractive Surgery Poll (October 1994): For high myopia (−8 to −12 D and above), what do you perform?*

Response	Percent
No treatment	25.8
RK	5.5
PRK	25.0
PRK + RK	8.6
ALK or LASIK	23.4
Epikeratophakia	0
Phakic lenses	3.9
Clear lens extracap + IOL	7.0

RK = radial keratotomy; PRK = photorefractive keratectomy; ALK = automated lamellar keratoplasty; LASIK = laser in-situ keratomileusis; IOL = intraocular lens.
*Total responses = 128

Table 3-5. ISRS procedure preferences

Myopia range (D)	Surgeons' preference
−1 to −3	RK, 66%; PRK, 31%
−3 to −6	PRK, 64%; RK, 33%
−6 to −9	PRK, 89%; RK, 9%
−6 to −9	LASIK* 89%

*Includes only those performing LASIK.

patient's age and other factors (e.g., gender, intraocular pressure), however, an argument can be made to treat up to −6 D with incisional techniques. Obviously, there is some overlap in determining which procedures work best in which ranges of myopia. The results of a poll of 150 refractive surgeons attending the 1994 ISRS meeting are summarized in Table 3-5.

Would the beginning refractive surgeon suffer from adopting conservative limits for procedure selection? We think not. Achieving "success" in refractive surgery involves meeting patients' realistic expectations. If a particular procedure challenges or exceeds a given surgeon's skill and experience, for example, degree of attempted correction with a particular procedure or the surgical technique, a judicious referral may be preferable. Give the patient the "intentional pass" (i.e., refer to an appropriately skilled colleague) and you will maintain a higher "batting average." This is true of all surgery but is particularly important in refractive surgery, where best corrected visual acuity is generally excellent initially; the surgeon cannot afford a less-than-optimal result if the best corrected visual acuity is very good initially.

Hyperopia

A word of caution should be given for attempted surgical correction of hyperopia. Although some techniques may work adequately in the hands of some surgeons, widely accepted procedures yielding reproducible results are not yet available. As new surgical procedures are being developed, it is useful to review the evolution and decline of past surgical techniques.

Incisional techniques for treating hyperopia have been in use since the early 1980s. Mendez introduced the concept of corneal steepening by hexagonal keratotomy for hyperopia in 1984. By shortening or lengthening the sides of the hexagon, the surgeon could decrease or increase the effective optical zone, thus modulating the degree of induced corneal steepening. Unfortunately, the original procedure called for incisions that intersected. Crossing or intersecting radial or astigmatic incisions are known to cause serious problems in corneal wound healing, irregular astigmatism, and refractive instability. Although attempts have been made by Grandon and others to reduce irregular astigmatism by avoiding intersecting sides of the hexagon, problems persist [5]. Most refractive surgeons agree that results of incisional techniques for treating hyperopia do not compare favorably to those for treating myopia in terms of safety (loss of best corrected visual acuity from irregular astigmatism) and predictability (achieving the target correction).

The development of techniques to steepen the cornea with non-incisional methods has yielded similar difficulties. Although many surgeons had attempted to reshape the corneal surface by the application of thermal energy, it was Fyodorov who popularized the technique. His procedure, named radial thermokeratoplasty, used thin wire probes to generate stromal temperatures of 600° C. Such extreme temperatures caused not only the desired effect of collagen shrinkage but also unintended collagen necrosis [26]. Corneal steepening was excessive in the immediate postoperative period but often decreased over time. The loss of effect over time did not always stabilize at the intended target correction. Most early proponents of radial thermokeratoplasty for hyperopia abandoned Fyodorov's apparatus but not his idea. It was felt that hyperopia could be treated more accurately if collagen shrinkage, rather than collagen relaxation and necrosis, could be promoted.

Current methods of laser thermokeratoplasty (LTK) utilize a holmium laser (wavelength = 2.06 µm) to deliver thermal energy via either a contact probe or a noncontact slit-lamp system, both of which heat stromal collagen to 60° C, thereby preferentially shrinking collagen without necrosis. Early clinical trials of LTK have shown efficacy in the range of 1–3 D of hyperopia [27, 28]. The effect may be more stable in patients older than age 40 and more pronounced in over-corrected patients after PRK, perhaps because of the absence of Bowman's layer in these individuals. Problems encountered in early LTK studies include a gradual regression of effect over 2 years and loss of BCVA of 2 lines in 25% of eyes. Continuing studies of LTK for treatment of hyperopia will reveal whether results can match FDA standards set for treatment of myopia by the excimer laser.

What about excimer PRK for treatment of hyperopia? Theoretically, it should be possible to flatten the peripheral cornea while maintaining the central cornea, thereby creating a relative increase in central corneal curvature. The problem created by such an ablation is how to prevent scar tissue from filling in the peripheral ablation thereby causing the loss of the desired effect. Dausch [4], Anschutz [unpublished data, 1994], and others have struggled with the problem of hyperopia treatment utilizing various marking techniques. Regression of effect over time has prevented a major breakthrough in such treatments. In a recent phase I blind eye study by VISX, a total of 10 amblyopic eyes underwent hyperopic PRK [29]. All eyes had an attempted correction of 4 D and a treatment zone diameter of 8 mm or 9 mm. As with myopic PRK, early data suggest that larger treatment zone diameters may yield a more stable refractive result. All corneas remained clear 2 years after treatment. Most eyes showed between 2.5 D and 3 D of increased corneal steepening, either by retinoscopy, autorefraction, or topography. As of this writing, VISX still awaits FDA approval to begin phase II studies of excimer laser treatment of hyperopia in sighted eyes. Anecdotal reports suggest that LASIK for hyperopia may be more promising than PRK, perhaps because of the more limited stromal remodeling that occurs beneath a corneal flap. However, even LASIK may not be able to effectively correct more than 4 to 5 D of hyperopia.

Safety, efficacy, predictability, and stability of outcome for the various treatments for hyperopia have been less reliable than those for myopia. Hexagonal keratotomy and radial thermokeratoplasty (Fyodorov method) are limited by their associated high rates of irregular astigmatism and loss of BCVA. The jury is still out regarding LTK and excimer laser treatment of hyperopia. Holmium LTK appears to have a short-lived effect in most patients. Early data suggest that the best long-term results may be in older patients (> 40 years) with thin corneas (< 500 µ central thickness) or those in whom Bowman's layer has been removed by PRK. The maximum obtainable, lasting effect appears to be in the range of 3–5 D [J Alio, personal communication, 1995]. ALK has been advocated for primary hyperopia and for consecutive hyperopia following overcorrected RK. The major concern with such a procedure, however, is with its mechanism of action: the cornea is steepened by creating a "controlled" ectasia from a deep lamellar cut with the microkeratome. More longitudinal follow-up is needed before the possibility of progressive, keratoconus-like, central corneal ectasia following such a procedure can be excluded. Despite the efforts of many refractive surgeons, we are still waiting for a hyperopia treatment procedure that offers consistently reliable results.

Astigmatism

Incisional Techniques

Heretofore, we have discussed the surgical correction of spherical refractive errors. Now we will consider radial asymmetry of the cornea and the correction of astigmatism.

The early 1980s provided some imaginative, though not always successful, incisional techniques for the treatment of astigmatism. Variations on Fyodorov's radial keratotomy included multiple radial or semiradial incisions over a steep sector of the cornea.

Another approach tested during this period utilized the oval optical zone marker. In a 3-mm by 4-mm oval central optical zone marker, the long axis of the oval marker was placed perpendicular to the steep axis of the cornea. Radial incisions were then made in standard fashion, so that longer radial incisions were made over the steep corneal meridian. This technique could correct low degrees of astigmatism (1–1.5 D of cylinder) when associated with RK for correction of myopia. Other incisional techniques were used to treat higher degrees of astigmatism. Short, straight incisions were made tangential to a large optical zone, perpendicular to the steep corneal meridian. One might have thought that these so-called T incisions were named for the teardrop appearance they caused in the keratometric mires in the early postoperative period. Although the appearance of the mires improved over time, surgeons continued to look for better methods than T cuts to correct astigmatism.

The risk of inducing irregular astigmatism with straight, tangential incisions may be reduced if they are made in an arc rather than in a line. The development of arcuate keratotomy (AK) for treatment of astigmatism relies heavily on the work of Lindstrom [7] and Thornton [25], who described a detailed nomogram for dealing with both naturally occurring and surgically induced astigmatism.

All incisional methods for correcting astigmatism recognize the phenomenon of coupling. Astigmatic cuts that flatten the steep axis induce some degree of relative corneal steepening in the opposite meridian. Various formulas have been proposed to estimate the an-

Table 3-6. ASCRS poll on arcuate keratotomy (AK) use

Response	Percent
How often do you perform AK? (total responses = 245)	
Never	20.8
Occasionally	27.8
On a regular basis	48.2
How do you rate predictability for high congenital astigmatism? (total responses = 106)	
Very low	22.6
Low	17.9
Medium	41.5
High	7.5
How do you rate predictability for high postoperative astigmatism? (total responses = 84)	
Very low	7.1
Low	38.1
Medium	42.9
High	9.5

ticipated result of these coupling forces when astigmatism alone is treated. In general, it is agreed that results after correction of myopic astigmatism are more predictable than the results of incisional techniques for treating astigmatism alone. This conclusion holds for enhancement procedures as well as for primary surgery.

In 1994, the participants in an ASCRS symposium were polled on their use of AK to correct astigmatism (Table 3-6). The general consensus of those actually performing the procedure was that AK is moderately predictable for astigmatism but not as predictable as RK is for myopia.

Photoastigmatic Refractive Keratectomy

Excimer laser techniques may avoid some of the problems associated with corneal coupling and induced astigmatism associated with incisional techniques for treatment of astigmatism. Since the early 1990s, compound myopic astigmatism has been treated by means of toric surface ablation using either a software ablation algorithm to control the shape of the laser beam within the laser itself or an appropriately oriented mask of variable thickness interposed between the laser and the patient.

The first series of sighted eyes treated in an FDA protocol (phase II-A of photoastigmatic refractive keratectomy [PRKa; PARK] with the VISX 20/20 laser system) employed the progressive separation of a pair of slits over an iris diaphragm [8]. As the slits parted, the corneal meridian perpendicular to the slits would receive progressively greater exposure to the laser beam. More tissue was removed in the center, creating a PRK-type ablation in the steep axis of the cornea while maintaining a PTK flat cut in the axis parallel to the slits. This program, called the *sequential method,* is employed when the magnitude of the cylinder exceeds the magnitude of the sphere in the target correction. In the case where the magnitude of the sphere exceeds the magnitude of the cylinder, an elliptical pattern is employed, using a combination of the slits and iris diaphragm. Because tissue is removed rather than incised, less coupling tends to occur. These techniques are illustrated in Chapter 4.

Tissue is subtracted from the cornea by surface ablation, and thus it is inevitable that some hyperopic shift will occur when astigmatism is corrected. At the present time PARK should be limited to patients who have a myopic spherical equivalent. While ablation algorithms do exist for correction of compound hyperopic astigmatism, a patient with a spherical equivalent of plano or slightly greater may be better served by incisional keratotomy, at least until more experience is gained with PARK. As laser software and hardware continue to evolve, the surgeon's ability to effectively treat a wider variety of astigmatic refractive errors with PARK should increase.

Pender reported greater accuracy in PRKa phase II-B results compared to phase II-A due in part to an astigmatic alignment system [8]. This device combines the properties of a lensometer and a potential acuity meter, allowing the patient to "rock the cylinder" in a supine position to align the laser immediately prior to the treatment. These results are not surprising, as it has been demonstrated that real or apparent positionally induced ocular cyclotorsion can occur when a patient is moved from the seated to the supine position [9]. Outside the United States, VISX excimer laser users have successfully treated up to 6 D of cylinder with this technique. This range of cylindrical correction by PRK is higher than the range that can be reliably corrected by AK. Preservation of BCVA after PRK for myopic astigmatism appears equal to that after PRK for myopia alone for the same spherical equivalent.

Another approach to astigmatism correction with the excimer laser is the erodible mask system developed by Summit Technology (Waltham, MA). Few human studies have been done of the erodible mask for treatment of astigmatism. Besides the addition of disposal cost, it remains unclear how the additional variable of a stationary mask in the PRK delivery system will affect the final result. A phase III clinical trial of this technique is scheduled to begin in late 1996.

The pattern of the excimer laser treatment for irregular astigmatism is more complex than that for regular astigmatism. An excimer laser with a scanning beam may offer an advantage over a broad beam in such cases. The future may bring a link in real-time between corneal topography devices and a scanning excimer laser. Eye-tracking devices may provide the necessary ingredient for treatment of irregular astigmatism, which can occur after decentered PRK ablations, trauma, infection, or penetrating keratoplasty.

Other Considerations

Any application of clinical results for common refractive surgical procedures needs to consider factors other than the degree and type of ametropia. Although the following list of variables is not intended to be exhaustive, it places in perspective, and perhaps further qualifies, any choice of procedure for an individual patient:

Age
Pupil size
Other ophthalmic or systemic condition
Lifestyle and occupation
History of prior procedure(s)
Need for future procedure

Age is a significant factor in determining the ultimate outcome of incisional techniques. The older the patient, the greater the surgical effect. All modern surgical algorithms for RK and AK planners now factor in the age of the patient. For example, Lindstrom's "mini-RK" nomogram recommends less aggressive surgery (larger optical zones) for patients older than age 35, compared to the original PERK technique, which made no allowance for age [6]. Table 3-7 shows an expected 2-D greater effect for 8-incision RK for a 45-year-old versus a 25-year-old at the same optical zone (3 mm). An age-dependent effect has yet to be conclusively demonstrated for PRK, but at least two studies suggest that this may be the case [23, 24].

Besides the universally accepted factors of refractive error and age, other factors may play a significant role in the success of keratorefractive surgery. Pupil size tends to be larger in younger patients. When pupil diameter exceeds the effective optical zone of the cornea, symptoms of halos and other visual complaints may result. In general, the bigger the better as far as effective optical zones are concerned. When performing RK, the risk-benefit ratio for optical zones smaller than 3 mm has not been accepted as tolerable by most refractive surgeons. Similarly, problems with halos and glare occurred when small PRK treatment zones were employed. The frequency and severity of symp-

Table 3-7. The effect of age on expected correction: Mini-RK

Age	Correction (3-mm optical zone)
25	4.5 D
35	5.5 D
45	6.5 D

Source: RL Lindstrom. Minimally invasive radial keratotomy. *J Cataract Refract Surg* 21 : 27–34, 1995. © *Journal of Cataract and Refractive Surgery.*

toms diminished with larger ablation zone sizes, but such aberrations may be more noticeable at night, when the pupil enlarges.

Some patients are simply not good candidates for any kerato-refractive procedure. Patients with severe keratoconjunctivitis sicca, connective tissue disorders, or a past history of herpes simplex keratitis should be discouraged from refractive surgery due to their increased risk of wound healing problems. Reports of delayed re-epithelialization, stromal melting with corneal perforation, and re-activation of herpes simplex have occurred in such high-risk patients following PRK. For a more complete discussion of inclusion and exclusion criteria for patient selection, please refer to Chapter 2.

The occupation and lifestyle of the patient should be carefully considered as part of the keratorefractive surgery evaluation. Certain jobs in the military and in law enforcement exclude patients who have undergone radial keratotomy, presumably because of the potential for wound rupture. Recently, Pinheiro and co-workers [10] reported that the rupture threshold of mini-RK incisions is not significantly different from that of normal eyes under experimental conditions, but at the present time it is prudent to assume that RK is potentially hazardous to patients at increased risk for blunt ocular trauma. Patients seeking RK who engage in contact sports should be warned about the possibility of wound rupture. Eyes are much less likely to rupture after PRK because only about 10% of the central corneal thickness is removed in a −5-D treatment. In contrast, a target depth of 80–90% of central corneal thickness is required of RK incisions, regardless of the degree of myopia being corrected.

Enhancement Procedures

A history of prior procedures should be carefully noted in the workup of refractive surgery candidates. If the patient has achieved what the surgeon believes is an optimal result and he or she remains unsatisfied, additional surgery should not be undertaken. Some patients may push hard for enhancements that their primary surgeon rightfully refused to perform. Other patients have become "addicted to plano" and have subsequently undergone mild regression. Beware of such patients and resist demands for additional surgery that may fail to meet unrealistic patient expectations.

Entire texts devoted solely to enhancement strategies in refractive surgery could be written. Although enhancements have played an important role in avoiding overcorrections after RK and in achieving greater gains in uncorrected visual acuity, they have some inherent limitations. For instance, an 8-incision RK at an optical zone of 3 mm with an achieved depth of 85% has given nearly maximal effect. An additional 10–20% effect might be obtained with 8 more incisions placed between the original 8 incisions. Is it worth it? Maybe. Will a 16-incision case be more unstable over time than an 8-incision case? Possibly. Most refractive surgeons avoid RK for high myopia because of the instability of such corneas and the likelihood of undercorrection that cannot be enhanced effectively by incisional methods.

Unless the primary procedure has achieved maximum effect, enhancements in kind are quite reasonable. That is, undercorrected RK is enhanced by longer or more numerous incisions, whereas PRK undercorrections are retreated by the excimer laser. If RK has given maximal effect and significant undercorrection persists, then PRK over RK may be a viable option. The 10-year PERK study reported a successful PRK over the original RK several years after the primary surgery [12]. However, problems can occur if PRK is attempted before the RK incisions have adequately healed. Increased rates of corneal scarring and loss of BCVA have been reported in PRK following undercorrected RK. Perhaps the excimer treatment itself stimulates keratocytes within the radial incisions. Perhaps mechanical debridement done in preparation for PRK disrupts the integrity of the RK wounds, leading to increased scarring, and transepithelial ablation over a previous RK surgery might minimize future wound healing problems. Excimer laser removal of the epithelium in such cases appears to be less traumatic than mechanical removal and therefore may cause less scarring. LASIK may provide a more promising alternative than PRK for undercorrection after RK, but this too awaits confirmation in the peer-reviewed literature.

Regardless of the type of enhancement surgery contemplated, it is best to wait until the eye is stable from the primary surgical procedure. How long is long enough? It varies. Avoid reoperating on an eye that exhibits changing refraction or topography over several visits over the course of 2–3 months. Eyes showing irregular astigmatism by keratometry and topography are poor candidates for enhancement procedures. The patient should return to preoperative BCVA before additional surgery is performed. The exception to this general recommendation may be the treatment of central islands (discussed below), which severely reduce BCVA.

The waiting time may range from 2 weeks to 6 months before enhancements are performed using incisional techniques, but 6 weeks is typically long enough for the refraction and topography to stabilize. With PRK, the wait may be even longer and little data are available on retreatments performed less than 6 months after the primary procedure. When treating high myopia with the excimer laser, corneal haze and regression of effect have been found to improve spontaneously in many cases [15].

Central islands are local areas of relative corneal steepening in a "sea" of corneal flattening. These topographic abnormalities have been observed in up to 20% of PRK cases in the first 3 months postoperatively, but nearly all are gone by 6–12 months. The etiology of and recommended treatment for central islands remain controversial. Further study is required to prove whether alteration of ablation algorithms will improve the results of PRK, particularly in the treatment of high myopia, where the incidence of central islands is increased. For a more complete discussion of central islands, see Chapter 5.

Before leaving the subject of enhancements, we should briefly discuss the subject of monovision. Many refractive surgeons have encountered the "successful" patient with good distance vision in one eye and good near vision in the other. Sometimes it was part of the preoperative plan; sometimes not. A monovision result is hepful in some presbyopes but less tolerated by pilots, athletes, and others requiring excellent stereopsis. Sometimes, the patient has a history of successful contact lens monovision and asks if you can do the same thing with surgery. Examples abound where very satisfied patients had only one eye treated (RK or PRK) and they concluded that they had the best of both worlds with good distance and near vision. Although it is more likely to be the motivated presbyope who will tolerate it, monovision should be discussed with all prospective surgical candidates.

Surgical Planning

The issue of timing between eyes for refractive surgery warrants some comment. The FDA has suggested a 3-month waiting period between initial PRK and treatment of the fellow eye. Our international colleagues do not have to abide by such restrictions. Some Canadian surgeons treat their patients bilaterally with PRK over a single weekend. The patient receives treatment on the first eye on Friday, recovers on Saturday and Sunday, then has the fellow eye treated on Monday. The assumption is that the epithelium will heal from the first operation in time to provide some useful vision during the recovery period for the fellow eye. In Europe and Latin America, LASIK is often performed in a bilateral simultaneous or rapidly sequential fashion (1–2 days). The idea is to achieve what the patient wants (better uncorrected vision in both eyes) with a minimum of inconvenience and expense (e.g., lost time from work, travel cost). Although such timing has its advocates, we believe that safety, not convenience, should govern timing issues.

It is estimated that 60% of all RK surgery is performed by 26% of all refractive surgeons, much of it in a bilateral simultaneous fashion. These surgeons cite the low risk of overcorrection and the extremely low risk of infection. The problem is that such complications can be disastrous when they do occur. The more conservative approach is to do one eye at a time; after all, the patient has lived with his or her myopia for 30 years on average. If a PRK patient does not wear contact lenses, it is worth considering whether to fit the fellow eye while the first recuperates from surgery. Temporary anisometropia may be bothersome to some patients who are contact lens–intolerant, but if the rationale behind this approach is explained, few patients will disagree. Evaluate how the first eye responds to your procedure before doing the fellow eye. Operating on one eye at a time protects you against repeating the same mistake when a patient responds in a fashion considered to be outside of normal surgical expectations. This is particularly important in avoiding overcorrections in the older (presbyopic) population.

There is general agreement among refractive surgeons that surgery for the second eye may be done any time after the patient has achieved adequate visual function in the first eye. The surgeon should recognize that the definition of such may vary among individual patients. There is less agreement, however, on the issue of staging a procedure for a given eye. Most refractive surgeons would advocate doing the one procedure that will give the best chance for optimal correction with the least risk of overcorrection. Studies of incisional techniques for treating myopic astigmatism show no advantage to staging; it is preferable to perform both the radial and arcuate incisions at the same encounter [7, 14, 25]. The same argument may prove true for PRK in the treatment of myopic astigmatism. Treatment of high myopia with primary RK followed by PRK enhancement should be questioned. Why subject the cornea to potential instability from RK? The RK will not do the job alone, and additional surgery may still require a maximal response from PRK. Results after combined RK-PRK should be analyzed critically and compared to other available (or soon-to-be-available) technologies such as LASIK. Ideally, the subject of staging procedures would not be complicated by the limitations of a given surgeon's equipment, experience, and, in the case of the FDA clinical trials, by protocol restrictions. In general, recommendations for staged procedures await the results of carefully designed and executed clinical trials.

Conclusions

Recommended guidelines for procedure selection by range of refractive error are summarized in the accompanying flowcharts (see Figs. 3-1 and 3-2). It seems fair to suggest that the surgeon starting out confine himself or herself to ranges of ametropia for which the proper equipment, support, and expertise exist and to refer to patients when they are unavailable. Select the surgical procedure that is most likely to meet the goals of both patient and surgeon while minimizing problems, including the need for more surgery.

References

1. American Society of Cataract and Refractive Surgery. First interactive symposium on refractive surgery (Suppl.). *J Cataract Refract Surg* 1995.
2. Assil KK, et al. One-year results of the intrastromal corneal ring in non-functional human eyes. *Arch Ophthalmol* 113:115–167, 1995.
3. Brint SF. What they don't tell you about ALK. *Review Ophthalmol* 2(3):70–76, 1995.
4. Dausch D, Klein R, Schroder E. Excimer laser photorefractive keratectomy for hyperopia. *Refract Corneal Surg* 9:20–28, 1993.
5. Grandon SC, et al. Clinical evaluation of hexagonal keratotomy for the treatment of primary hyperopia. *J Cataract Refract Surg* 21:140–149, 1995.
6. Lindstrom RL. Minimally invasive radial keratotomy. *J Cataract Refract Surg* 21:27–34, 1995.
7. Lindstrom RL. The surgical correction of astigmatism. *J Refract Corneal Surg* 6:441–454, 1990.
8. Pender PM. Photorefractive keratectomy for myopic astigmatism. *J Cataract Refract Surg* 20:262–264, 1994.
9. Smith EM, et al. Comparison of astigmatic axis in the seated and supine positions. *Refract Corneal Surg* 10:615–620, 1995.
10. Pinheiro MN, et al. Corneal integrity after refractive surgery. *Ophthalmology* 102:297–301, 1995.
11. Salz JJ, Salz JM, Jones DJ. Ten years experience with a conservative approach to radial keratotomy. *J Refract Corneal Surg* 7:12–22, 1991.
12. Waring GO, McDonnell PJ, Lynn MJ. Results of the prospective evaluation of radial keratotomy (PERK) study 10 years after surgery. *Arch Ophthalmol* 112(10):1298–1308, 1994.
13. Werblin TP, Stafford GM. The casebeer system for predictable keratorefractive surgery. *Ophthalmology* 100:1095–1102, 1993.

14. Verity SM, et al. The combined (Genesis) technique of radial kerato-tomy: A prospective multicenter trial. *Ophthalmology* 102:1908–1917, 1995.
15. Seiler T, McDonnell PJ. Excimer laser photorefractive keratectomy. *Survey Ophthalmol* 40:89–118, 1995.
16. Salz JJ, et al. A two-year experience with excimer photorefractive keratectomy for myopia. *Ophthalmology* 100:873–882, 1993.
17. Talamo JH, et al. Multicenter study of excimer PRK for moderate myopia of −6 to −8 D. *J Refract Surg* 11:238–247, 1995.
18. Krueger RR, et al. Clinical analysis of photorefractive keratectomy using a multiple zone technique for severe myopia. *Am J Ophthalmol* 119:263–274, 1995.
19. Ibrahim O, et al. Automated in situ keratomileusis for myopia. *J Refract Surg* 11:431–441, 1995.
20. Pallikaris IG, et al. A corneal flap technique for laser in situ kera-tomileusis. *Arch Ophthalmol* 109(12):1699–1702, 1991.
21. Pallikaris IG, Sigamos DS. Excimer laser in situ keratomileusis and photorefractive keratectomy for correction of high myopia. *Refract Corneal Surg* 10(5):498–510; 1994.
22. Salah T, et al. Excimer laser in situ keratomileusis under a corneal flap of 2 to 20 diopters. *Am J Ophthalmol* 121:143–155, 1996.
23. Dutt S, Steinert RF, Raizman MB. One-year results of excimer laser photorefractive keratectomy for low to moderate myopia. *Arch Ophthalmol* 112:1427–1436, 1994.
24. Kornstein HS, Filater VV, Talamo JH. The influence of age at 1-year results of excimer laser photorefractive keratectomy for moderate myopia. *Invest Ophthalmol Vis Sci* 36(Suppl.):S983, 1995.
25. Thornton SP, Sanders DR. Graded non-intersecting transverse incisions for correction of idiopathic astigmatism. *J Cataract Refract Surg* 13:27–31, 1987.
26. Aquarella JV, et al. Alterations in corneal morphology following thermokeratoplasty. *Arch Ophthalmol* 94:2082–2085, 1976.
27. Seiler T, et al. Laser thermokeratoplasty by means of a pulsed hol-mium:YAG laser for hyperopic correction. *Refract Corneal Surg* 6:355–359, 1990.
28. Thompson VM, et al. Holmium:YAG laser thermokeratoplasty for hy-peropia and astigmastism: An overview. *Refract Corneal Surg* 9:5134–5137, 1993.
29. Macy JI, et al. Laser Correction of Hyperopia: Results from the United States. In JJ Salz (ed), *Corneal Laser Surgery.* St. Louis: Mosby–Year Book, 1995. Pp. 256–260.

Photorefractive Keratectomy (PRK)

4 PRK Surgical Techniques

General Considerations

Berthold Seitz and Peter J. McDonnell

Guided by popular notions of refractive surgery or enticed by radio or television commercials, people often expect laser refractive surgery to be a quick and painless procedure with attendant risks no greater than spectacles or contact lenses. It is important that photorefractive keratectomy (PRK) not be inappropriately trivialized. All patients should understand that they may experience significant pain during the immediate postoperative period (24–48 hours) after cessation of the effect of the local anesthetics, and that their vision may be poor for weeks. The patient also should be made aware of the risk of undercorrection, overcorrection, and regression, and of the possibility of problems such as haze, glare, and halos (most pronounced in the first 4 months after the procedure).

Preoperative patient counseling regarding presbyopia is required for all potential patients, although it is very difficult for a young adult to grasp the significance of presbyopia. Monovision is a viable option for presbyopic and prepresbyopic myopic patients. The patients are likely best served by a slight undercorrection (Table 4-1).

Patients should understand that, although the process may be inconvenient for them, surgical techniques and results can only be as accurate as preoperative measurements permit. Soft or hard gas-permeable contact lenses should be removed for at least 2 weeks and hard polymethylmethacrylate (PMMA) contact lenses for at least 3 weeks before obtaining baseline measurements. Keratometry or central corneal topography should demonstrate that the power in both

Table 4-1. Counseling prior to excimer laser PRK

Patient's expectations
Stability of refraction
Stability of corneal topography (contact lens users)
Refractive accuracy of the procedure and results of clinical trials
Presbyopia
Postoperative pain
Visual recovery
Complications
Need for sedation
Informed consent

Table 4-2. Evaluations prior to excimer laser PRK

Uncorrected visual acuity
Manifest refraction
Cycloplegic refraction (corrected to corneal plane)
Best corrected visual acuity
Keratometry
Corneal topography
Specular endothelial microscopy (optional)
Biomicroscopy
  Tear film assessment
  Lids
  Lacrimal system
  Dilated funduscopy
Tonometry

meridians does not differ by more than 0.5 diopter (D) between two measurements taken at different times. Previous refraction needs to be evaluated to ensure stability for at least 1 year (Table 4-2).

Because severe dry eye syndrome may result in a higher probability of corneal haze and regression, a Schirmer's test and the break-up time of the precorneal tear film should be assessed routinely. Patients with keratoconjunctivitis sicca should be excluded from PRK, or at least be treated preoperatively, as should patients with other external diseases and surface pathologies (e.g., blepharitis). If silicone punctal plugs are not placed prior to surgery, the use of temporary intracanalicular collagen implants before or at the time of surgery may be a good option in dry eye syndrome. If plugs are not placed, patency of the lacrimal system should be ensured before surgery. If pressure over the lacrimal sac results in reflux from the inferior punctum, the risk of postoperative infection is increased.

Autoimmune or connective tissue diseases known to be associated with corneal melting disorders are considered absolute contraindications for PRK. Diabetes and other conditions known to influence wound healing should be considered and discussed with the patients preoperatively in terms of the potential for a nonroutine postoperative course. Clearly, however, experience has shown that diabetics can successfully undergo excimer PRK.

Preoperative Medication

Sedation

The patient should have a light meal on the day of surgery. The need for a mild tranquilizer, such as 5–10 mg of diazepam (Valium), should be determined on an individual basis. Some surgeons utilize such medications routinely, while others do so only rarely. The patient should be escorted to and from the laser center by friends or relatives.

Miotics

Performing the laser procedure the day after a cycloplegic refraction carries the risk of a persistent mydriasis, which could make centration of the laser application more difficult. It remains controversial whether the center of the pupil is substantially displaced when mydriatic or miotic drugs are applied. Some surgeons instill 1 drop of 1% pilocarpine 30 minutes before the procedure to induce a "mild" miosis, believing that this minimizes the possibility of severe decentration. Alternatively, the light of the operating microscope can be used to produce a physiologic miosis.

Anesthesia

All procedures are performed under topical anesthesia. A drop of anesthetic, such as proparacaine or tetracaine, is applied to the ocular surface. After the procedure, an oral analgesic such as acetaminophen with codeine, oxycodone, demerol or vistaril is typically prescribed for the first 24–48 hours postoperatively.

Laser Maintenance, Calibration, and Programming

Laser beam homogeneity is crucial because the energy profile of the beam is projected directly onto the surface of the cornea, leaving its "fingerprint." The beam is homogenized as it passes through several optical components. These optical elements may degrade over time, the beam profile can change between pulses, and the beam intensity may become less uniform as the gases in the active medium become degraded, resulting in hot and cold spots.

At regular intervals, a careful assessment of the effective beam profile on the cornea is mandatory. There are at least two different approaches to external calibration of laser output. One method adjusts the laser energy until a calibrated gelatin filter (Wratten gelatin filter no. 96; Kodak, Rochester, NY) or blackened photographic paper of a defined thickness is perforated by a given number of pulses. Alternatively, test ablations using an appropriate test material, such as PMMA, can be performed and read using a lensometer or profilometer. The quality and dioptric power of the lens created by the laser is a measure of the uniformity and fluence of the beam as well as of the alignment of the optics and scanning or masking system.

In addition, some surgeons recommend keeping the temperature and humidity in the laser room constant to maintain a more stable beam profile. In case of an unsatisfactory beam profile, the gases or the optical components, or both, need adjustment before proceeding with any treatment.

Ideally, real-time analysis of the final pulse energy, homogeneity, and shape of the beam would be linked to a computer-controlled feedback mechanism. This could modulate both the output from the laser and the beam management in the delivery system to ensure that each pulse meets exact specifications.

Newer lasers are now available that utilize fluences less than those applied in earlier clinical trials (160–180 mJ/cm^2) of wide-area ablation; these lasers are capable of ablating tissue while producing thinner electron-dense pseudomembranes on the corneal surface. However, the relationship between pseudomembrane thickness and clinical factors, such as re-epithelialization or postoperative haze, remains to be determined.

Safety Considerations

People with cardiac pacemakers must keep a distance of about 2 meters from the laser. Appropriate measures to contain possible leaks of toxic gases should be ensured. It may be prudent for observers to wear eye protection in the laser room, although no harmful ocular effects have been reported from unprotected exposure. Surgical masks may also be advisable to protect the surgeon and his or her assistants from photoablated cornea tissue, which may cause respiratory irritation.

Myopia

Berthold Seitz and Peter J. McDonnell

PRK is based on the 193-nm excimer laser's unique ability to remove submicron amounts of corneal tissue by corneal surface ablation while causing minimal changes to the subjacent tissue. This results in a change in corneal curvature and thus in the refractive properties of the eye (Fig. 4-1). To make this clinically useful, a computer-generated algorithm relating diameter and depth of ablation to the required dioptric change has been refined by each manufacturer. The desired change of refraction is entered into the computer program that controls both the laser operation and the pattern of laser exposure on the corneal surface. Table 4-3 outlines intraoperative considerations during PRK.

In principle, there are three different approaches to PRK: the scanning slit, flying spot, and wide-area ablation techniques. Specific operating parameters and instructions for most currently available lasers are outlined in Part II, Technical Considerations.

With the original wide-beam technique, the laser beam has a fluence of 160–180 mJ/cm^2 within a circular area of 5–7 mm. The laser

Fig. 4-1. Computer-aided design of a spherical myopic correction with a central flattening of the cornea. (Courtesy of Fa. Aesculap-Meditec GmbH, Heroldsberg, Germany.)

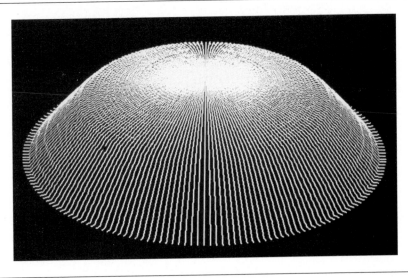

Table 4-3. Intraoperative considerations during excimer laser PRK

Computer data entry
Patient positioning
Anesthesia
Fixation
Centration
"Training" procedure
Epithelial removal
Focus and centration
Maintaining corneal hydration
Cylinder axis alignment

generally runs at a repetition rate of 5 or 10 pulses/sec (Hz) and ablates about 0.2 µm per pulse.

There are several approaches to shape the excimer laser beam for myopic wide-area ablation.

Optical shaping of the beam by variable irradiance lenses can distribute energy over the corneal surface in desired patterns.

An *ablatable mask* may be used, formed in the shape of the tissue to be removed; as the mask ablates, the beam passes through to ablate corneal tissue.

A *multiple disc mask* with multiple different-sized apertures from large (7 mm diameter) to small (1 mm diameter) rotates to create successively smaller or larger ablation zones, thus inducing a negative lens effect on the cornea.

A *diaphragm mask* expands or contracts so that the outer portion of the ablation is shallower than the continuously exposed inner portion. The diaphragm edge is etched onto the corneal surface with each pulse, creating some irregularity; the greater the number of steps, the smoother the resultant surface. Use of an expanding iris aperture when performing ablations to correct myopia may be preferable to use of contracting apertures because the former produces a pseudomembrane with fewer discontinuities, although clinical benefits in terms of speed of epithelial wound healing, amount of stromal haze, and amount of corneal flattening could not be demonstrated in a rabbit model. A slightly defocused laser beam results in less prominent, slightly wavy lines rather than sharply demarcated concentric ridges. This effect is even more pronounced when an expanding aperture is used.

Patient Positioning

Before the procedure, the patient is instructed on the proper head and body position to maintain during surgery and told about the sights, sounds, and smells that may be perceived while in the laser room.

Once the patient is seated in the chair, a surgical head bonnet is used to prevent hair from approaching the surgical field. At this point, the patient should be made as comfortable as possible, with armrests adjusted for maximum comfort. The patient is then placed supine under the laser delivery system while the surgeon centers and focuses the eye to be treated through a surgical microscope.

The cornea of the patient's eye must be accurately located along the vertical ultraviolet laser beam axis (*z axis*). The reference for positioning the eye is a microscope that allows the ophthalmologist to look along the axis of the ultraviolet beam through a beam splitter. The microscope is adjusted to the proper pupillary distance and the ophthalmologist's prescription. In some machines, a cross-hair reticle pattern in the microscope, seen superimposed on the image of the eye, can be centered with respect to the ultraviolet beam so that alignment of the eye with this pattern ensures proper centering of the ablation while the patient fixates on the target.

Especially with eyes that lie deep in the orbit, the patient's neck should be hyperextended using a specially formed pad to prevent the superior orbital rim and upper lid from interfering with the beam during the procedure. This is particularly important if a fixation handpiece is used.

Speculum and Patching of the Fellow Eye

When not using a fixation handpiece, proper centration depends on the patient correctly fixating on the target. Therefore, the fellow eye should be patched, lightly but completely, to prevent inadvertent cross-fixation during the procedure, which would cause the ablation zone to be decentered. Another patch may be placed on the cheek of the treated side to prevent irrigation fluid from running into the ear. A lid speculum is placed between the upper and lower lids. Additional topical anesthetics may be applied, or an annular sponge soaked in topical anesthetic may be placed at the limbus.

Patients often complain of anisometropia during the postoperative period after the first eye is treated, causing some surgeons to consider bilateral surgery. This approach raises the possibility of bilateral infection, and it may prevent the patient from experiencing monovision.

It is possible that an over- or undercorrection in the first eye might necessitate modifying the procedure in the other eye after assessment of the wound-healing response in the first eye. If bilateral surgery is performed, we recommend careful informed consent, as well as the use of a separate set of topical drugs and operating instruments (including lid speculum) for the second eye to minimize the small but real risk of bacterial contamination of both eyes.

Fixation (Manual vs. Self)

There are different ways to fixate the eye during the procedure, which takes between 20 and 100 seconds for a −5 D ablation, depending on the laser system used. The patient may self-fixate on a coaxial target light during the procedure, or the surgeon may maintain fixation, using a handpiece with or without suction, a fine-toothed forceps, or a fixation ring. Experience has shown that most patients are capable of voluntarily maintaining fixation on the target light, even through-out relatively prolonged procedures. Patients should be told that the clarity of the fixation target will decline during the ablation procedure, but they should still be able to see it.

To start the ablation, the surgeon presses down the foot switch until the ablation is completed. The surgeon monitors the progress of the procedure through the operating microscope. The ophthalmologist must ensure the correct position of the eye to avoid a "drifting" ablation with resultant irregular astigmatism and unpredictable out-come. If fixation is broken, the ablation is interrupted by releasing the foot switch. After fixation and centration are re-established, the pro-cedure can be resumed. The tendency to ignore patient fixation losses in an effort to complete the procedure is a common error of beginning surgeons (Table 4-4).

Table 4-4. Common errors in PRK

Decentration
Cross fixation
Misalignment of the eye
Excessive removal of epithelium
Dehydration
Not stopping ablation when patient loses fixation
Bell's phenomenon
Not confirming refractive data planned and programmed into the computer
Not confirming axis of astigmatism
Improperly converting from "plus" to "minus" cylinder

PTK Training

To aid the patient's self-fixation, a low myopic ablation or a shallow phototherapeutic keratectomy (PTK) ablation can be done as an optional "training program" prior to mechanical epithelial removal. This allows the surgeon to evaluate the patient's response to the noise, the odor of the ablation products, and the change in appearance of the fixation light during the procedure. A blocking film of methylcellulose (1%) or similar viscous lubricant may be used to protect the corneal epithelium during this training phase.

Epithelial Removal

Numerous strategies exist for removal of the epithelium, but proper centration is the initial key step.

For centration of the epithelial defect, the patient is asked to look directly at the fixation light, which is coaxial with the excimer laser beam. For mechanical removal of the epithelium, the surgeon may first mark the center with an instrument (blunt hook, radial keratotomy clear zone marker). Although some surgeons argue that the procedure is best centered on the fixation light reflex, most maintain that the appropriate reference is the center of the entrance pupil (Fig. 4-2). Varying the level of illumination induces different pupil diameters without miotics and may help to improve exact centration. A large optical zone marker (e.g., 6.5–7.0 mm) of the same size or somewhat larger (e.g., 0.5 or 1.0 mm) than the desired ablation zone may be used with or without methylene blue. The cross hairs on the marker are placed over the centration mark created earlier, and the ring is carefully pressed onto the cornea to delineate the area of the epithelium to be removed.

The area of epithelial removal should not markedly exceed the area of the consecutive refractive laser ablation, because the greater the defect, the longer the period required for the epithelium to heal. In addition, epithelial adhesion problems may occur within the region of epithelial debridement that is not treated with the laser. During and after the epithelial removal, a tear substitute can be used to moisten the cornea. To ensure uniform surface hydration, excess tear substitute should be gently wiped from the cornea with a moistened sponge before the treatment procedure.

Whatever technique is used to remove the epithelium, the surgeon should attempt to minimize extreme drying or wetting of the corneal surface and to avoid leaving residual islands of epithelium.

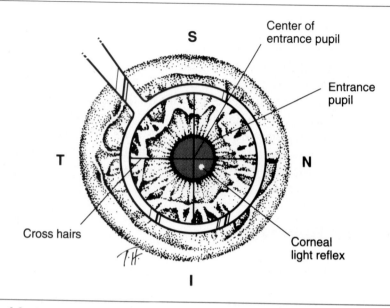

Fig. 4-2. Centration procedure. Cross hairs of a large (e.g., 6.5-mm) optical zone marker are centered on the center of the entrance pupil. S = superior; T = temporal; I = inferior; N = nasal.

Laser

To remove the epithelium with the laser, a PTK mode is used to an ablation depth of 50 μm, using a diameter equal to the diameter of the refractive treatment and centering the laser as with the refractive treatment. As seen through the operating microscope, a change in fluorescence arising from the laser-cornea interaction can indicate the transition from epithelium (bluish) to Bowman's layer (black), a difference that is especially prominent with the coaxial light turned down (see Chap. 5).

All methods of de-epithelialization produce, at least in the rabbit and monkey model, a significant decrease in superficial stromal keratocyte density. De-epithelialization with the laser may be associated with a greater inflammatory response. Furthermore, the corneal epithelium is an inhomogeneous structure and ablates at a faster rate than the corneal stroma. Within the epithelium, the nuclei are more resistant to ablation than is the cytoplasm. The irregular ablation of the multilayered epithelium could create an irregular surface on the stroma. In addition, after laser removal of the epithelium, some surgeons perceive a higher incidence of central islands.

When performing PRK in corneas with previous incisions (e.g., radial keratotomy, hexagonal keratotomy), laser removal of the epithelium may have the advantage of avoiding trauma that may induce gaping of the radial keratotomy incisions. Furthermore, in cases of retreatment of PRK (for haze, regression, or decentration of the original procedure), mechanical debridement may be difficult to complete because of the tight adhesion between basal epithelium and underlying stromal tissue.

Blade or Spatula

Removal of the epithelium appears to be more complete when a sharp instrument (such as a surgical blade or a hockey knife) is used rather than a dull instrument (such as a Paton spatula). This is of clinical relevance because residual epithelium and basement membrane after de-epithelialization may influence the depth of ablation and the regularity of the surface subsequently achieved with the excimer laser. Original surface irregularities of the tissue as well as all kinds of "fuzzes" are imprinted as "shadows" during the ablation process.

Rotating Brush

Some surgeons recommend use of a rotating brush with soft plastic bristles, 6–7 mm in diameter, for rapid (required time < 5 seconds) and exact removal of a circular area of epithelium of defined diameter (Fig. 4-3). This method is reported to prevent the dehydration that may occur after prolonged scraping and to produce a smooth and homogeneous stromal surface without epithelial remnants or stromal

Fig. 4-3. Rotating brush. The corneal epithelial remover consists of a pencil-type motor device, a plastic brush, and a metal stick fixated in both the motor device and the brush so as to constitute the axis around which the brush rotates. The insert in the lower left corner represents the brush piece (7 mm in diameter). (From IG Pallikaris. Rotating brush for fast removal of corneal epithelium. *J Refract Corneal Surg* 10 : 439–442, 1994.)

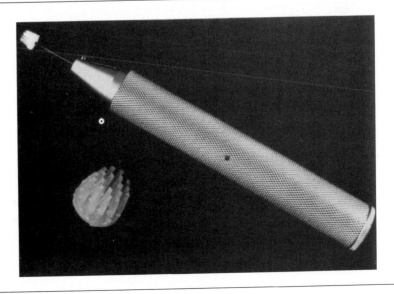

alteration. It may also contribute to a decreased re-epithelialization time.

Chemical

One drop of cocaine 4% applied 15 minutes preoperatively facilitates epithelial removal with a blunt instrument and is reported to have no adverse effect on re-epithelialization after PRK, although all epithelium may be loosened. Some surgeons use 10%, 15%, or 30% ethanol, left for a short time (e.g., 15–30 seconds) in contact with the central corneal epithelium. The alcohol is confined to the center with a radial keratotomy marker or a trephine firmly attached to the corneal surface and can be completely removed with a cellulose sponge. The epithelium can then be quickly and elegantly peeled away as a single sheet with a fresh, dry cellulose sponge. The advantages of this technique include (1) a well-circumscribed epithelial defect with a clear, well-circumscribed edge; (2) rapid and reproducible operating time, which may help standardize the hydration status of the underlying stroma; and (3) lack of surgical trauma to areas of the corneal surface not undergoing photoablation. Some surgeons have noted increased patient comfort and more rapid recovery of visual acuity when ethanol debridement techniques are used. There is some concern, however, that residual toxicity of such a chemical might delay postoperative closure of the epithelial defect and that uneven hydration might cause the stromal ablation rate to increase or become inhomogeneous. Clinical trials are currently under way to assess the safety and predictability of epithelial removal with dilute ethanol solutions.

Laser-Scrape

A technique combining laser and mechanical techniques of epithelial removal includes use of the laser to ablate the anterior 40 μm of the epithelium at the diameter to be used for stromal ablation, followed by mechanical scraping of the residual basal epithelial cells and basal membrane. This technique results in the smallest possible defect size, avoids possible chemical toxicity, and minimizes the amount of time during which corneal dehydration may occur.

Tracking Systems

Precise concentric overlapping of successive laser pulses onto the cornea during PRK procedures seems to be of paramount importance to avoid irregular ablation. The basic principle of a tracking system is to recognize eye movements and quickly (in < 100 ms) reposition the laser beam. Such a tracker can be based on computer imaging of the pupil position or other anatomical landmarks. After the ablation is started, the software repeatedly determines the current position of the eye with respect to the initial position. This value is processed and results in automated beam repositioning. A tracking system might be of help to compensate for unintended eye movements during the procedure and may improve the accuracy and safety of PRK procedures, particularly when longer treatment times are employed to correct higher refractive errors.

Centration

After epithelial removal, the laser is focused again precisely on the surface of Bowman's layer. Alignment is achieved with an optical reticle or paired laser spots, where two crossed helium-neon pilot beams merge on the center of the ablation zone at the outer surface of the cornea. With the patient fixating on the coaxial target, the surgeon centers the laser over the entrance pupil or the fixation light reflex (see Epithelial Removal above). It is important that the limbal plane be horizontal so that the laser beam is orthogonal (perpendicular to the corneal apex). Each brand of excimer laser has different technology to assist with ablation centration. The reader is encouraged to consult the laser-specific chapters that follow in Part II, Technical Considerations.

Single vs. Multizone Ablations

Original clinical studies of PRK for myopia indicated a greater tendency for regression of refractive effect if the preoperative refractive error was greater than −6 D. Treating myopia of this magnitude with a 1.5-mm-wide tapered transition zone bordering the refractive zone of 4 mm (overall diameter of treatment 7 mm) might result in less regression because the transition from the optical zone to the untreated area is smoother and avoids abrupt changes, presumably inducing less stimulation of postoperative wound healing.

The maximal central depth of an ablation to correct myopia can be approximated using the following equation:

$$\text{Central ablation depth } [\mu m] = \frac{(\text{diopters of myopia } [D]) \times (\text{ablation zone diameter } [mm^2]}{3}$$

It is clear from this formula that increasing the ablation zone diameter substantially increases central ablation depth. On the other

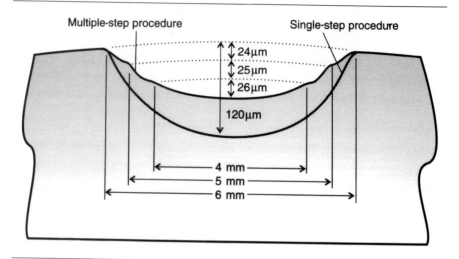

Fig. 4-4. Multistep, variable-diameter spherical ablation for high myopia. In the 6-mm zone, 20% of the ametropia is corrected; in the 5-mm zone, 30% is corrected; and in the 4-mm zone, 50% is corrected. The ablation depths for an intended −10 D correction are 75 μm with a multiple-step procedure and 120 μm with a single-step procedure.

hand, an ablation zone of at least 5.0–5.5 mm seems to be necessary to avoid glare and halos, especially during nighttime driving, when the pupils are relatively dilated.

One surgical strategy to avoid a very deep stromal ablation in high myopia may be the application of a multi-step procedure during the same session, using decreasing optical zone diameters (for example, 6.0 mm [20%], 5.0 mm [30%], 4.0 mm [50%]) (Fig. 4-4). A planned two-step, time-delayed (6 months later) PRK with a larger second ablation zone may be another approach to the problem of undercorrection and regression in high myopia. While theoretically advantageous, the value of multizone approaches to PRK awaits confirmation in prospective clinical trials.

Hydration

Because the ablation rate increases as the cornea dries, marked dehydration of the cornea before ablation might lead to relative overcorrection of myopia. Surgeons should use a technique that minimizes changes in hydration to maximize the predictability of excimer laser PRK.

To speed epithelial healing and minimize reparative response and consecutive superficial stromal haze, it seems reasonable to strive for the smoothest possible postablation surface. Superficial corneal deturgescence produced by nitrogen gas results in a rougher surface immediately postoperatively with undesirable effects on surface healing and corneal haze. Because dehydration causes irreversible changes in surface morphology, it is not sufficient to simply rehydrate the cornea after allowing desiccation to occur.

The blowing of humidified gas (such as nitrogen or helium) during excimer laser corneal ablation for myopia produces a smoother surface than does the blowing of dry gas, comparable to that produced under ambient (no blowing) conditions. If blowing gas is necessary to remove debris from the surface, the gas should be humidified. At the present time, those laser systems with effluent removal capabilities utilize debris aspiration rather than gas blowing.

Another way to improve the smoothness of the ablated surface is to use a masking fluid. The fluid protects the low points of an irregular surface from photoablation. Thus, a leveling procedure during photoablation may lead to a smoother surface afterwards. Wetting the debrided central cornea with a sponge soaked in methylcellulose (e.g., 0.3%) or balanced salt solution can help meet both requirements: prevention of deturgescence and masking of surface irregularities. Care must be taken, however, not to allow excess fluid from the sponge to pool on the corneal surface, as this will result in focal stromal elevations (central islands) or undercorrection.

After the ablation is complete, the eye is irrigated with balanced salt solution, the lid speculum is removed immediately and the lids are closed promptly, thus preventing or minimizing surface desiccation under the light of the operating microscope. Some surgeons apply a semipressure patch to the treated eye after instillation of a cycloplegic (e.g., homatropine 5%), nonsteroidal anti-inflammatory drug (NSAID) (e.g., diclofenac or ketorolac) and a combination steroid and antibiotic ointment (e.g., dexamethasone-tobramycin). Alternatively, many surgeons use the combination of a therapeutic soft contact lens and topical NSAID to blunt the postoperative rise in prostaglandin E_2, a main mediator of pain, thereby reducing postoperative discomfort.

Bibliography

Campos M, et al. Corneal wound healing after excimer laser ablation. Effects of nitrogen gas blower. *Ophthalmology* 99(6):893–897, 1992.

Campos M, et al. Corneal wound healing after excimer laser ablation in rabbits: Expanding versus contracting apertures. *Refract Corneal Surg* 8(5):378–381, 1992.

Campos M, et al. Corneal surface after deepithelialization using a sharp and a dull instrument. *Ophthalmic Surg* 23(9):618–621, 1992.

Campos M, et al. Keratocyte loss after different methods of de-epithelialization. *Ophthalmology* 101(5):890–894, 1994.

Campos M, et al. Keratocyte loss after corneal deepithelialization in primates and rabbits. *Arch Ophthalmol* 112(2):254–260, 1994.

Campos M, Trokel SL, McDonnell PJ. Surface morphology following photorefractive keratectomy. *Ophthalmic Surg* 24(12):822–825, 1993.

Campos M, et al. Ablation rates and surface ultrastructure of 193nm excimer laser keratectomies. *Invest Ophthalmol Vis Sci* 34(8):2493–2500, 1993.

Dausch D, et al. Excimer laser photorefractive keratectomy with tapered transition zone for high myopia. A preliminary report of six patients. *J Cataract Refract Surg* 19(5):590–594, 1993.

Dougherty PJ, Wellish KL, Maloney RK. Excimer laser ablation rate and corneal hydration. *Am J Ophthalmol* 118(2):169–176, 1994.

Förster W. Time-delayed, two-step excimer laser photorefractive keratectomy to correct high myopia. *Refract Corneal Surg* 9(6):465–467, 1993.

Gobbi PG, et al. Automatic eye tracker for excimer laser photorefractive keratectomy. *Invest Ophthalmol Vis Sci* 35(Suppl. 4):2017, 1994.

Heitzmann J, et al. The correction of high myopia using the excimer laser. *Arch Ophthalmol* 111(12):1627–1634, 1993.

Krueger RR, et al. Corneal surface morphology following excimer laser ablation with humified gases. *Arch Ophthalmol* 111(8):1131–1137, 1993.

Krueger RR, et al. Clinical analysis of excimer laser photorefractive keratectomy using a multiple zone technique for severe myopia. *Am J Ophthalmol* 119(3):263–274, 1995.

Krueger RR, et al. Diffractive smoothing of excimer laser ablation using a defocused beam. *J Refract Corneal Surg* 10(1):20–26, 1994.

Pande M, Hillman JS. Optical zone centration in keratorefractive surgery: Entrance pupil center, visual axis, coaxially sighted corneal reflex, or geometric corneal center? *Ophthalmology* 100(8):1230–1237, 1993.

Seiler T, Wollensak J. Myopic photorefractive keratectomy with the excimer laser: One year follow-up. *Ophthalmology* 98(8):1156–1163, 1991.

Sinbawy A, McDonnell PJ, Moreira H. Surface ultrastructure after excimer laser ablation: Expanding vs. contracting apertures. *Arch Ophthalmol* 109(11):1531, 1991.

Talamo JH, Vidaurri-Leal JS. Abad JC. Refractive effects of 18% ethanol versus mechanical epithelial removal before excimer PRK. *Ophthalmology* 102:154, 1995.

Tavola A, et al. Photorefractive keratectomy for myopia: Single vs double-zone treatment in 166 eyes. *Refract Corneal Surg* 9(Suppl. 2):S48–S52, 1993.

Astigmatism

Berthold Seitz and Peter J. McDonnell

Astigmatism can occur either congenitally or after ocular surgery, especially after penetrating keratoplasty. The astigmatism is defined as regular when specific criteria are met: (1) two principal meridians are identifiable by refraction and keratometry; (2) these meridians are 90 degrees apart; (3) the end point of keratometry is distinct; (4) the photokeratoscope or computerized videokeratography (CVK) mires are regular ovals; and (5) maximal quality visual acuity can be obtained by spectacle correction. With current CVK analysis, regular astigmatism is typically represented by a symmetric bowtie pattern (see Chap. 2).

The excimer laser was first employed as an improved "scalpel" for creating narrow linear excisions of corneal tissue. As experience was gained with the laser for creation of linear radial keratotomies (for myopia) or transverse keratotomies (for astigmatism), it became clear that this approach did not improve on results obtained with the diamond blade, and the concept of wide-field ablation for photorefractive astigmatic keratectomy (PARK) was born.

Ablation Parameters and Options

To correct astigmatism with wide-area surface ablation, a different profile of tissue is ablated in the steep and flat meridians, so that the preoperatively steep meridian is selectively flattened or the preoperatively flat meridian is selectively steepened relative to the other meridian. The flat meridian can be protected from further flattening by a metal mask system or an erodible (ablatable) mask.

Metal Mask System

The most widely used strategy for PARK at the present time is that employed by VISX excimer laser systems (Santa Clara, CA). With this technique, the laser beam is passed through a set of blades that expand or contract with successive pulses (VISX). A cylindrical or elliptical ablation can be performed, with elliptical ablations used to correct simultaneously spherical myopia and myopic astigmatism. The long axis of the ellipse or slit must be aligned with the flat preoperative meridian.

With cylindrical ablations, the entire optical zone of the flat meridian is exposed to each pulse. In the steep meridian, the ablation becomes progressively shallower, moving to the periphery (Fig. 4-5).

Erodible (Ablatable) Mask

An alternative approach that has yet to be proved clinically valuable is the use of an erodible or ablatable mask employed in the beam path. The mask consists of a polymer that is progressively ablated with successive excimer laser pulses. It has an optical zone similar to that of a toric hard contact lens. The excimer laser beam penetrates the mask and ablates corneal tissue initially at its thinnest area (i.e., in the

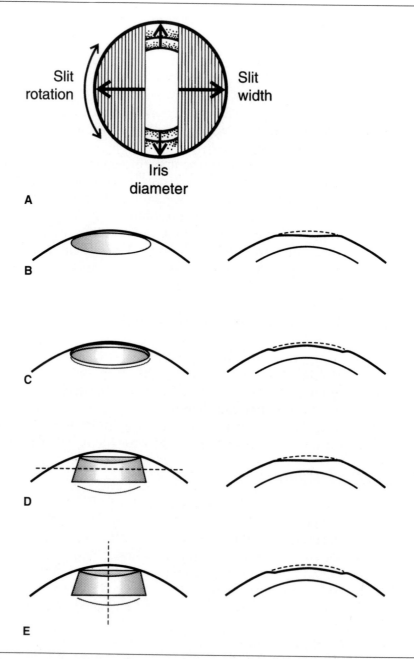

A

B

C

D

E

Fig. 4-5. Schematic illustration (**A**) of the method of creating cylindrical ablations by progressively widening the separation between parallel blades during the ablation. Variables that can be controlled include depth of ablation, width of ablation zone, and orientation of the slit. With blades oriented as shown, the cornea would be flattened in the horizontal meridian to correct an against-the-rule astigmatism. Comparison of myopic ablation (**B**), in which the greatest amount of tissue is removed centrally, with progressively less removed toward the periphery; a phototherapeutic keratectomy with a small transition zone (**C**), in which a uniform amount of tissue is ablated without intended refractive change; and cylindrical ablation (**D** and **E**) for correction of against-the-rule astigmatism. Cross section through the originally steep meridian after ablation (D) is identical to myopic ablation (B), whereas a cross section through the originally flat meridian (D), in which no refractive change is intended, is identical to phototherapeutic keratectomy (C).

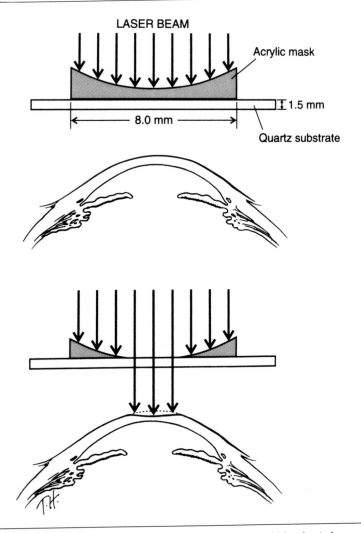

Fig. 4-6. Principle of the erodible mask technique. The erodible plastic button adheres to a quartz substrate (transparent for 193-nm radiation). The shape of the mask is transferred by the wide-area laser beam inversely onto the cornea underneath the mask. When the mask is completely eroded, the greatest amount of tissue will have been ablated centrally, with progressively less tissue removed toward the periphery of the ablation zone, and more tissue ablated in the original steep meridian.

steep meridian); the later pulses progressively ablate the thicker areas of the mask (Fig. 4-6).

Difficulties with centration, correct alignment of the axes, and tissue effluent plume removal may limit the practicality of this approach. An advantage of the erodible mask, however, is the lack of diaphragmatic "steps" on the corneal surface.

Patient Positioning and Axis Marking

Patients are placed in a supine position under the excimer laser, as for myopic PRK. Centration and epithelial removal are performed as for spherical myopia. Unique to astigmatic treatment is the requirement that the ablation be properly oriented relative to the steep and flat corneal meridians to avoid astigmatic undercorrection. The patient's preoperative corneal topographic map is positioned so that the surgeon can readily double-check the correct alignment of the axis. Correct centration and exact alignment of the axes are most critical in astigmatic correction with the excimer laser because the magnitude of correction is very sensitive to misalignment. An axial error of 15 degrees can induce an astigmatic undercorrection of 50% (Fig. 4-7). Through the use of limbal landmarks (e.g., prominent vessel, hyperpigmentation) (Fig. 4-8), or a mark at the limbus placed at the slit lamp, the proper orientation is ensured in the event of some cyclotorsion of the globe intraoperatively. A summary of axial alignment errors that may produce undercorrection is provided in Table 4-5.

Using the VISX laser, the blades are oriented by the computer to be parallel to the axis of the refractive minus cylinder, thereby flattening the cornea in the perpendicular (steep) meridian. To avoid an abrupt step at the end of the spherically ablated (flatter) meridian, a transition zone is created. The patient fixates on a coaxial fixation light during the entire procedure. Should a patient make any movements during the procedure that result in loss of proper centration, the procedure

Fig. 4-7. Astigmatic undercorrection by axis alignment error. An axial error of 15 degrees can induce an astigmatic undercorrection of 50%.

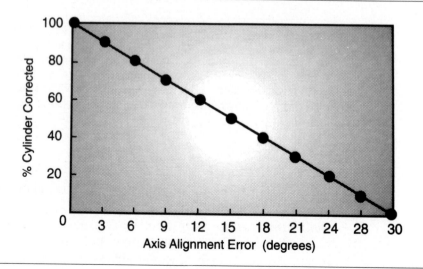

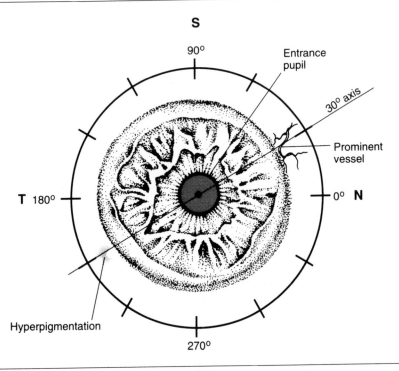

Fig. 4-8. Landmarks for correct axis alignment in astigmatic photorefractive keratectomy. A prominent vessel and a hyperpigmentation at the limbus, as determined at the slit lamp, are used to find the 30-degree flat axis intraoperatively with the patient in the supine position. S = superior; T = temporal; I = inferior; N = nasal.

Table 4-5. Astigmatic undercorrection by axial alignment errors

Axis measurement errors in preoperative refraction
Misalignment of the patient's head on the operating table
Misalignment of the laser beam
Cyclotorsion of the patient's eye (real or apparent)
Angular motion during treatment

is interrupted immediately. Centration is then re-established, and the procedure completed.

Combining PARK with Myopic or Hyperopic Treatment

Cylindrical and spherical refractive errors commonly coexist, and an ablation may be designed to correct both components of ametropia. Compound myopic astigmatism can be corrected by sequential cylindrical ablation for astigmatism and circular ablation for spherical

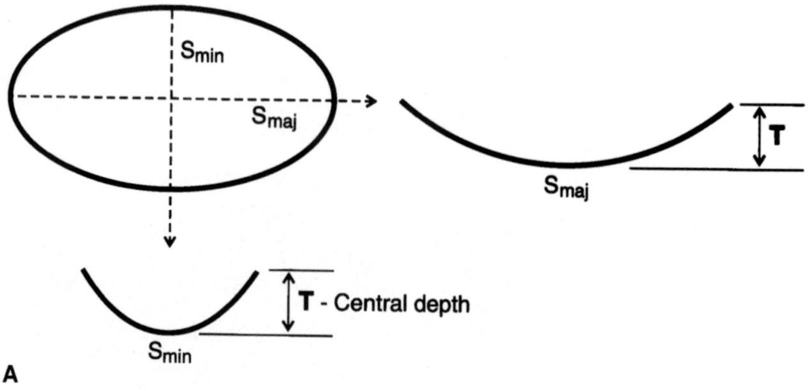

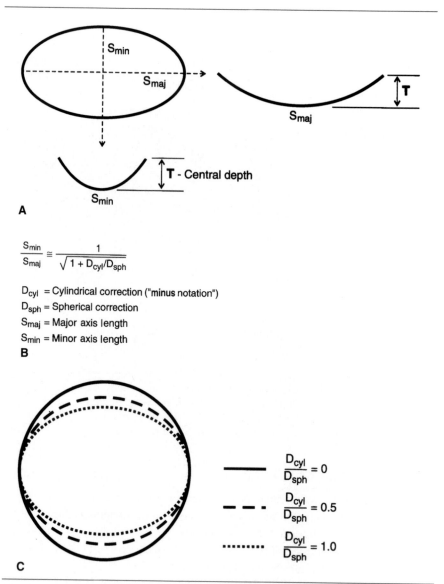

$$\frac{S_{min}}{S_{maj}} \cong \frac{1}{\sqrt{1 + D_{cyl}/D_{sph}}}$$

D_{cyl} = Cylindrical correction ("minus notation")
D_{sph} = Spherical correction
S_{maj} = Major axis length
S_{min} = Minor axis length
B

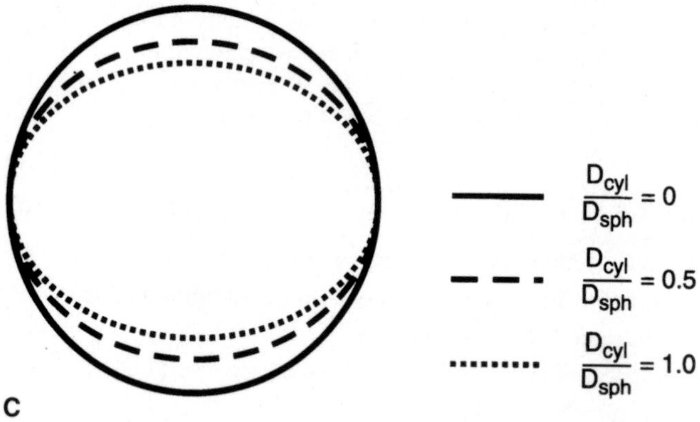

Fig. 4-9. Illustration of elliptical ablation for simultaneous correction of myopia and astigmatism. Unlike the concentric circular ablation for spherical myopia, a series of concentric elliptical ablations are created. (Drawing after graphics provided by VISX, Santa Clara, CA) **A.** The narrowest width (S_{min}) of the ellipse is oriented parallel to the preoperatively steep meridian. The cross section through the vertical meridian shows greater removal of tissue per cross-sectional area than does the cross section through the horizontal meridian. Because the central depth (T) is identical, greater corneal flattening is achieved in the vertical meridian. Formula for (**B**) and examples of (**C**) elliptical ablation, including the ellipse geometry and refractive correction. In the case of no refractive cylinder, S_{min} and S_{maj} should be equal, and a spherical ablation is achieved. In case of an equal amount of refractive cylinder (minus notation) and spherical ametropia, S_{min} should be about $0.7 \times S_{maj}$.

myopia, or simultaneously by a "simple" elliptical ablation (Fig. 4-9). Both approaches have been successful clinically.

In another strategy, the Meditec laser (Heroldsberg, Germany) scans a slit-beam across the corneal surface (diameter of the treatment zone is 5 or 7 mm) through an hourglass-shaped opening in a rotating metal mask at each nonequidistant step (see Chap. 15).

The ideal patient for the techniques described above has regular compound myopic astigmatism. A full astigmatic correction is attempted, with a slight undercorrection of spherical myopia, avoiding overcorrection with consequent hyperopia. Residual myopic ametropia can be corrected later if necessary.

With astigmatic ablations, histologically evident alterations in epithelial thickness and new collagen production are correlated with ablation depth only in the axis that was originally steep. This suggests that the radially asymmetric stromal ablation produces quantitatively asymmetric wound healing, presumably followed by partial regression of the effect in some patients.

Unlike ablations for myopic astigmatism, in which the steep meridian is selectively flattened, treatment for hyperopic astigmatism selectively steepens the flat meridian. One method (Meditec) uses a rotating hyperopic template with an 8.5-mm ablation zone and a 6-mm optical zone to create a circular, furrowlike ring-zone ablation; this is achieved by utilizing unequal rotating angle steps and angle distances due to differences in rotation speed of a hyperopic mask (see Chap. 15). The ablation depth varies from the center to the periphery in each desired meridian. In hyperopic PRK, this ablation depth is intensified in the periphery.

To correct mixed astigmatism, the hyperopic spherical refractive error may be treated in the same session, switching to the hyperopic handpiece after correction of the astigmatic error, with the suction device staying in place (Meditec). Other examples of strategies for correction of hyperopic astigmatism are described in the chapters on individual laser systems (see Part II, Technical Considerations).

Treating Irregular Astigmatism

Astigmatism is said to be irregular when the principal meridians, as detected by keratometry or CVK studies, are (1) separated by an angle of other than 90 degrees; (2) when the end point of keratometry is not distinct; (3) when the circular mires of the photokeratoscope are distorted; and (4) when better visual acuity can be obtained with a rigid contact lens than with spectacles. With CVK analysis, corneal dioptric power measurements are variable and often asymmetrically distributed around the apex of the videokeratograph. The steep hemimeridians, which should be oriented 180 degrees apart, may be separated by 170 degrees or less. In addition, the amount of dioptric power in the steep and flat hemimeridians may be markedly different. In severe cases of irregular astigmatism, there may be multiple steep and multiple flat hemimeridians.

Using the CVK map as a guide, excimer ablation can be used to create a more regular surface contour with improved visual function. Using strategies that combine phototherapeutic and photorefractive ablation patterns, the amount of tissue to be removed is calculated on the basis of the diameter and steepness of the irregular areas of the corneal surface. The amount of tissue to be excised in a localized steep region can be estimated by the following formula:

$$\text{Depth } (\mu m) \ = \ \frac{(\text{diameter } [mm])^2 \ \times \ (\text{relative steepness } [D])}{3}$$

To flatten the steeper corneal zones defined by CVK maps, multiple PTK ablations may be placed in the midperiphery of the appropriate hemimeridians. In the same session residual spherical refractive error may be corrected by a PRK ablation in the center of the cornea (Fig. 4-10, Plates 6 and 7).

Fig. 4-10. Treatment plan based on biomicroscopic observation and topographic analysis. To flatten local steep areas, three confluent 4-mm circular zones (A, B, C) in the inferior portion are ablated (each PTK mode; no intended refractive power change; intended depth 20 μm; 0.35-mm transition zone). The edges of the zones are barely touching. The final ablation (D in figure) to correct residual myopia (PRK mode; 6-mm circular zone; intended refractive power change −1.5 D; intended depth 20 μm) is centered over the entrance pupil. (From R Gibralter, SL Trokel. Correction of irregular astigmatism with the excimer laser. *Ophthalmology* 101:1310–1315, 1994.)

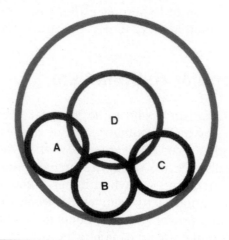

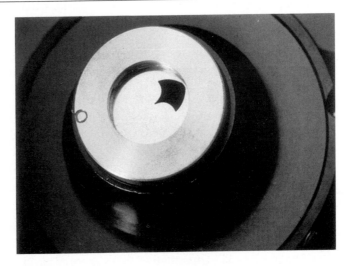

Fig. 4-11. Spearhead-shaped opening of a rotating metal mask for the correction of presbyopia or highly irregular astigmatism. (Courtesy of Fa. Aesculap-Meditec GmbH, Heroldsberg, Germany.)

To steepen the flat hemimeridian when highly asymmetric astigmatism is present, a rotating metal mask with a spearheadlike aperture and a scanning beam can be used (Fig. 4-11).

In the near future, irregular astigmatism might be treated by a computer-controlled small-diameter laser beam that scans as a "flying spot" across the corneal surface according to a software program, which incorporates the data from preoperative and possibly intra-operative corneal topographic analysis and depicts true corneal tissue elevations and depressions rather than a Placido disk–based image reflection.

For a discussion of decentration, see Chapters 5 and 6.

Bibliography

Brancato R, et al. The erodible mask in photorefractive keratectomy for myopia and astigmatism. *Refract Corneal Surg* 9(Suppl. 2):S125–S130, 1993.

Campos M, et al. Photorefractive keratectomy for severe postkeratoplasty astigmatism. *Am J Ophthalmol* 114(4):429–436, 1992.

Campos M, McDonnell PJ. Photorefractive Keratectomy: Astigmatism. In FB Thompson, PJ McDonnell (eds.). *Color Atlas/Text of Excimer Laser Surgery: The Cornea.* New York: Igaku-Shoin, 1993.

Colliac J-P, Shammas HJ, Bart DJ. Photorefractive keratectomy for the correction of myopia and astigmatism. *Am J Ophthalmol* 117(3):369–380, 1994.

Dausch D, et al. Photorefractive keratectomy to correct astigmatism with myopia or hyperopia. *J Cataract Refract Surg* 20(Suppl.):252–257, 1994.

Gibraltar R, Trokel SL. Correction of irregular astigmatism with the excimer laser. *Ophthalmology* 101(7):1310–1315, 1994.

McDonnell PJ, et al. Photorefractive Keratektomie zur Korrektur von myopem Astigmatismus. *Klin Monatsbl Augenheilkd* 202(3):238–244, 1993.

McDonnell PJ, et al. Photorefractive keratectomy for astigmatism—Initial clinical results. *Arch Ophthalmol* 109(10):1370–1373, 1991.

McDonnell PJ, et al. Photorefractive keratectomy to create toric ablations for correction of astigmatism. *Arch Ophthalmol* 109(5):710–713, 1991.

Seiler T, et al. Excimer laser keratectomy for correction of astigmatism. *Am J Ophthalmol* 105(2):117–124, 1988.

Shieh E, et al. Quantitative analysis of wound healing after cylindrical and spherical excimer laser ablations. *Ophthalmology* 99(7):1050–1055, 1992.

Smith EM, et al. Comparison of astigmatic axis in the seated and supine positions. *J Refract Corneal Surg* 10(6):615–620, 1994.

Spigelman AV, et al. Treatment of myopic astigmatism with the 193nm excimer laser utilizing aperture elements. *J Cataract Refract Surg* 20 (Suppl.):258–261, 1994.

Taylor HR, et al. Comparison of excimer laser treatment of astigmatism and myopia. *Arch Ophthalmol* 111(12):1621–1626, 1993.

Hyperopia

Berthold Seitz and Peter J. McDonnell

To correct hyperopia, a minimal amount of tissue is removed centrally, and progressively more stroma is ablated toward the corneal periphery so that the central cornea is steepened (Fig. 4-12). Visual performance after hyperopic PRK depends heavily on excellent centration of the central optical zone, which in most cases is of a significantly smaller diameter than that created after myopic PRK. As with astigmatism, a variety of software and hardware approaches are available to correct hyperopia. We will outline only two approaches in this chapter (Meditec and Summit), but other strategies are covered in individual systems chapters elsewhere in the book (see Part II, Technical Considerations).

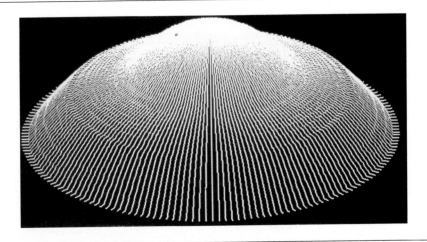

Fig. 4-12. Computer-aided design of a hyperopic correction with a central steepening of the cornea. (Courtesy of Fa. Aesculap-Meditec GmbH, Heroldsberg, Germany.)

Rotating Mask System

Using the Meditec laser, the photoablation pattern for hyperopic corrections is achieved by masks mounted on a suction ring fixed on the patient's globe. The metal diaphragm with double-heart–like perforations (Fig. 4-13) is rotated by a fixed angle between subsequent laser exposures, depending on the amount of intended correction. Initially, an optical zone of 4 mm and an overall ablation diameter of 7.5 mm were employed, and the small transition zone seemed responsible for the high amount of regression, especially as observed in higher corrections (i.e., > + 5.0 D).

Unfortunately, the predictability of hyperopic corrections of less than 5 D seems to be significantly less than that of myopic correction of similar magnitude. Presumably, the specific changes of corneal contour for hyperopic correction, requiring both relative flattening of the more peripheral treated area and relative steepening of the central portion, are prone to filling in by epithelial hyperplasia or new collagen formation, or both.

The problems of regression may be overcome by a larger transition area from the optical zone to the untouched periphery (e.g., 5-mm optical zone, 8- to 10-mm diameter of overall treatment zone). This can be achieved by eccentrically rotating a lens about a mechanical center, thereby offsetting the image of a rotating, variable-width slit (Plate 8). Wound healing after these large ablations seems to result in less refractive regression. Some surgeons recommend that the patient

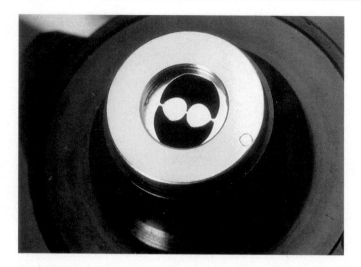

Fig. 4-13. Photoablation of cornea through a double-heart–shaped opening of a rotating metal mask for the correction of hyperopia. (Courtesy of Fa. Aesculap-Meditec GmbH, Heroldsberg, Germany.)

wear a therapeutic soft contact lens for several weeks, as this may reduce the severity of ring-shaped haze and regression after hyperopic PRK; this effect has not been validated by clinical trials.

Erodible Mask System

The erodible mask (Summit Technologies, Waltham, MA) consists of a precisely shaped plastic button that exhibits an ablation rate similar to that of corneal stroma. The mask is held a short distance above the eye on a thin quartz substrate that is transparent at 193 nm. The laser beam is designed to illuminate the entire mask. During the first few pulses, the radiation is totally absorbed by the mask material. As the thinner, peripheral portions of the mask material are photoablated, laser light eventually penetrates this region, reaches the surface of the eye, and removes corneal tissue. With subsequent pulses, the area of removed mask material increases, leading to ever-increasing areas of photoablation on the cornea. When the mask material is totally removed, the shape of corneal ablation approximates inversely the original shape of the mask.

To align the mask on the eye, a special eye cup has been developed that includes internal illumination and a humidified air flow to prevent corneal ablation by-products from condensing underneath the mask, where they could affect the transmission of 193-nm radiation.

Technically, fixation and especially centration of the mask can be difficult. Using small ablation zones, regression is a major problem in the long-term follow-up. Furthermore, erodible hyperopic masks can produce paradoxical myopic corrections due to a lack of transition zone at the edge of the mask.

To address the technical problems associated with the erodible mask, the manufacturer is making an effort to place the mask within the delivery system of the laser itself rather than close to the cornea.

Bibliography

Amann T, et al. Wound healing after excimer PRK for hyperopia in rabbits. *Invest Ophthalmol Vis Sci* 36(Suppl. 4):S711, 1995.

Dausch D, Klein R, Schröder E. Excimer laser photorefractive keratectomy for hyperopia. *Refract Corneal Surg* 9(1):20–28, 1993.

Gobbi PG, et al. A simplified method to perform photorefractive keratectomy using an erodible mask. *J Refract Corneal Surg* 10(Suppl. 2):S246–S249, 1994.

Goes F. Short term results with excimer laser-photorefractive keratectomy. *Bull Soc Belge Ophthalmol* 245:69–74, 1992.

Maloney RK, et al. A prototype erodible mask delivery system for the excimer laser. *Ophthalmology* 100(4):542–549, 1993.

McDonald MB, et al. Excimer laser hyperopia PRK phase I: The blind eye study. *Invest Ophthalmol Vis Sci* 35(Suppl. 4):1488, 1994.

McDonnell PJ. Excimer laser corneal surgery: New strategies and old enemies. *Invest Ophthalmol Vis Sci* 36(1):4–8, 1995.

Ramirez-Florez S, et al. Correction of hyperopia with excimer laser PRK. *Invest Ophthalmol Vis Sci* 35(Suppl. 4):2023, 1994.

Seiler T. Photorefractive Keratectomy: European Experience. In FB Thompson, PJ McDonnell (eds.). *Color Atlas/Text of Excimer Laser Surgery: The Cornea*. New York: Igaku-Shoin, 1993.

Shimmick JK, et al. Analysis of an offset slit excimer laser delivery system for the treatment of hyperopia. *Invest Ophthalmol Vis Sci* 35(Suppl. 4):1487, 1994.

Uozato H, Guyton DL. Centering corneal surgical procedures. *Am J Ophthalmol* 103(3):264–275, 1987.

Presbyopia

Berthold Seitz and Peter J. McDonnell

It is well known that a minority of patients achieve an unintended, multifocal lens effect after myopic PRK or radial keratotomy that enables them to maintain reasonable uncorrected visual acuity over a large range of defocus. After multifocal ablations, a greater spread of surface powers over the entrance pupil is observed, often with a bimodal distribution. These observations suggest that in some patients undergoing PRK for myopia, it may be possible to reduce symptoms of presbyopia, although a decrease in image contrast or monocular diplopia may complicate this approach. The development of these techniques is in its infancy, and many leaders in the field consider them investigational. The reader is advised to consult both the literature and experienced colleagues prior to attempting to correct presbyopia by surface photoablation.

The optical performance of a multifocal cornea is analogous to that of multifocal intraocular lenses, which is based on the reception of simultaneous images at the retina through various regions of the lens. The ability to process these different images is a form of pseudo-accommodation. Postulating that this is true for a multifocal cornea as well, the aim has been to create distinct refraction zones by asymmetrically sculpting the cornea with the laser (Fig. 4-14).

To reduce presbyopic symptoms in a *myope* who is undergoing PRK, after a defined amount of conventional myopic correction, a sectorial or central mask can be inserted and the ablation completed (Meditec). In this manner, an inferior steepening ("shoulder effect," pupil size of larger than 2 mm required) or central steepening (artificial central island) is produced.

Fig. 4-14. Computer-aided design of a presbyopic correction with a segmental steepening of the cornea. (Courtesy of Fa. Aesculap-Meditec GmbH, Heroldsberg, Germany.)

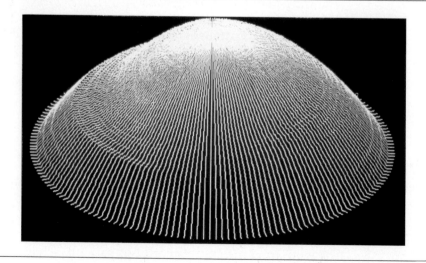

To correct presbyopia combined with *hyperopia,* after a defined amount of conventional hyperopic correction using a double-heart–shaped rotating mask, a nonrotating template with an inferior oval opening can be inserted and the ablation completed. This results in a semilunar area of relative inferior steepening. This approach is not recommended in combination with a hyperopic treatment of more than + 4 D.

To correct *emmetropic* presbyopia or highly asymmetric astigmatism, a rotating mask with a spearheadlike aperture (see Fig. 4-11) and a scanning beam system can be used. This technique produces a defined, partial aspherical steepening on the cornea in any desired meridian. Clinical experience suggests that the treated area must cover an arc length of at least 130 degrees to minimize regression of the effect with loss of the improved unaided near vision over time (Fig. 4-15). As a consequence of the initial markedly asymmetric corneal steepening, loss of one or two lines of best corrected distant vision, and subjective phenomena, such as ghost images and monocular diplopia, are experienced by about one-third of these patients for 3–6 months; longer follow-up data are not available at this time.

Fig. 4-15. Correction of presbyopia or highly irregular astigmatism with segmental flattening. Schematic illustration of segmental hyperopic correction in the 270-degree hemimeridian, including a transition zone. An overall treatment zone of about 130 degrees seems to be necessary to minimize regression of the effect. (Drawing after a graphic provided by Fa. Aesculap-Meditec GmbH, Heroldsberg, Germany.)

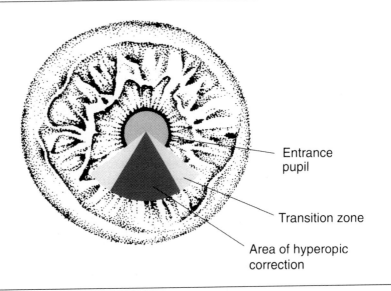

Entrance pupil

Transition zone

Area of hyperopic correction

Bibliography

Anschutz T. Laser Correction of Hyperopia and Presbyopia. In ON Serdarevic (ed.). Refractive Surgery. *Int Ophthalmol Clin* 34(4):107–137, 1994.

Holladay JT, et al. Optical performance of multifocal intraocular lenses. *J Cataract Refract Surg* 16(4):413–422, 1990.

Krueger RR, McDonnell PJ. New Directions in Excimer Laser Surgery. In FB Thompson, PJ McDonnell (eds.). *Color Atlas/Text of Excimer Laser Surgery: The Cornea.* New York: Igaku-Shoin, 1993.

McDonnell PJ, Garbus JJ, Lopez PF. Topographic analysis and visual acuity after radial keratotomy. *Am J Ophthalmol* 106(6):692–695, 1988.

Moreira H, et al. Multifocal corneal topographic changes with excimer laser photorefractive keratectomy. *Arch Ophthalmol* 110(7):994–999, 1992.

Pallikaris IG, et al. Rotating brush for fast removal of corneal epithelium. *J Refract Surg* 10:439–442, 1994.

Schröeder E, et al. Multicenter clinical trial to evaluate presbyopic excimer laser PRK. Unpublished data. Symposium on Cataract, Intraocular Lens, and Refractive Surgery, San Diego: April 1–5, 1995.

PRK After Other Corneal Surgical Procedures

Shu-Wen Chang, Suhas W. Tuli, and Dimitri T. Azar

Although refractive surgery has been commonly used to correct ametropia, the existing keratorefractive procedures are far from perfect. All types of refractive keratotomy procedures share one weakness—the inability to predict the outcome of surgery for an individual patient. This problem results from variability in technique among surgeons and from variability in corneal biomechanical properties and wound healing among patients. Under- and overcorrection are frequent outcomes, and as many as 33% of patients may undergo repeated keratorefractive procedures (enhancements).

The development of pulsed lasers, particularly the argon-fluoride (193-nm) excimer laser, offers a potential solution to these problems because these lasers can create accurate and precise excisions of corneal tissue to an exact length and depth with minimal disruption of the remaining tissue. In addition, this minimal tissue disruption and the smooth edges may allow more uniform stromal wound healing. Laser surgery can make cuts in almost any conceivable configuration. Using computers to control these lasers may improve the precision of refractive surgery, allowing the surgeon to reproducibly perform the desired operation repeatedly [1–4]. PRK may be of great value in treating residual or consecutive refractive errors following other refractive surgical procedures. However, to avoid inaccuracy in the preoperative assessment and undesired wound healing processes, it may be prudent to wait for at least 6 months to 1 year before proceeding with PRK as a second refractive surgical procedure.

PRK Following Radial Keratotomy

Radial keratotomy (RK) remains a commonly used surgical technique to correct myopia [5]. Although it is not as serious a complication as overcorrection, undercorrection following primary RK procedures is common. In the multicenter prospective evaluation of radial keratotomy (PERK) study, 43% of patients experienced a hyperopic shift of 1.0 D or greater 10 years after treatment [6]. As a safeguard against the development of hyperopia, several investigators advocate conservative RK, leaving the patient with intentional undercorrection. However, significant undercorrections may occur in some patients even if a conservative approach is not employed. Undercorrections following RK traditionally have been treated with reoperations that involve adding, deepening, or lengthening incisions, which may reduce the optical zone size. If a component of the RK procedure that explains the undercorrection can be identified (i.e., inadequate incision depth or length), it may be logical to repeat the surgery. Reoperations are more difficult, however, and less predictable. The alternatives include the use of nonsurgical techniques or different keratorefractive procedures.

RK acts indirectly through peripheral radial incisions that cause flattening of the central cornea, but the nonlinear characteristics of corneal biomechanics often limit the amount of central flattening that can be achieved [7, 8]. PRK, on the other hand, acts by ablating tissue directly from the central cornea [9, 10]. Thus, performing PRK after RK theoretically combines the advantages of the two methods. Several authors have reported good results with this approach [11–15], but Ribeiro et al. [16] reported a patient who experienced significant haze, increased astigmatism, and three-line loss of best corrected visual acuity when PRK was performed after RK. Maloney et al. [17] found that PRK on eyes after RK was less accurate than excimer laser PRK as a primary procedure for eyes with a similar range of myopia. They reported a higher incidence and persistence of corneal haze and a significant loss of visual function 1 year after PRK in eyes with residual myopia following RK. The authors attributed this loss of visual function to either corneal haze or irregular astigmatism. We retrospectively analyzed the visual outcomes of 55 eyes of 45 patients (unpublished data) undergoing PRK for residual myopia after RK. Case examples are illustrated in Figure 4-16 and Plate 9.

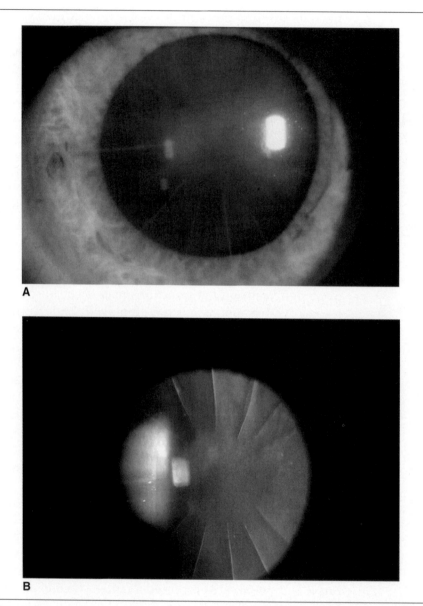

Fig. 4-16. **A.** One-year postoperative clinical appearance of a 47-year-old female who underwent PRK for residual myopia after 16-incision radial keratotomy (RK). The refractive error prior to RK was −13.0 + 2.00 × 88. She received a 16-incision RK with an optical zone of 2.75 mm. Her visual acuity was 20/20 with −8.5 + 2.25 × 170 1 year postoperatively. She received photoastigmatic refractive keratectomy with a correction of −3.95 × −2.15 × 180. The ablation zone was 6.0 mm with no transition zone. **B.** One year after laser treatment, the visual acuity could be corrected to 20/20 by −3.0 + 0.5 × 60. The corneal haze was graded as + 0.5.

Refraction data from this series reveal an initial mean overcorrection, which gradually regressed toward emmetropia. The percentage of eyes within ± 1.00 D of intended correction increased from 44.4% at 1 month to 65% at 12 months. The procedure in patients with lower refractive errors tended to have more predictable and stable results than in those with higher refractive errors. We could not find a definite correlation between the RK response and the PRK response. In terms of efficacy, stability, and safety, PRK after RK as a planned two-stage procedure in treating high myopia is not commonly performed. However, in the unexpectedly undercorrected eye after maximal RK, we believe excimer laser PRK may prove a viable option in well-informed patients. Further study is warranted.

Overcorrection after RK may be more difficult to manage. Noninvasive techniques to rectify this problem include glasses and contact lenses. The cornea is more difficult to fit with a contact lens after RK because of the changes in peripheral corneal topography and the potential for corneal neovascularization and ulceration. PRK and laser in-situ keratomileusis (LASIK) are appealing alternatives, but their safety, efficacy, and stability are yet to be established in this setting. Large-area ablation for the correction of hyperopia must involve removal of tissue in the midperiphery in order to increase the curvature of the optical zone. In principle, this change in contour may be particularly prone to filling in by regenerating epithelium and new collagen formation [18]. Clinical experience with this approach is limited, but the early studies of large-area ablation indicate that the attempted hyperopic correction will be prone to regression because of epithelial hyperplasia as well as new collagen formation. In the correction of myopia, the new surface contour follows the original corneal contour with flattening of the central zone. In contrast, the hyperopic correction is biphasic, requiring both relative flattening of the more peripheral treated zone and relative steepening of the more central zone.

The best approach for overcorrection following RK is to suture the wounds using interrupted or purse-string sutures. Other alternatives include hexagonal keratotomy, laser thermokeratoplasty (LTK), epikeratoplasty, and LASIK. Of these options, only LTK and LASIK appear to hold much promise at the present time. The interrupted-suture approach stabilizes the ocular surface by correcting excessive wound gape and promotes wound healing, which corrects hyperopia. Purse-string sutures steepen the central cornea uniformly by an encircling-band–like effect but may not appose gaping wound edges as well as multiple pairs of interrupted sutures [19–22]. The disadvantages of hexagonal keratotomy include cutting across previous incisions, which further weakens the cornea, and the unpredictability and instability of the procedure. Hyperopic LASIK is a possibility, and it may work well if two conditions are met. First, the patient must be at least 1 year post-RK. Secondly, the RK incisions must be very well healed, without gaping or epithelialization. If these conditions are not observed, hyperopic LASIK may lead to incision rupture during lamellar keratectomy and/or yield unpredictable results, often with large amounts of astigmatism. Thermokeratoplasty is known to cause recurrent erosions, corneal scars, and necrosis. Intrastromal pulsed holmium:YAG LTK, which focuses the laser beam and causes a cone-shaped coagulation of stroma, is less invasive. LTK leads to more pronounced shrinkage of the collagen fibrils and may result in greater refractive effect and stability. The best approach with this procedure is to treat over the incision area rather than between incisions to avoid gaping of the RK wounds. Epikeratoplasty can add mass to a potentially compromised cornea and also facilitate contact lens fitting by the improved corneal topography following epikeratoplasty [19]. Nevertheless, epikeratoplasty requires a homoplastic donor, and it has historically produced unpredictable results.

PRK Following Astigmatic Keratotomy

Up to 95% of myopic eyes may have clinically detectable astigmatism, and approximately 10% of the population can be expected to have astigmatism greater than 1.00 D, which affects the quality of uncorrected visual acuity [20]. Most patients with refractive errors that need astigmatic keratotomy (AK) receive surgical correction of the ametropia at the same time. An unanticipated undercorrection, however, may require a second refractive surgical procedure. Early PRK series limited the preoperative astigmatism to 1.00 D or less, as this is the maximum amount of astigmatism that will not excessively influence refractive results after aspherical PRK treatment. Ring et al. [21] attempted to correct compound myopic astigmatism utilizing PRK following transverse keratotomy. They found a coupling effect, whereby the increase in myopia is half the loss in astigmatism, which was reliable enough in patients with up to 2.00 D of astigmatism to proceed with PRK within 2 days. For astigmatism greater than 2.00 D, they found that the cornea took longer to stabilize, and they allowed at least 3 weeks between the AK and PRK. Because these eyes have had recent incisional corneal surgery, they may have a propensity to scar due to activated fibroblasts in the cornea [22, 23]. The rationale to treat residual refractive errors following AK or RK is similar, but special consideration should be given to the topographic change following PRK. In AK, there is usually a flattening of the central optical zone in the meridian of the incision(s) and an area of slight steepening just peripheral to the astigmatic incision. If the previous AK surgery has an optical zone of 5 mm and one would like to correct residual refractive errors using an excimer laser ablation zone of 6 mm, it is possible that the astigmatic correction may change after PRK. However, if the previous AK surgery has an optical zone larger than the intended photoablation zone, it is less likely that astigmatism may change after PRK. In Ring's series [21], in which transverse keratotomy was performed in conjunction with spherical PRK, 75% achieved 20/40 or better uncorrected visual acuity at 6 months. Presently, the preferred timing of AK is unclear. Much will be learned from clinical trials examining AK prior to, concurrent with, and following excimer PRK.

PRK Following Automated Lamellar Keratectomy

Automated lamellar keratectomy (ALK), or keratomileusis in situ, has been used for the treatment of high myopia. It involves making a primary cap or flap followed by resection of a refractive lenticule to achieve the desired refractive effect. When replaced, the cap or flap conforms to the shape of the resected bed, thus altering the anterior curvature of the cornea. It is the thickness and the diameter of the second resection that dictates the power of the correction. The thickness partially depends on the accuracy of the microkeratome, which in turn depends on the speed with which the unit is passed across the corneal surface. Although several efforts have been made to improve microkeratome technology, the precision of the second pass, or refractive cut, remains poor. Overcorrection and undercorrection are to be expected, and secondary procedures to correct residual refractive errors are often needed.

The alternatives available for the correction of residual myopia following myopic ALK include RK, repeat ALK, LASIK, and laser PRK. Treatment of residual myopia should be based on the spherical equivalent of the cycloplegic refraction to determine the parameters of the enhancement treatment. If the residual myopia is high and the eye is not a candidate for RK, revision surgery can be performed at 1 month or less. In this situation, comparison of the desired thickness of the lenticule obtained at the primary surgery to the actual thickness may be informative. If the lenticule is thin by an amount that corresponds to the residual myopia, the new lenticule may be cut soon, provided that the eye is very quiet and the cap and interface are clear. If the relationship between the thickness of the lenticule and the residual myopia do not correspond well or no measurements are available, a waiting period of 3 months or until the refraction is stable may be necessary before repeating the procedure. Similarly, the flap can be lifted and the residual myopia treated by excimer photoablation. In low residual myopia, RK or surface PRK can be performed on top of the flap when corneal wound healing is complete and the refractive status is stable.

When considering PRK following ALK, the refractive surgeon must decide whether the laser treatment should be on top of the corneal surface (surface PRK) or in the corneal bed underneath the corneal flap or cap (LASIK). Surface PRK has the advantage of avoiding revision of the flap, yet it has the disadvantage of ablation through Bowman's layer and inciting the resultant interaction between keratocytes and corneal epithelium, increasing the possibility of haze and/or regression of effect. Before making a final decision, the surgeon should first take several measurements. Using optical pachymetry, corneal epithelial thickness and the depth of the lamellar wound can be estimated from previous lamellar surgery. Second, the surgeon should estimate the ablation thickness of the intended correction. Third, it is necessary to consider factors such as measurement error, corneal dehydration, and stromal edema during surgery to avoid creating a hole in the flap.

If the intended correction is high and there is a risk of ablation through the flap or cap (i.e., creating a hole in the corneal flap or cap), it is better to treat underneath the corneal flap. A corneal flap that is less than 6 months from previous surgery can be elevated again. If more than 6 months have passed since surgery, creating a new flap is an alternative if the flap cannot be elevated. Flap elevation may be the better choice; the cap can be reposited manually to avoid the risk of shredding by the microkeratome. Flap elevation can be done within the first year after surgery by finding the temporal edge of the cap with a Colibri forceps that is dragged from the limbus centrally until it engages the edge of the cap. Movement at the junction of the cap and peripheral cornea inferiorly and superiorly opens a space into which a Kimura spatula can be inserted and pushed across the interface to the nasal side. By rotating the spatula superiorly and inferiorly, the healed peripheral area can be dissected. The thickness of the residual corneal bed is measured using ultrasonic pachymetry. Care should be taken to avoid extensive tissue removal from the corneal bed, which may render the cornea too thin, resulting in corneal ectasia. It is best to leave at least 250 μm on the corneal bed after the intended photoablation and to avoid going deeper than 70% of the preoperative corneal thickness. While it is possible to ablate deeper, it is likely to increase the risk of progressive corneal ectasia and result in a paradoxical increase in myopia. Treatment of overcorrection after myopic ALK is difficult. Options include hyperopic PRK, LASIK, and keratophakia.

Astigmatism may also occur after ALK. Regular astigmatism following ALK may be due to regular astigmatism that was present before the procedure and not altered by the procedure or due to astigmatism induced by the procedure. Irregular astigmatism, more frequently present after ALK than LASIK, may occur when there is inaccuracy in manipulating and replacing the cap during ALK or as a result of a decentered stromal section. It may also occur during replacement of the corneal cap or flap. When the wound healing is complete, regular astigmatism can be treated by arcuate keratotomy close to the limbus [24]. Alternatively, photoastigmatic keratectomy (PARK) can be used to treat regular astigmatism. Irregular astigmatism, however, may require manipulation of the cap before PRK, and the surgeon should be convinced that refractive error and corneal topographic findings have stabilized before proceeding with any surgical intervention.

Management of overcorrected hyperopic ALK (consecutive myopia) is more controversial. It can be treated as residual myopia following myopic ALK. Flattening the central cornea using surface PRK seems the most reasonable approach. However, because the previous hyperopic ALK works via producing central corneal ectasia, excessive removal of central stromal tissue under the ALK flap may risk producing more ectasia, which results in central corneal steepening instead of the expected central flattening.

The alternatives for managing undercorrected hyperopic ALK (residual hyperopia) include a second hyperopic keratomileusis 6 months after the first procedure, hyperopic PRK, or hyperopic LASIK. Large degrees of residual hyperopia usually result from inadequate depth and, therefore, fail to induce anterior bowing of the posterior stroma. Smaller degrees of residual hyperopia (less than 30% of preoperative refraction) may result from the optical zone being too large. It is pointless to attempt another ALK because of the unpredictability of the procedure and the added risks of the secondary procedure. Surface PRK has a potential role in treating residual hyperopia in such situations, but the need for such interventions should decrease markedly in the future as most surgeons have abandoned the technique.

PRK Following Penetrating Keratoplasty

Residual refractive errors following penetrating keratoplasty occur frequently. High myopia and astigmatism often complicate penetrating keratoplasty, making it difficult to rehabilitate the patient's vision. In the past, high astigmatism was the only refractive error following penetrating keratoplasty that required surgical intervention. Conventional surgical procedures to treat astigmatism following penetrating keratoplasty include wedge resection, relaxing incision, and astigmatic keratotomies. Refractive outcomes following these procedures are often unpredictable, and the residual spherical ametropia following penetrating keratoplasty is usually remedied by prescribing spectacles or contact lenses. Contact lenses, however, may not be tolerated by patients who have had a penetrating keratoplasty and may have deleterious effects on the graft [25]. With improvements in PRK and PARK results, the indications for these procedures may be extended to include patients who are unhappy with spectacle or contact lens correction after penetrating keratoplasty. Refractive surgery should be delayed until all sutures are removed and stability of the refractive status has been established. The effect of PRK or other refractive surgical procedures may be even less predictable following penetrating keratoplasty than usual because corneal wound healing may vary in different meridians [26–28]. Complex corneal biomechanical changes resulting from 360-degree, full-thickness wound healing may predispose these eyes to the development of irregular astigmatism. Other treatment options include epikeratoplasty over penetrating keratoplasty [29], repeat transplantation, lens implant exchange in pseudophakic eyes, and RK. Although RK is the most widely employed keratorefractive procedure, using it to correct myopia after penetrating keratoplasty raises the concerns of performing incisional surgery on already surgically compromised eyes [30, 31]. In addition to weakening the structural integrity of the graft, other potential complications following RK in the keratoplasty patient include vascularization and recurrent epithelial erosions. Young et al. [28] have reported vascularization of the radial incisions, which can trigger an acute allograft rejection in the keratoplasty patient. Keates et al. [29] performed epikeratophakia on a patient with postkeratoplasty myopia.

Although the efficacy and safety of 193-nm excimer laser PRK in correcting physiologic refractive errors continues to be established, there is clearly some potential benefit from treating residual ametropia following previous ocular surgery [32–34]. Such surgery for refractive errors is still in the early stages of evaluation [35–41]. Early experience of excimer laser treatment following penetrating keratoplasty stressed its phototherapeutic potential [34, 38, 39]. The phototherapeutic keratectomy procedure was successful in clearing and smoothing the cornea, thus obviating the need for repeated penetrating keratoplasty. However, one episode of graft rejection following excimer laser treatment was observed [39].

Using PRK, John et al. [34] treated a case of recurrent granular dystrophy following penetrating keratoplasty with concomitant myopia, and the subepithelial haze was judged to be of similar magnitude to that observed after primary PRK procedures. Georgaras et al. [35] reported slightly more haze 6 months after surgery.

Before performing refractive surgery following penetrating keratoplasty, corneal topographic maps should be examined carefully. Contact lenses may sometimes be the only method of correcting irregular astigmatism after surgery. If the residual ametropia is small but the patient is intolerant to the anisometropia and contact lens correction, PRK should be considered. Clinical experience in excimer laser treatment after penetrating keratoplasty for refractive purposes is limited. Based on a small series of cases, it appears that eyes with corneal transplants respond to PRK similarly to eyes undergoing primary PRK procedures. When the excimer laser has been used to perform toric ablations in patients with severe astigmatism after penetrating keratoplasty, the refractive effect has been observed to regress substantially in some patients, typically at about 3 months or later. If there is high myopia with small regular astigmatism, LASIK might be an alternative [42]. Special attention should be paid to the integrity of the transplant wound bed because the high intraocular pressure required during lamellar resection may threaten the circumferential wound of penetrating keratoplasty.

References

1. Absten GT, Joffe SN. Lasers in medicine. New York: Chapman, 1985.
2. Koch JW, Lang GK, Naumann GOH. Endothelial reaction to perforating and non-perforating excimer laser excisions in rabbits. *Refract Corneal Surg* 7(3):214–222, 1991.
3. Krauss JM, Puliafito CA, Steinert R. Laser interactions with the cornea. *Surv Ophthalmol* 31:37–53, 1986.
4. Loertscher H, et al. Preliminary report on corneal incisions created by a hydrogen fluoride laser. *Am J Ophthalmol* 102:217–221, 1986.
5. Waring GO. *Refractive Keratotomy for Myopia and Astigmatism*. St. Louis: Mosby, 1992.
6. Waring GO, Lynn MJ, McDonnell PJ, and the PERK Study Group. Results of the Prospective Evaluation of Radial Keratotomy (PERK) study 10 years after surgery. *Arch Ophthalmol* 112:1298–1308, 1994.
7. Villasenor RA, Cox KO. Radial keratotomy: Reoperations. *J Refract Surg* 1:34–37, 1985.
8. Salz JJ. Radial Keratotomy. In FB Thompson (ed.). *Myopia Surgery: Anterior and Posterior Segments*. New York: Macmillan, 1990. Pp. 31–65.
9. Marshall J, et al. Photoablative reprofiling of the cornea using an excimer laser: Photorefractive keratectomy. *Lasers Ophthalmol* 1:21–48, 1986.
10. Taylor DM, et al. Human excimer lamellar keratectomy. *Ophthalmology* 96:654–664, 1989.
11. Meza J, et al. Photorefractive keratectomy after radial keratotomy. *J Cataract Refract Surg* 20:485–489, 1994.
12. McDonnell PJ, Garbus JJ, Salz JJ. Excimer laser myopic photorefractive keratectomy after undercorrected radial keratotomy. *Refract Corneal Surg* 7:146–150, 1991.

13. Frangie JP, et al. Excimer laser keratectomy after radial keratotomy. *Am J Ophthalmol* 115:634–639, 1993.

14. Durrie DS, Schumer DJ, Cavanaugh TB. Photorefractive keratectomy for residual myopia after previous refractive keratotomy. *Refract Corneal Surg* 10(Suppl. 2):S235–238, 1994.

15. Seiler T, Jean B. Photorefractive keratectomy as a second attempt to correct myopia after radial keratotomy. *Refract Corneal Surg* 8:211–214, 1992.

16. Ribeiro JC, McDonald MB, Klyce SD. Photorefractive keratectomy after radial keratotomy in a patient with severe myopia. *Am J Ophthalmol* 118:106–108, 1994.

17. Maloney RK, et al. A multicenter trial of photorefractive keratectomy for residual myopia after previous ocular surgery. *Ophthalmol* 102: 1042–1053, 1995.

18. Steinert RF. Human Application. In RS Brightbill (ed.). *Corneal Surgery: Theory, Technique and Tissue* (2nd ed.). St. Louis: Mosby, 1993.

19. Carlson KA, Goosey JD. Epikeratoplasty following overcorrected radial keratotomy. *Invest Ophthalmol Vis Sci* 29(Suppl.):390, 1988.

20. Lindstom RL. The surgical correction of astigmatism: A clinician's perspective. *Refract Corneal Surg* 6:441–454, 1990.

21. Ring CP, Hadden OB, Morris AT. Transverse keratotomy combined with spherical photorefractive keratectomy for compound myopic astigmatism. *J Refract Corneal Surg* 10:S217–S221, 1994.

22. Hanna KD, et al. Corneal wound healing in monkeys 18 months after excimer laser photorefractive keratectomy. *Refract Corneal Surg* 6: 340–345, 1990.

23. Hanna KD, et al. Corneal wound healing in monkeys after repeated excimer laser photorefractive keratectomy. *Arch Ophthalmol* 110: 1286–1291, 1992.

24. Hollis S. Astigmatism Correction for Lamellar Keratoplasty. In GW Rozakis (ed.). *Refractive Lamellar Keratoplasty.* Thorofare, NJ: Slack, 1994. Pp 101–108.

25. Matsuda M, et al. The effect of contact lens wear on the keratoconic corneal endothelium after penetrating keratoplasty. *Am J Ophthalmol* 107:246–251, 1989.

26. Gothard TW, et al. Four-incision radial keratotomy for high myopia after penetrating keratoplasty. *Refract Corneal Surg* 9(1):51–57, 1993.

27. Shapiro MB, Harrison DA. Radial keratotomy for intolerable myopia after penetrating keratoplasty. *Am J Ophthalmol* 115:327–331, 1993.

28. Young SR, Lundergan MK, Olson RJ. Late complications of combined radial and transverse keratotomy after penetrating keratoplasty associated with atopic keratoconjunctivitis. *Refract Corneal Surg* 5:194–197, 1989.

29. Keates RH, Watson SA, Levy SN. Epikeratophakia following previous refractive keratoplasty surgery: Two case reports. *J Cataract Refract Surg* 12:536–540, 1986.

30. Compos M, Lee M, McDonnell PJ. Ocular integrity after refractive surgery: Effects of photorefractive keratectomy, phototherapeutic

keratectomy, and radial keratotomy. *Ophthalmic Surg* 23:598–602, 1992.

31. Bloom HR, Sands J, Schneider D. Corneal rupture from blunt trauma 22 months after radial keratotomy. *Refract Corneal Surg* 6:197–199, 1990.

32. Seiler T, Wollensak J. Results of a prospective evaluation of photorefractive keratectomy at 1 year after surgery. *Ger J Ophthalmol* 2: 135–142, 1993.

33. Salz JJ, et al. A two-year experience with excimer laser photorefractive keratectomy for myopia. *Ophthalmology* 100:873–882, 1993.

34. John ME, et al. Photorefractive keratectomy following penetrating keratoplasty. *J Refract Corneal Surg* 10(Suppl. 2):S206, 1994.

35. Geogaras SP, et al. Correction of myopia anisometropia with photorefractive keratectomy in 15 eyes. *Refract Corneal Surg* 9(Suppl.):S29, 1993.

36. Wu WCS, Stark WJ, Green WR. Corneal wound healing after 193-nm excimer laser keratectomy. *Arch Ophthalmol* 109:1426–1432, 1991.

37. Lawless MA, Cohen P, Rogers C. Phototherapeutic keratectomy for Reis-Bucker's dystrophy. *Refract Corneal Surg* 9(Suppl.):S96–S98, 1993.

38. Hersh PS, Jordan AJ, Mayers M. Corneal graft rejection episode after excimer laser phototherapeutic keratectomy (letter). *Arch Ophthalmol* 111:735–736, 1993.

39. Stark WJ, et al. Clinical follow-up of 193-nm ArF excimer laser photokeratectomy. *Ophthalmology* 99:805–812, 1992.

40. Hersh PS, et al. Phototherapeutic keratectomy: Strategies and results in 12 eyes. *Refract Corneal Surg* 9(Suppl.):90–95, 1993.

41. Campos M, et al. Photorefractive keratectomy for severe postkeratoplasty astigmatism. *Am J Ophthalmol* 114:429–436, 1992.

42. Kermer F, Kermer I. Postkeratoplasty myopia treated by keratomileusis. *Ann Ophthalmol* 25:370–372, 1993.

5 PRK Postoperative and Complications Management

Ronald R. Krueger and Theo Seiler

Surgical technique during a commonly performed procedure is subject to change and variability among surgeons and even for the same surgeon at different times. The postoperative management following a procedure is also subject to change. Intraoperatively as well as postoperatively, change and variability is what allows a given surgical procedure to evolve and be perfected until it becomes a work of art in the hands of a master surgeon.

When considering excimer laser photorefractive keratectomy (PRK), skill and artistry in pressing the laser foot switch is a matter of speed and alignment. The goal of the procedure is to remove the corneal epithelium and initiate stromal ablation in a rapid but predictable time interval while achieving and maintaining centration of the laser beam. Although intraoperatively the steps are few, careful postoperative follow-up and time-specific intervention make excimer laser PRK a challenging procedure. The effects of corneal wound healing with regard to re-epithelialization, early stromal remodeling, and late regression and haze make the management of postoperative changes and complications nearly as important as that of intraoperative techniques. Consequently, both surgical procedure and postoperative management require the expertise and astute observation of a physician trained and experienced in refractive surgery.

For the new refractive surgeon and the surgeon who is inexperienced with excimer laser PRK, this chapter sets guidelines for routine postoperative management and management of complications. Any individual with a firm grasp of ophthalmology, corneal wound healing, and the management concepts suggested here will likely be able to manage safely any complication or postoperative result following excimer PRK.

Routine Postoperative Management

Immediate Postoperative Period

Once the surgeon takes his or her foot off the excimer laser foot switch, the procedure is complete and the postoperative period begins. The immediate postoperative period is typically the time from the end of the procedure until the beginning of the next day. It also can include the first few days following surgery and, for the purpose of organizing this chapter, we consider the immediate postoperative period to include the first postoperative week or the time until the epithelium is closed. Management is most crucial during this time because it includes the period of corneal re-epithelialization, inflammatory cell infiltration [1], and keratocyte activation [2].

First Day

Immediately following the procedure, the patient is brought up from the supine position and seated at the edge of the treatment bed, where he or she is then given instructions regarding postoperative care. Although a great deal of variation exists between investigators with regard to the steps of early postoperative care, there are basically two distinctly different pathways by which current investigators and surgeons from around the world treat the de-epithelialized excimer laser–treated eye. Both pathways for managing excimer laser PRK prior to re-epithelialization appear to have their own distinct advantages, which have proved to be acceptable for the patient population being considered. For simplicity, we refer to the two pathways according to the geographic area of their greatest use in treatment.

The North American Experience. Many individuals in North America are oriented toward comfort and convenience when having a refractive procedure performed. Postoperative pain following excimer laser PRK can be a major limiting side effect [3–5]. Management that minimizes the symptom of postoperative pain is a highly selected modality for patients concerned with postoperative discomfort.

Although early clinical trials with the VISX (Santa Clara, CA) excimer laser in the United States utilized a pressure patch following PRK surgery, significant pain following the procedure during the first 24–36 hours compelled investigators to consider an alternate method by which the patient could have rapid visual recovery with re-epithelialization and with minimal to no postoperative pain. Their alternative utilizes a bandage soft contact lens together with a topical corticosteroid, topical antibiotic, and cycloplegic agent. Tobramycin-dexamethasone (TobraDex) is a topical corticosteroid and antibiotic often taken in combination and has been used frequently in both the

United States and Canada. More recently, as an alternative, ofloxacin (Ocuflox) or ciprofloxacin (Ciloxan) has been used with a topical steroid to avoid the epithelial toxic response of tobramycin. Typically, disposable contact lenses (e.g., Accuvue, Protec) can be used and cycloplegic agents, such as homatropine 2%, are considered effective (Fig. 5-1).

In addition to these medications and this intervention, many investigators also use topical nonsteroidal agents, such as diclofenac sodium (Voltaren) or ketorolac (Acular), to help minimize some of the pain sensation. Corneal pain sensation appears to be associated with the level of prostaglandin in the cornea, which may act as a mediator of stimulation for the corneal nerves. Medications that reduce the prostaglandin levels in the eye following an insult, such as a corneal abrasion or excimer laser PRK, are highly useful. Topical diclofenac sodium has been shown to reduce prostaglandin levels following excimer laser PRK, but it does not inhibit the leukotriene pathway. Increased polymorphonuclear cell infiltration has been seen following excimer PRK in the rabbit model (Fig. 5-2). For this reason, as well as a reported increased incidence of clinical sterile corneal infiltrates after excimer laser PRK [6], topical corticosteroid use has been advocated together with nonsteroidals in the early postoperative period.

Patients are generally given oral analgesics, such as acetaminophen (Tylenol) with codeine or oxycodone and acetaminophen (Percocet), with the instruction to take these tablets once every 4 hours, as

Fig. 5-1. Eye with disposable contact lens 1 day following excimer laser PRK. Notice the partially closed epithelium, mild conjunctival injection, and moderately dilated pupil.

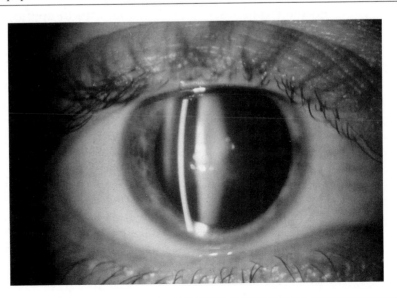

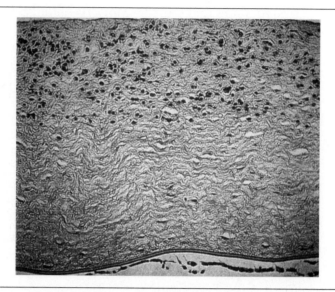

Fig. 5-2. Marked polymorphonuclear cell infiltration in the anterior third of a rabbit cornea 10 hours after excimer laser PRK and treatment including hourly topical diclofenac sodium without a bandage contact lens or topical steroid. (From AF Phillips et al. Arachidonic acid metabolites after excimer laser corneal surgery. *Arch Ophthalmol* 111:1273–1278. Copyright 1993, American Medical Association.)

needed. Patients are told that they may not experience any significant pain, in which case it is not necessary to take the tablets, but if pain does occur, the tablets are available for use.

At present, some Canadian surgeons using the VISX excimer laser are the strongest proponents of this postoperative treatment modality. Additionally, many of these also advocate transepithelial laser ablation and "laser scrape" as the form of epithelial removal during the procedure. In laser scrape, the epithelium is first ablated to nearly its full thickness, and the remainder is then removed with a blunt spatula and sponge. They claim that both rapid and limited epithelial removal by the laser together with the minimal discomfort of a contact lens, topical corticosteroid, and nonsteroidal agent results in a more comfortable postoperative recovery with equally fast re-epithelialization compared to patching and topical antibiotics alone [6a].

The European Experience. In contrast to the frequent use of topical steroids and bandage contact lenses in North America, the European excimer laser surgeon has generally adopted an alternate method whereby topical steroid medication is not given until the epithelium has completely repopulated the corneal surface. Additionally, some immobilize the eye with a pressure patch until re-epithelialization has occurred, or at least for the first postoperative day. Not all investigators and surgeons in Europe adhere to this postoperative treatment modality, but it appears that a significant number of surgeons prefer this method. Typically, immediately following treatment, antibiotic ointment is placed into the operative eye with or without a cycloplegic agent. Often the eye is covered with a pressure patch, although in some cases only ointment without patching is used.

Many European surgeons believe that topical corticosteroids can impede re-epithelialization and avoid their use until the epithelium is intact. Some feel that patching further speeds the process by immobilizing the lid. The issue of postoperative pain and discomfort is less stringently addressed by this group. Although topical nonsteroidals are frequently used, the use of bandage soft contact lenses are discouraged because of their increased risk of infection and the possibility of delayed re-epithelialization [7]. When topical diclofenac sodium or ketorolac is used by European surgeons, it is often without the concurrent use of topical corticosteroids. Patients are told to remove their patch temporarily and apply the nonsteroidal agent up to every 4 hours during the first postoperative day.

Recently, use of topical tetracaine 0.1% has been tested in a prospective randomized clinical study of 100 patients in London [8]. It was shown to reduce post-PRK pain effectively when given in half-hourly doses for the first 2 days. Significant delay of corneal re-epithelialization and impaired clinical outcome was not observed when using tetracaine for this limited postoperative period. Although we do not personally advocate the use of topical tetracaine after PRK, due to epithelial toxicity and increased risk of undetected early infection, we should also note that topical nonsteroidals may be toxic to the epithelium, and recommendations have been made to use them no more frequently than every 4 hours and for no more than 2 or 3 consecutive days [6].

First Week

After the first postoperative night, the patient should be evaluated the next day and every other day until re-epithelialization is complete. This is important because early postoperative problems can occur in the de-epithelialized cornea that can be detected and appropriately managed before serious complications arise. Early postoperative inflammation, infection, or nonhealing conditions can be found in a significant number of patients, warranting close postoperative follow-up.

With regard to the use of soft contact lenses, some investigators suggest their discontinuation after the first day because most of the benefit of pain relief is achieved in the first 24 hours. This helps to minimize any risk of infection associated with contact lens use. Others advocate their use until re-epithelialization is complete.

Advocates of patching either limit patching to the first postoperative day or continue its use until re-epithelialization is complete, often depending on the needs and wishes of the patient. When using an ocular patch, removal and replacement by the patient is necessary several times a day when applying topical medication. Follow-up and careful instruction is necessary to ensure that the patient is properly performing these steps for adequate lid immobilization. Patients not using a patch or contact lens beyond the first postoperative day may experience some delay in re-epithelialization due to the movement of the lid over the cornea. This is why patching or contact lens use is often recommended until re-epithelialization is complete.

Typically, re-epithelialization following myopic PRK should take 3–5 days [9–11]. Any patient requiring 1 week or more for re-epithelialization to occur is subject to wound healing problems and may experience increased haze and regression during the later postoperative period. If delayed re-epithelialization occurs in any patient with a given postoperative management scheme, an alternate scheme or treatment should be employed.

As the epithelium resurfaces the cornea, epithelial adhesion complexes form to secure the multiple-cell layer to the corneal surface and its basement membrane. The cell layer progressively thickens over the first week, leaving the epithelium hyperplastic, with more than the usual number of cells [12]. The increased number of central epithelial cells gradually becomes more uniform in time, as the epithelium further stabilizes. The corneal epithelium, however, nearly always remains more hyperplastic centrally relative to the periphery, as can be verified during excimer laser retreatment procedures performed late in the postoperative period [13].

The re-epithelialized cornea provides a smooth surface on which corneal topography can be imaged and through which refraction can be performed. Although some feel that videokeratography performed after the first postoperative week may not yield any useful information, early detection of steep central islands, decentration, and baseline corneal shape before regression may warrant its use. Manifest autorefraction with visual acuity also can be performed at the first postoperative week; however, the reader should be aware that this is optional as it will not alter the postoperative management. Slit-lamp biomicroscopy verifies stabilization of the epithelial surface and allows for assessment of corneal haze.

Treatment following re-epithelialization has been recommended by most to include a topical corticosteroid medication, such as fluorometholone 0.1% or 0.25% [14, 15]. Use of a corticosteroid at least 4 times a day is believed to reduce postoperative inflammation, keratocyte activation, and stromal wound healing postoperatively.

Wound Healing Phase

First Month

Because of the variability of healing response between patients, wound healing modulation with the use of topical corticosteroids demonstrates some benefit to the overall refractive outcome of myopic patients receiving excimer laser PRK. By manipulating the postoperative treatment, refractive predictability at 1 year within < 1 D may improve by as much as 20% [16]. This makes careful postoperative management of excimer laser PRK nearly as important as the actual laser treatment itself.

For purposes of simplicity, the variability of corneal stromal wound healing after excimer PRK can be categorized into three major types: (1) normal wound healing, (2) inadequate wound healing, and (3) aggressive wound healing. These types are not meant to be rigidly defined, nor are they to be strictly enforced as categories by which the same eye or fellow eye must respond on subsequent treatments. Rather, they are arbitrarily defined based on the patient's refraction (deviation from intended correction) and return of best spectacle-corrected visual acuity (BSCVA) because these are the objective measures by which we quantify our outcome.

The criteria for each of the three types vary depending on the type of excimer laser used, the diameter of the ablation zone, and the level of preoperative myopia. All three parameters influence the amount of regression and refractive overshoot experienced during the early postoperative period. Even with this in mind, there is a general range of refractions at 1 month that define overcorrection and undercorrection and can be loosely correlated to wound-healing type. They are not meaningful, however, unless there is a return to preoperative BSCVA or a significant percentage return to preoperative BSCVA [Marc Odrich, personal communication, January 1996]. In general, patients who are corrected to their intended level or slightly overcorrected (plano to + 1.0 D) are considered *normal healers*. Those who are moderately or markedly overcorrected (> + 1.0 D) are considered *inadequate healers*. Finally, those who are undercorrected at 1 month postoperatively are considered *aggressive healers*.

At the 1-month postoperative visit, a corrected and uncorrected visual acuity, manifest refraction, tonometry, slit-lamp examination, and corneal topography should be performed. As mentioned above, the refraction has the greatest impact on decisions of postoperative management. These decisions, however, can only be made reliably if the BSCVA is no worse than 1 line from the preoperative reading. In cases of poor BSCVA, an attempt should be made to define the nature of the BSCVA loss rather than that of the refraction. Slit-lamp examination with assessment of corneal haze and corneal topography can also be helpful in determining the wound-healing response. In general, normal healers have trace to 1.0 grade corneal haze and minimal topographic change over the ensuing months. Patients treated with topical steroids, such as fluorometholone, may be tapered off the medication over the next several postoperative months. Further follow-up may be scheduled for the 3-month post-operative visit, at which time an even better assessment of healing type can be made. Plate 10 shows a patient with trace corneal haze at the 1-month postoperative visit, corresponding to normal wound healing.

In an inadequately healing cornea, the stroma is usually crystal clear or has trace haze at the first postoperative month. Topographically, there will be little or no change over the ensuing months, and in some cases the intraocular pressure may be elevated, as this group tends to have a higher number of corticosteroid responders [13]. Patients receiving topical steroids should discontinue or rapidly taper off their medication, and in some cases be fitted with a soft contact lens. The contact lens has been anecdotally reported to serve as a stimulant for further wound healing, and it can be used for temporary refractive improvement of overcorrection if necessary. Because these inadequately healing patients fall outside the realm of normal wound healing, they should return again in 1 month for a 2-month post-operative visit. Plate 11 shows the cornea of a patient with inadequate wound healing. Note the crystal clear cornea with an absence of any haze.

Aggressive corneal healing may look much like normal healing at the 1-month visit, revealing mild haze and refractive regression. This is because the aggressive phase of healing may be more evident at 2 or 3 months postoperatively, which warrants monthly follow-up in patients suspected of aggressive corneal wound healing. Conditions suggestive of this type of healing include corneal haze greater than trace, topographic regression, and an undercorrected refraction together with a BSCVA within 1 line of the preoperative value. Patients who may already be taking fluorometholone 0.1% can be switched to fluorometholone 0.25% (FML forte) or even dexamethasone 0.1% if a significant moderate haze of grade 2.0 is observed. The topical corticosteroids can be continued at 4 times daily and then slowly tapered over several months. Close follow-up is necessary to check for steroid responders as well as to monitor for early signs of myopic regression. An obvious example of aggressive healing at 1 month after excimer is shown in Plate 12. Here the cornea shows grade 2.0–3.0 stromal haze, demonstrating the need for more potent treatment of longer duration with topical steroids.

Although we have presented a way of titrating corneal wound healing with topical corticosteroids, some investigators may choose not to use corticosteroids at all during the postoperative period. Evidence from double-blind, randomized, prospective studies reveals that postoperative treatment with topical corticosteroids for 3 months does show a greater refractive effect at 3 months when compared to a placebo control [17], and a greater refractive effect and less corneal haze at 3 and 6 months when compared to no topical drops as a control [18]. In both studies, however, there was no statistically significant difference after 3 and 6 months, when the drops were discontinued. Although these results suggest that the long-range outcome may be no different whether topical steroids are used or not, the relatively small sample size, small ablation-zone diameters, and lack of titration of steroids all limit the potential impact that topical steroids can have in clinical practice.

Part of the reason for the difference in early outcome between these studies is the fact that the placebo drop used as a control in the first study [17] served as a wetting or lubricating agent, thus helping to minimize the wound-healing effect. Keeping the cornea moist and well lubricated during the postoperative period seems to have a beneficial effect in the prevention of corneal haze and regression. This is especially true in patients with dry-eye symptoms, often secondary to chronic contact lens wear. In a review of results with the VISX laser, patients with a decreased Schirmer's test had greater refractive variability and corneal haze than did patients with normal tear production [Stephen Trokel, personal communication, April 1995]. This stresses the importance of keeping the cornea moist with artificial tears or wetting drops, especially if topical corticosteroids are not used.

Whether topical corticosteroids will continue to play a role in the postoperative management of excimer laser PRK in the future is uncertain. At this point, they do appear to have a beneficial effect in wound healing modulation, and they still are used by the vast majority of surgeons. Although topical nonsteroidal anti-inflammatory agents and other medications have been used in an attempt to modulate corneal wound healing after excimer laser surgery, none has been proved to be effective in a clinical setting [19–22].

Subsequent Months

In the routine postoperative management of patients undergoing excimer laser PRK, those who are moderately overcorrected (inadequate healers) or undercorrected (aggressive healers) at 1 month should return for a 2-month visit. Patients with higher preoperative refractive error or BSCVA greater than 1 line from the preoperative reading also should return at this time because the true impact of their wound healing is yet unknown. Patients with a normal healing response following PRK for low myopia are safe to return 2 months later, for a 3-month visit. Patients returning at 2 months should also return at 3 months, followed by a visit at 6 months and 1 year. During these visits, as at 1 month, a corrected and uncorrected visual acuity, manifest refraction, tonometry, slit-lamp examination, and corneal topography should be performed. The classification of wound healing type assessed during the 1-month visit and the trend associated with this type can be verified by noting the refraction, topography, and level of haze at the 2- and 3-month points and at the 6-month visit.

Patients who are still significantly overcorrected at the 2- or 3-month visits should have their corticosteroids discontinued and, if it has not already been done, can be fitted with a bandage contact lens. The expectation for inadequate wound healers is for an increase in corneal haze to the level of trace (grade 0.5) or mild (grade 1.0) and a corresponding myopic shift in refraction. Usually, this therapy allows the inadequate healer to convert to a more normal healing response. Follow-up for the patient receiving a contact lens should be 1 week rather than 1 month and progressively longer thereafter.

Aggressive corneal wound healers who appear further under-corrected at the 2-month visit require continuation of their corticosteroid drops. A slowly tapering dosing schedule should be continued over the course of 3–4 months using fluorometholone 0.25%, with discontinuation prior to the 6-month visit. Patients still on corticosteroids at 3 months should be seen again at 4 months and, if necessary, at 5 months. The expectation for this healing type with the above therapy is a stabilization of the refraction between the 3- and 6-month visits and a decrease in corneal haze.

At the 6-month visit, stabilization of refraction should be achieved in most patients. Patients who are still significantly overcorrected, appreciably undercorrected, or who develop late corneal haze in a previously clear cornea should consider further management, as outlined under Management of Complications. Prior to excimer laser retreatment, a stable refraction should be recorded over a 3-month period [24]. If stabilization is not achieved, retreatment should be postponed, and reinstitution of topical corticosteroids can be considered. The effect of late reinstitution of topical steroids for undercorrection is further outlined in the complications section.

Management of Complications

Intraoperative Complications

Although many mistakes and errors can be made during excimer laser PRK, there are only three major intraoperative complications that bear significance and have been experienced clinically: (1) eccentric ablation, (2) inadequate or prolonged epithelial removal, and (3) laser system malfunction. When these problems occur intraoperatively, they may not be noticed or appreciated by the surgeon until their consequences are observed postoperatively.

Eccentric Ablation

Proper corneal centration of a refractive surgical procedure along the line of sight is extremely important in producing a regular and symmetric change in corneal curvature. This is just as important in excimer laser PRK as it is in other refractive procedures, and errors may occur for two major reasons: (1) decentered alignment and (2) patient or eye movement.

Decentered Alignment. The line of sight or corneal intercept of the visual axis is an impossible point to locate and has generated some controversy regarding the best method for centering refractive surgical procedures. At least when performing excimer laser PRK, most refractive surgeons agree that the optical zone should be defined around the center of the entrance pupil [25]. For most commercially available excimer lasers this is easily achieved by alignment of two or three HeNe laser spots on the cornea or underlying pupil margin. An optical reticle used by the VISX system achieves centration by aligning concentric rings around the pupillary center. Whatever the method of alignment by the surgeon, the patient plays an equally important role in maintaining fixation on a coaxial light source within the laser delivery system (light filament, light-emitting diode [LED], or laser). This fixation should be maintained not only during initial alignment but also throughout the procedure. Carefully patching the patient's nonoperative eye helps to prevent distraction or loss of fixation.

The use of pilocarpine during the procedure may introduce the possibility of nonconcentric constriction of the pupil. Although this phenomenon has been observed, especially in high myopes, it is usually of insignificant magnitude when only mild miosis is targeted. We recommend only 1 or 2 drops of pilocarpine 1%.

Patient or Eye Movement. Once proper alignment has been achieved, it must be maintained throughout the procedure. This is primarily the responsibility of the surgeon. Recently, active and passive tracking systems have been implemented in some systems to maintain the alignment initially established by the surgeon. Passive tracking locks in on the alignment of a high-contrast interface, such as the limbus, and automatically stops subsequent pulsing of the laser when the eye moves outside an established tolerance level, usually approximately 500 μm. It then resumes treatment when the eye comes back into alignment without the surgeon needing to take his or her foot off the foot switch. Active tracking goes beyond this by allowing the beam to follow subtle eye movements, maintaining ablation even with horizontal eye movements. The surgeon must observe gross eye movements, however, because loss of patient fixation may allow ablation within the pupillary axis, not along the line of sight but with the beam oblique to the normal surface.

For excimer lasers without a tracking system, maintenance of fixation and centration can be sufficiently approximated, but this is generally true only of wide field–ablating lasers. The surgeon must maintain the alignment around the pupil and be trained to interrupt the procedure as soon as he or she recognizes a systematic or abrupt movement of the treated eye. Small irregular movements can be tolerated. If the surgeon must interrupt the procedure, the patient can be asked to refixate on the fixation light source, and the procedure can be continued at the point where the surgeon stopped.

Anecdotal reports have been made of anxious patients suddenly looking away from the fixation light and the surgeon continuing the treatment for several seconds. In these patients, an eccentric ablation resulting in irregular astigmatism has been observed, and increased symptoms of glare are reported [26]. In one prospective study with the Summit laser (Waltham, MA), 1 of 120 patients "moved bodily slightly down the operating table during the treatment." This ablation was eccentric by approximately 1 mm and resulted in 1–2 D of astigmatism with an asymmetric halo effect [26]. The actual incidence of optical zone decentrations and their postoperative management are discussed under Postoperative Optical Complications.

Inadequate or Prolonged Epithelial Removal

Inadequate epithelial removal may occur when an overly small or decentered area of epithelium is marked and debrided. Because an excessively large area of epithelial debridement is discouraged, most surgeons remove a zone of epithelium approximately 1 mm larger than the ablation zone diameter. Epithelial removal can also be inadequate when small cell remnants adhere to Bowman's layer and remain undetected by the surgeon. This can be particularly true of contact lens wearers, where the epithelium adheres more strongly to Bowman's layer. Coaxial illumination is usually sufficient to detect these tiny islands of epithelium, but dim illumination used to minimize patient discomfort may lead to overlooked fragments. Before starting laser treatment, the illumination should be momentarily brightened to check the corneal stromal surface. If tiny islands remain during photoablation, the irregularity will be reproduced in the corneal stroma, resulting in irregular astigmatism. Although there have been no reports of excimer PRK being performed with incomplete epithelial removal, patients with localized paracentral areas of undercorrection that were likely due to incomplete epithelial removal have been observed [13].

Prolonged epithelial removal may also be a problem during excimer laser PRK because localized stromal hydration changes can occur in segmentally de-epithelialized cornea and under the influence of the microscope light. Stromal hydration plays an important role in the ablation rate of corneal tissue, with areas of relative dehydration showing more stromal tissue removal than hydrated areas [27]. Nitrogen gas blowing performed during early ablations with the VISX excimer laser demonstrated increased corneal haze and surface roughness due to excessive corneal drying [28–32]. Although nitrogen gas blowing is no longer performed, prolonged epithelial removal with corneal drying under the microscope light can result in poorer, less predictable results. Some surgeons prefer carefully removing the epithelium, hydrating the surface with cool balanced salt solution and then lightly drying the surface with a cellulose sponge. When this practice is performed repeatedly in the same fashion, it seems to produce good results. Equally good is the rapid technique of debridement or laser ablated de-epithelialization because this maintains the hydration level of the native corneal stroma. Some Canadian surgeons prefer transepithelial laser ablation with a PTK algorithm followed immediately by myopic PRK of the underlying stroma. This seems to be a regional preference, with most PRK surgeons in the rest of the world preferring manual epithelial debridement. A final alternative for removing the corneal epithelium is use of a rotating plastic brush [33]. This motorized brush completely removes the zone of corneal epithelium within 3 seconds and produces a microscopically smoother surface than does the rounded blade or spatula technique.

Laser System Malfunction

The hardware and software reliability of a given commercially available excimer laser system in large part depends on the reputation and reliability of the manufacturer producing the laser. Hardware and software malfunctions can occur unexpectedly, but should they occur as a systematic error in multiple systems or multiple times in the same system, the laser manufacturer may be doing a substandard job in troubleshooting and servicing its system. This is why preoperative calibration and testing of the laser is so important. What if, after preparing and training the patient, removing the epithelium, and cleaning the surface, the laser shuts down due to an electrical or software problem, or simply does not test properly because of low energy output? It may require an additional 5 minutes or more to reestablish a working laser system. If this is the case, it may be best to postpone the laser treatment due to the excessive time of corneal de-epithelialization with resultant hydration changes. Should a system malfunction occur during the laser treatment, however, every attempt should be made to correct the problem as quickly as possible and complete the laser treatment.

Preoperative gas filling, energy calibration, homogeneity checking, and even a refractive check in polymethylmethacrylate (PMMA) plastic has been established to ensure that the laser system is fully functional for clinical PRK surgery. Checking the laser terminal display to verify the programming and ablation parameters is important to ensure that the correct optical zone and attempted refractive correction is selected. Periodic maintenance checking of cavity alignment and degradation of the optics is necessary to ensure the energy and homogeneity of the beam is upheld. An error in any one of these parameters could lead to a dramatic shift in results. An example of a laser system error leading to an undercorrection in five consecutive patients was reported by Sher et al. [34]. They report a defect in the energy measuring device associated with the Taunton/VISX laser (now no longer available) that led to a 30–35% lower fluence with subsequent undercorrection. Other anecdotal reports of laser system malfunction have been made, and they illustrate the continual need for system checking and awareness by the surgeon of the functional status of the laser [35].

Postoperative Optical Complications

Night Glare and Halos

A significant concern when reshaping an optically transparent cornea is creation of distortions of vision in the form of glare and halos. Intuitively, it might seem that corneal haze or scarring would be the major contributor to this symptom, but clinical experience has shown this not to be the case. The major contributor to symptoms of glare and halos is the effective spherical aberration of the centrally flattened cornea [36]; in other words, the deviation of spherical corneal shape within the effective optical zone, which results in degradation of the retinal image. Although other conditions, such as decentration and steep central islands, can contribute to this phenomenon, the main reason for glare and halos is an effectively small ablation zone diameter. Table 5-1 illustrates the reported incidence of night glare and halos for various ablation zone diameters and clinical investigators [9, 13, 32, 37–43]. As shown in Table 5-1, a 6-mm ablation zone diameter sufficiently minimizes halos and glare and, when present, these symptoms tend to resolve with time [9, 38, 41]. A higher myopic correction is associated with a higher percentage of halos and glare when using a small-diameter ablation zone [41]. Significant night-driving

Table 5-1. Incidence of night glare and halos after excimer PRK

Reference	Optical zone	Attempted correction	Postoperative examination	Night glare and halos	Significant night driving limitation
Seiler et al. [9]	3.5–5.0 mm	−1.4 to −7.25 D	3 mo	72% (184/255)	N/A
			6 mo	48% (65/136)	3% (4/136)
			9 mo	34% (18/53)	0%
Gartry et al. [37]	4.0 mm	−2.0 to −7.0 D	early mo	78% (94/120)	N/A
			1 yr	N/A	10% (12/94)
Tengroth et al. [38]	4.3 or 4.5 mm	−1.25 to −7.5 D	3 mo	82% (344/420)	N/A
			6 mo	44% (185/420)	
			1 yr	26% (109/420)	0%
Gimbel et al. [39]	4.5 or 5.0 mm	−4.0 ± 0.8 D	variable	50% (21/42)	12% (5/42)
Kim et al. [40]	5.0 mm	−2.0 to −7.0	6 mo	45% (91/202)	N/A
			1 yr	10% (20/202)	
Seiler et al. [41]	5.0 mm	−1.25 to −3.0	1 yr	16.7% (7/42)	N/A
		−3.1 to −6.0		36.5% (31/85)	
		−6.1 to −9.0		59% (10/17)	
		−9.1 and up		71.4% (5/7)	
		Total		35% (53/151)	0.7% (1/151)
O'Brart et al. [42]	5.0 mm	−3.0 and −6.0 D	6 mo	52.5% (21/40)	17.5% (7/40)
	6.0 mm			27.5% (11/40)	0%
Dello Russo et al. [43]	5.0 mm	N/A	6 mo	37.5% (59/157)	3.2 (5/157)
	5.5 mm			5.5% (6/109)	1.8% (2/109)
	6.0 mm			0% (0/128)	0%
Maguen et al. [32]	4.0 mm	N/A	N/A	75–80%	N/A
	4.5 mm			35–40%	
	5.0 mm			20%	
	6.0 mm			< 5%	
	7.0 mm			0.5%	
Seiler et al. [13]	6.0 mm	N/A	1 yr	< 1%	N/A

N/A = not available.

limitations do occur with smaller ablation zones [9, 37, 39, 41, 42], but so far this symptom has not been reported with ablation zones of 6 mm or more. Often, glare and halos disappear once the second eye is treated.

Glare and halo symptoms typically become worse at night, when the pupil dilates, and more peripheral light rays enter the eye from the untreated or peripheral transition zone. Roberts and Koester [44] have shown this relationship in ray tracing diagrams and conclude that the optical zone diameter must be at least as large as the entrance pupil diameter to prevent foveal glare and larger than the entrance pupil to prevent parafoveal glare (Fig. 5-3). An example of parafoveal glare in the form of a ghost image is seen in Fig. 5-4. Here the "ghost goose" image was photographed paracentrally using a modified camera simulating the effect of an ablation zone smaller than or equal to the pupil diameter. Although most investigators believe that a 6-mm ablation zone diameter is the clinical standard, some advocate using a 7-mm zone, stating that it is sufficiently large for even 9- or 10-mm pupil dilation in dim light [32]. Measurement of the pupillary diameter in both bright and dim light is suggested for all patients. Patients with very wide pupils should be advised preoperatively of this possible complication and be treated with an ablation zone diameter that is sufficiently wide.

Management. Management of symptoms of glare and halos from a sufficiently small effective optical zone (< 5.5 mm) should include excimer laser retreatment with transepithelial ablation. A phototherapeutic keratectomy (PTK) profile of 6.5 mm or larger should be used and the ablation continued until a midperipheral breakthrough of the epithelium is detected by a decrease in fluorescence (Plates 13

Fig. 5-3. Ray tracing diagram of an excimer laser treated eye demonstrating foveal glare (**A**) and parafoveal glare (**B**), when pupillary diameter is larger than ablation zone diameter. (From RR Krueger, P Binder, PJ McDonnell, The Effects of Excimer Laser Photoablation of the Cornea. In JJ Salz [ed], *Corneal Laser Surgery.* St. Louis: Mosby–Year Book, 1995.)

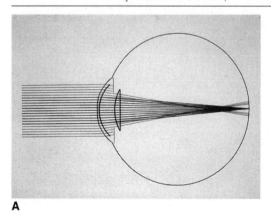
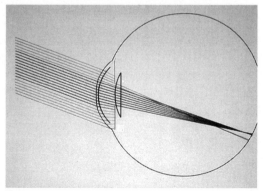

A   B

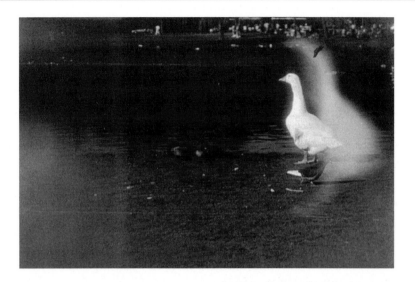

Fig. 5-4. Photographic example of parafoveal glare, as seen by a ghost image of a goose captured using a modified camera simulating the effect of an eye treated with a smaller ablation zone diameter than that of the pupillary diameter. (From RR Krueger, P Binder, PJ McDonnell, The Effects of Excimer Laser Photoablation on the Cornea. In JJ Salz [ed], *Corneal Laser Surgery.* St. Louis: Mosby–Year Book, 1995. P. 37.)

and 14). A similarly sized PRK should then be performed with the desired refractive change plus an additional −1.0 D depending on the system. This is done to compensate for the remaining hyperplastic epithelium centrally, which makes performing the PTK alone similar to performing a hyperopic PRK of 1.0 D.

Refractive Instability and Regression

Two types of refractive instability are of concern after refractive surgery: short-term instabilities (diurnal fluctuations) and long-term instabilities (regression or progression). Although a common complaint after radial keratotomy (RK), diurnal fluctuations do not appear to occur often after excimer laser PRK. One report in a very large series noted 10 patients who complained of diurnal fluctuations up to 6 months following PRK [45]. In this series, refractive shift toward myopia over the course of the day, as seen with RK, was not observed in any patient. There was, however, a diurnal shift toward hyperopia of + 0.3 D +/− 0.3 D, but this was not significantly different from a control group of 10 volunteer eyes. One possible explanation for this subtle, insignificant shift is accommodation, which decreases over the course of the day. This finding is in contrast to the diurnal myopic shift noted after RK, in which undercorrected patients see better in the morning than in the evening because of additional corneal flattening in the morning from eyelid compression while sleeping [46].

Long-term instability of refraction is a more significant complication after myopic PRK, but before refractive stability can be addressed postsurgically, it is important to note the variability of refraction measurements in normal control eyes. In the Prospective Evaluation of Radial Keratotomy (PERK) study, 156 patients had surgery in only one eye and were examined both preoperatively and 1 year postoperatively in the control eye under standardized conditions and by the same clinical examiner [47]. In this series, a change in refraction was noted of only 0.25 D or less in 44% and 0.5 D to 0.89 D in 56% of eyes, with no patient changing 1.0 D [47]. Others have recommended a variation of 1.0 D as the cutoff for stability of refraction [48]. With this in mind, progressive hyperopia after excimer PRK is considered a rare finding: it has been reported in only one patient [49] and anecdotally found in several others [Alan Spiegelmann, personal communication, 1992].

Myopic refractive regression, however, is a frequently seen finding within the first year after myopic PRK, and the amount of early regression depends on both the targeted attempted correction and the ablation zone diameter. With regard to ablation zone diameter, the smaller-sized zones of the early Summit laser led to a greater hyperopic overshoot with greater regression than the larger-sized VISX zones. This finding of early regression as well as decreased predictability of effect in relation to smaller ablation zone diameter was recently demonstrated in a prospective study of 5-mm and 6-mm ablations with the Summit laser [42, 50]. The 6-mm treatment group had less overshoot, less regression, and a smaller standard deviation around the targeted correction than both the 5-mm group and a 5-mm group with an additional 1-mm transition zone [50]. Patients with higher myopic refractive error and undergoing excimer laser PRK have a higher level of regression and decreased predictability as well [23, 31, 51–53]. In a study of excimer laser PRK for severe myopia, four patients with refractive error greater than −12.0 D had greater than 8.0 D of regression within 6 months after treatment [31]. One patient with PRK for −17.0 D of myopia had such severe regression that her refraction at 6 months was more myopic than it had been preoperatively. Plates 15 and 16 show the effect of this dramatic regression topographically. In these four patients, however, nitrogen gas blowing was used during the procedure and was believed to contribute to the regression of effect.

With regard to regression within the first 6 months or 1 year after PRK, nomograms have been established to predict the point of stability of refraction, and during this initial period the refractive outcome is more a matter of predictability. True long-term refractive stability

Table 5-2. Change in refraction between 1 and 2 years after excimer PRK

Myopia group	Refractive correction	Number of eyes	Optical zone	Change in manifest refraction during yr 2	% of eyes regressed 1.0 D during yr 2
Low	−1.25 to −3.0 D	35	5.0 mm	−0.03 ± 0.43 D	0%
Medium	−3.1 to −6.0 D	67	5.0 mm	−0.29 ± 0.59 D	8.6%
Moderate	−6.1 to −9.0 D	20	4.5–5.0 mm	−0.48 ± 0.64 D	20%
High	−9.1 D and up	4	4.5 mm	−2.63 ± 1.68 D	100%

Source: T Seiler, H Schmidt-Petersen, J Wollensak. Complications after Myopic Photorefractive Keratectomy, Primarily with the Summit Excimer Laser. In JJ Salz (ed.). *Corneal Laser Surgery.* St. Louis: Mosby, 1995.

should be evaluated between the first and second year and beyond. In Table 5-2, a summary of the change in refraction during the second year after PRK is recorded. Statistically significant differences in refraction between 1 and 2 years occur in patients with more than −6.0 D of correction (p < .02). The lack of stability in refraction for the higher myopic patients in the above series is in part due to the smaller ablation zone diameter [41].

Refractive Unpredictability

It is difficult to choose a standard for refraction above or below which a given procedure is considered to fall out of the range of predictability. Although many consider a standard for accuracy to be within 1.0 D of the targeted correction, this may be too rigid for higher myopic corrections, and yet for lower levels of myopia, 0.50 D may be appropriate. To keep things simple, we consider an unpredictable result one that falls outside of the range of 1.0 D of the intended outcome at 1 year after the procedure. Although any point between 6 months and 1 year could be considered, we have defined stability as a change between 1 year and 2 years, and so it seems appropriate that predictability should be reported at 1 year.

Overcorrection. For the myopic patient, overcorrection can be a symptomatically disturbing outcome, especially if the patient is presbyopic or nearly presbyopic and the overcorrection is more than + 1.00 D. For this patient, overcorrection might be experienced as a real complication that requires some sort of intervention.

Frequently, overcorrection results in patients with a minimal healing reaction after PRK, and many of them are also corticosteroid responders [54]. Usually at 1 month after the procedure, about 10% of eyes show some sign of overcorrection, with a perfectly clear cornea (no evidence of any haze) and an intraocular pressure (IOP) elevated by 5–10 mm Hg compared to the preoperative level. For these patients, we suggest immediate cessation of corticosteroids, which may allow some regression over the ensuing months. The incidence of overcorrection at 1 year is reported in Table 5-3 [55–58]. As expected, this finding is more frequent in patients with higher refractive correction and may be associated with other machine-related factors, such as optical zone size.

MANAGEMENT. For a patient who remains symptomatically overcorrected at 6 months to 1 year following surgery, epithelial debridement can be performed with no postoperative corticosteroid medication. A corneal healing response may be elicited with subsequent regression of effect of 1.0–3.0 D in the following months. Follow-up visits should be continued at monthly intervals until stabilization is achieved. In cases that do not respond, simple PTK through the hyperplastic epithelium can be performed in patients treated with a 5-mm optical zone primarily. Holmium laser thermokeratoplasty can be also considered because it stimulates corneal wound healing in addition to correcting hyperopia. Finally, hyperopic PRK, available in most systems, can be employed.

Undercorrection. Although the undercorrected patient may be accustomed to being myopic and may have some improvement of vision, a less than ideal result may be very disappointing. In contrast to overcorrection, undercorrection may be due to a more aggressive healing reaction, with early refractive regression and corneal haze formation. A patient who is undercorrected at 1 month postoperatively should continue corticosteroid medication in a slowly tapering dose for at least a 4-month period.

If the patient has further regression during this time and remains symptomatically undercorrected at 6 months or more, topical corticosteroid medication can be restarted in an attempt to elicit a reversal of myopic regression [59–61]. Topographic flattening with refractive improvement of 1–2 D can be seen several days after reinstituting corticosteroids, but this effect is sometimes lost after the medication is discontinued. The flattening effect with topical steroids occurs presumably by a reduction of hyaluronic acid (glycosaminoglycan) production by keratocytes, which decreases the water content of and thins the cornea. This is in contrast to the decrease in consumption of glycosaminoglycans in the trabecular meshwork by endothelial cells when using corticosteroids [62]. This phenomenon increases the trabecular meshwork outflow resistance with increasing IOP in patients who are steroid responders [63].

The incidence of undercorrection can be best assessed when early regression tends to stabilize at 6 months to 1 year postoperatively (the 1-year incidence is shown in Table 5-3) [55–58]. As with overcorrections, undercorrections of greater than −1.0 D are more frequently seen in higher myopic corrections. The difference between

Table 5-3. Overcorrection, undercorrection, and induced astigmatism 1 year following excimer PRK

Reference	Number of eyes	Refraction	Optical zone	Overcorrection	Induced undercorrection	Astigmatism
Maguen et al. [55]*	67	−1.0 to −3.5 D	5.5 mm	0	7.5%	9%
	81	−3.6 to −6.0 D	5.0 mm	2.5%	25.9%	
Seiler et al. [56]	42	−1.25 to −3.0 D	5.0 mm	0	2.4%	2%
	85	−3.1 to −6.0 D	5.0 mm	3.5%	4.7%	
	27	−6.1 to −9.0 D	4.5–5.0 mm	3.7%	52.5%	
Talley et al. [57]	23	−1.0 to −3.0 D	6.0–7.0 mm	0	0	N/A
	58	−3.1 to −6.0 D		1.7%	6.9%	
	4	−6.1 to −8.0 D		25.0%	25.0%	
Piebenga et al. [58]*	25	−1.25 to −3.0 D	5.0 mm	0	12.0%	1.6%
	45	−3.1 to −6.25 D		0	46.6%	

*Nitrogen gas blowing used during some or all procedures.

studies in the percentage of patients with undercorrection may be in part due to different laser algorithms during treatment, attempted corrections not aiming toward emmetropia, or environmental conditions, such as nitrogen gas blowing [30, 55, 58].

MANAGEMENT. Undercorrected eyes can be retreated with the excimer laser with good results. In a series of 30 undercorrected eyes treated with the Summit laser in Berlin, two-thirds of the patients were successfully retreated with refractions within 1.0 D of emmetropia at 6 months after retreatment [24]. During retreatment, transepithelial laser ablation is performed using a PTK pattern until an outer ring of decreased fluorescence is seen, signifying breakthrough of the epithelium. Because the epithelium is thicker centrally than paracentrally, further treatment with PRK must compensate for the residual remaining epithelium by adding a small value to the targeted retreatment correction. This is especially seen with ablation zone diameters smaller than 6 mm. The follow-up of repeat PRK should include fluorometholone 0.25% 4 times daily in a tapering dose over 4 months, with monthly visits until stabilization is achieved.

Induced Astigmatism. The induction of regular or irregular astigmatism after excimer laser PRK is an infrequent complication, but it can occur as a result of decentration, irregular ablation, or systematic errors in the laser system. The induction of more than 1.0 D of astigmatism is outlined in Table 5-3 [55, 58]. For most investigational series, this number is small. The reason for the higher percentage reported by Maguen et al. [55] (see Table 5-3) is the contribution of nitrogen gas blowing to an irregular ablation.

A more sensitive measurement of induced astigmatism would be an increase of more than 0.5 D. This level of induced astigmatism was reported by Seiler et al. [41, 56] in only 5.6% (10/178) of prospectively treated myopic eyes at 1 year and in 1.7% (3/178) at 2 years. In contrast, an equivalent reduction of preoperative cylinder was reported in 1.1% (2/178) at 1 year.

MANAGEMENT. Although infrequent, induced regular astigmatism or even unchanged preoperative astigmatism can be retreated with astigmatic excimer PRK if it is associated with myopia. If astigmatism alone exists, arcuate incisional keratotomy can be performed peripheral to the ablation zone.

Decentration

As mentioned earlier, decentration of the ablation zone can occur as a result of poor alignment with the patient's fixation or eye movement during the procedure. Postoperatively, this can be detected by a decentered zone of flattening on corneal topography and, if significant, by symptoms of monocular diplopia, glare, or halos. For ablation zone diameters up to 5 or 6 mm, clinically significant decentration appears to be associated with a displacement greater than 1 mm of the geometric center of the zone of flattening from the central point of fixation on videokeratography (Plate 17). This fact serves to introduce the importance of videokeratography in assessing postoperative findings of excimer laser PRK. Whenever a patient complains of symptoms of monocular diplopia, glare, halos, or decreased vision after any refractive procedure, videokeratography is essential to further management.

The incidence of decentration of the ablation zone is outlined in Table 5-4 [37, 51, 55, 56, 64, 65]. Usually only 1 or 2 cases of decentration greater than 1 mm are reported in a series, and the incidence is typically less than 1% [37, 56, 65]. When decentration greater than 1 mm is found in more than 1–2%, some concern may arise regarding the techniques of PRK employed. In a study by Maguen et al. [65], more decentration was observed when a suction ring was used to stabilize the eye than when patient fixation was used, but this was not found to be statistically significant due to small sample size. Also in this study, nitrogen gas blowing was used in some patients, perhaps contributing to the decentration. In a study by Schwartz-Goldstein et al. [65] of topographic centration analysis, decentration greater than 1 mm was significantly associated with higher attempted correction, presumably due to increased lasing time. Other factors, such as surgeon skill, may also play a role, contributing to the wide range of percentages reported in Table 5-4.

The clinical impact of decentration (see Table 5-4) is the presence of a higher grade of halos and glare in the opposite direction of the decentration, altered night driving, loss of uncorrected and best corrected visual acuity under glare conditions, and irregular astigmatism. In the series in Berlin [41, 56], two patients decentered greater than 1 mm had increased refractive astigmatism of 1.25–1.5 D at 1 year, which decreased to 1.0 D with associated myopia at 2 years. In contrast, 23% of treated eyes had a decentration between 0.5 and 1.0 mm with no impact on best corrected visual acuity or refractive astigmatism.

MANAGEMENT. When residual myopia exists, symptomatic decentrations of 1 mm or more can best be managed by excimer laser retreatment. The best strategy for such a retreatment would be to intentionally decenter an equal-sized ablation zone by an equal amount but opposite to the original decentration. The corneal topographic map should be carefully evaluated to determine both the amount of reablation (determined from the topographic undercorrection at the center of the pupil) as well as the distance and direction of eccentric reablation. The corneal epithelium should then be marked, and an excimer PTK performed until the peripheral zone of epithelial

Table 5-4. Incidence and impact of excimer ablation zone decentration

Reference	Optical zone	Attempted correction	Decentration > 1 mm	Decentration > 1.5 mm	Clinical symptoms
Garty et al. [37]	4 mm	−1.5 to −7.0 D	0.8% (1/120)	0%	Large inferior halo affecting night driving
Brancato et al. [51]	3.5–5.0 mm	−0.8 to −25.0 D	10.6% (117/1165)	N/A	Some irregular astigmatism and lost visual acuity
Seiler et al. [56]	4.5–5.0 mm	−1.25 to > −9.0 D	0.7% (2/281)	0%	Loss of best corrected vision under glare conditions
Schwartz-Goldstein et al. [64]	4.6–5.0 mm	−1.5 to −6.0 D	2.9% (5/173)[a]	0%	High-grade halos and glare; worse uncorrected acuity
Maguen et al. [55]	5.0–5.5 mm	−1.0 to −7.75 D	24.1% (7/29)[b]	13.8% (4/29)[b]	N/A
			4.8% (1/21)		
Lin et al. [65]	5.0–6.0 mm	−1.0 to −24.0 D	0.4% (2/502)	0.2%	N/A

[a]Worse decentration was correlated with higher attempted correction.
[b]Eyes were stabilized with a suction ring rather than patient fixation.

breakthrough (decreased fluorescence) is adequately visualized (Plate 18). The PRK can then be performed while the patient maintains fixation. This procedure may leave some residual regular astigmatism, but the asymmetric halos and undercorrection are improved significantly.

Steep Central Islands

In addition to decentration of the ablation zone, other topographic abnormalities have been observed following excimer PRK. Lin et al. [65] described four topographic patterns: (1) a uniform circular ablation, (2) a central island of topographic steepening in the ablation zone, (3) a keyhole of central steepening, and (4) a semicircular ablative pattern. The first and fourth patterns describe normal centration and decentration, respectively. The keyhole pattern is likely a variant of the steep central island, which, along with decentration, is the most significant pattern because of its associated symptoms. A steep central island is an area of topographic steepening ranging from 1–3 mm in diameter and from 1.0–3.0 D or more in height relative to the surrounding zone of corneal flattening. It can be seen immediately following PRK [66] and tends to reduce in magnitude over time (Plate 19). The symptoms associated with steep central islands are monocular diplopia, ghosting of images, and loss of best corrected visual acuity. These symptoms are typically reported in the first few postoperative months, and often resolve as the steep central island dissipates [65, 67].

The incidence of steep central islands is highly variable, mostly depending on the definition of size and power of the steep central island, type of laser, level of stromal hydration, ablation zone diameter, postoperative time of evaluation, and the type of corneal topography system used. Table 5-5 shows the incidence of steep central islands at several different time points following excimer PRK for various laser systems, steep central island criteria, ablation zone diameters, and topography systems [55, 57, 66–70]. In general, with the larger ablation zone diameters, the incidence of steep central islands at 1 month is greater than 50% and at 3 months is approximately 20%.

Early studies indicated that steep central islands were found mostly in the VISX 20/20 excimer laser system, and not in the Summit ExciMed UV-200. This was believed to be due to the larger diameter of the ablation zone of the VISX system, as well as the "top hat" beam profile of the VISX system, as compared to the gaussian profile of the Summit system. Some investigators thought that steep central islands were not a problem with the Summit system [69]. However, in a study of steep central island formation with use of the Schwind

Table 5-5. Incidence of steep central islands after excimer PRK

Reference	Laser	Optical zone	Criteria	Videokeratograph	Postoperative examination	Steep central islands
Parker et al. [68]	Taunton/VISX (Santa Clara, CA) VISX	N/A	1 mm, 1.0 D	Computed Anatomy (TMS-1) (New York, NY)	3 and 6 mo	29% (43/150)
Hersh et al. [69]	Summit (Waltham, MA)	4.5–5.0 mm	1 mm, 1.0 D	EyeSys (Houston, TX)	3 mo	27% (6/22)
						0% (0/112)
					1 yr	0% (0/181)
Maguen et al. [55]	VISX	5.0–5.5 mm	3 mm, 3 D	Computed Anatomy	3 mo	5% (12/240)
					6 mo	1.2% (3/240)
Lin et al. [65]	VISX	5.0–6.0 mm	2.5 mm, 1.5 D	Computed Anatomy (TMS)	1 mo	26% (131/502)
					3 mo	18% (58/322)
					6 mo	8% (16/203)
					1 yr	2% (2/92)
Talley et al. [57]	Taunton/VISX	6.0–7.0 mm	1 mm, 1 D	Computed Anatomy (TMS)	3 mo	15% (14/91)
					6 mo	3% (3/91)
					1 yr	2% (2/91)
Krueger et al. [67]	VISX	6.0 mm	1.5 mm, 3.0 D	Computed Anatomy (TMS)	1 wk	71% (25/35)
					1 mo	51% (18/35)
					3 mo	20% (7/35)
					6 mo	11% (4/35)
				Excluding nitrogen gas blowing	1 wk	88% (22/25)
					1 mo	64% (16/25)
					3 mo	24% (6/25)
					6 mo	16% (4/25)
Schmidt-Petersen et al. [70]	Summit and Schwind (Kleinostheim, Germany)	6.0 mm	3 mm, 3.0 D	EyeSys	1 mo	35% (22/62)
				Technomed (Baesweiler, Germany)	1 mo	81% (50/62)

Keratom I (Kleinostheim, Germany) as well as the Summit OmniMed laser, both using ablation zone diameters of at least 6.0 mm, an incidence of 81% (50/62) was found in the first postoperative month [70]. This incidence was further divided according to preoperative refraction, with steep central islands being seen in 55% (< −3 D), 89% (−3 to −6 D), and 100% (> −6 D). This incidence was noted with the Technomed C-scan topography unit (Baesweiler, Germany), whereas the EyeSys topography unit (Houston, TX) found an overall incidence with both laser systems of only 35% (22/62) in the first month [70]. This is not to say that somehow the Summit and Schwind laser systems have a higher incidence of steep central islands; rather, these islands are present to a similar degree following treatment with all wide-field excimer laser systems but vary in presentation based on the corneal topography system used.

The theories of steep central island formation include (1) the vortex plume theory, (2) the epithelial thickening theory, (3) the optics/homogeneity theory, and (4) the stress wave/fluid theory [67]. The fact that nitrogen gas blowing, although not recommended, actually reduces the incidence of steep central islands suggests that theories 2 and 3 do not play a significant role in the formation of islands [67]. Also, steep central islands have been seen immediately following ablation, before the epithelium can play a role [66]. The vortex plume theory was first proposed when steep central islands began to be noticed in association with the discontinuation of nitrogen gas blowing [68]. The gas blowing was thought to remove the vortex plume from the surface, and when gas blowing was discontinued, the vortex plume remained and attenuated the central beam, creating a steep central island. Although this theory is plausible, the most likely theory contributing to steep central island formation is the stress wave/fluid theory, which assumes that stress waves generated with large-area ablation result in central fluid accumulation, which attenuates the amount of stromal tissue ablated centrally. Jeffrey Machat [32] has shown the impact of the accumulation of this central fluid by comparing the incidence of steep central islands under regular conditions with those of a "stall-and-wipe" pattern of treatment, where fluid is wiped clear with a blunt spatula or cellulose sponge every few seconds intraoperatively and allowed to evaporate. The incidence of islands decreased from 16.7% under regular conditions to 10.3% with the stall-and-wipe method.

Although steep central islands are a frequent problem with wide-field ablating lasers, they are nearly unknown with scanning slit and flying spot lasers. Also, the symptomatic complaints experienced by some are rarely permanent. Steep central islands tend to resolve with time, and only a small percentage persist beyond 1 year. Recently, we have observed a 2.0-mm central iron ring at 1 year following PRK, indicating the presence of a persistent steep central island. A persistent steep central island is unlikely to undergo any further resolution and often, when symptomatic, will require retreatment.

Management. The management of steep central islands is first a matter of prevention. Several strategies currently exist to prevent or minimize the formation of steep central islands. VISX excimer laser users are currently employing a new central island factor (CIF) software program (version 2.92). The software program implements a simultaneous addition of 1.5 μm/D of tissue removal within the central 2.5-mm optical zone. In contrast, the Schwind laser routinely employs a central overcorrection of 80% using its aspheric software. Both strategies have effectively reduced the incidence of steep central islands.

When steep central islands do occur and persist beyond 6 months or 1 year, they can be managed by excimer laser retreatment. A 7.0-mm transepithelial PTK ablation is performed until a central and far peripheral breakthrough of the epithelium is noted by a decrease in fluorescence (Plates 20 and 21). A 6.5-mm myopic PRK set at the pre-retreatment level of myopia can then be performed on the central bare stroma and small residual midperipheral epithelium. This retreatment not only significantly reduces the magnitude of the central island but also eliminates any residual myopia associated with steep central island formation.

Postoperative Medical Complications

The medical complications of excimer laser PRK include not only complications purely related to the laser's effect on the cornea itself but also complications related to the postoperative management. Perhaps the most significant medical complication is corneal haze or scar formation, which is due to a corneal wound-healing effect. Because of the potential for modulation of corneal haze, as well as that of refractive regression, topical corticosteroids have been used to minimize their significance. This has contributed to a second group of medical complications related, at least in part, to topical corticosteroid use. The difficulty of postoperative pain in some patients has led many North American surgeons to use contact lenses with topical nonsteroidal agents to minimize patient discomfort. This practice has contributed to a third group of medical complications related, at least in part, to contact lens use. We review the medical complications related to wound healing and other systemic conditions first, followed by those seen more frequently in association with topical steroid and contact lens use.

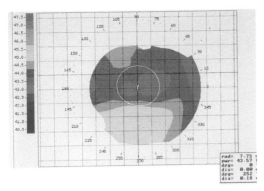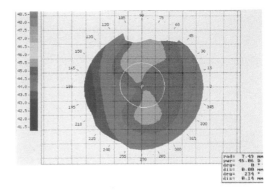

Plates 1*(left)* **and 2** *(right)***.** Corneal warpage from gas-permeable contact lenses with inferior steepening **(Plate 1)** and after resolution **(Plate 2)**. (See Chap. 2.)

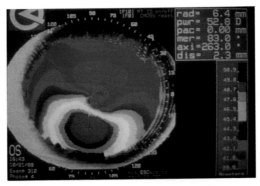

Plate 3. Clinical keratoconus. (See Chap. 2.)

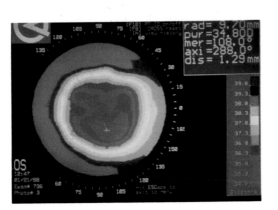

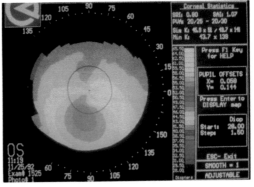

Plate 4. Preclinical keratoconus. (See Chap. 2.)

Plate 5. Postoperative excimer laser PRK. (See Chap. 2.)

▼**Plates 6** *(bottom left)* **and 7** *(bottom right)*. Preoperative topographic map of irregular astigmatism and optical distortion resulting from penetrating keratoplasty **(Plate 6)**. Postoperative topographic map showing a more regular corneal surface after treatment **(Plate 7)**. (From R Gibralter, SL Trokel. Correction of irregular astigmatism with the excimer laser. *Ophthalmology* 101:1310–1315, 1994.) (See Chap. 4.)

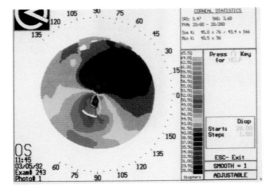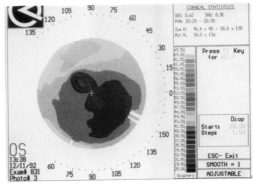

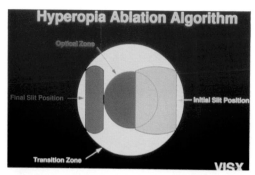

Plate 8. Correction of hyperopia by eccentrically rotating a lens about a mechanical center, thereby offsetting the image of a rotating variable-width slit. (Courtesy of VISX, Inc., Santa Clara, CA.)(See Chap. 4.)

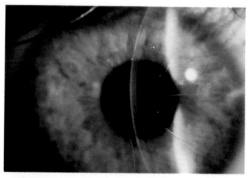

Plate 9. One-month postoperative clinical appearance of a 28-year-old female who underwent PRK for residual myopia 3.5 years after RK. Her refractive error before RK was −7.25 + 2.25 x 85. She received 8-incision RK with an optical zone of 3.5 mm. Her visual acuity before laser was 20/20 with −3.25 − 3.25 x 177. She received a laser photoastigmatic correction of −3.13 − 2.90 x 180. The ablation zone was 6.0 mm with no transiton zone. Her unaided visual acuity 1 month after the laser treatment was 20/25 and could be corrected to 20/20 with −0.5 − 1.25 x 165. The corneal gaze was graded as +0.5. (See Chap. 4.)

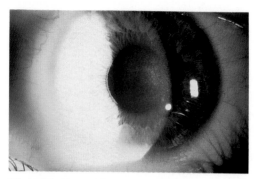

Plate 10. Eye with trace corneal haze 1 month following excimer laser PRK (normal corneal wound healing). (See Chap. 5.)

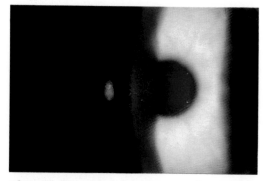

Plate 11. Eye with a clear cornea and no stromal haze 1 month following excimer laser PRK (inadequate wound healing). This patient also had an elevated intraocular pressure of 22 mm Hg and a hyperopic refraction of +1.5 D. (See Chap. 5.)

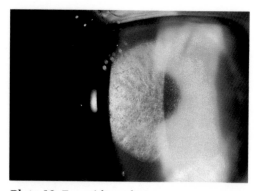

Plate 12. Eye with grade 2.0 − 3.0 corneal haze 1 month following excimer laser PRK (aggressive wound healing). (See Chap. 5.)

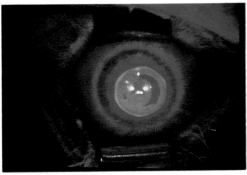 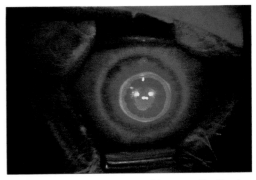

Plates 13 *(left)* **and 14** *(right)*. Excimer laser retreatment of undercorrection with a small effective optical zone. Initially, a PTK of the epithelium demonstrates breakthrough (decreased fluorescence) seen in the midperiphery **(Plate 13)**, which results in a midperipheral annulus of epithelial breakthrough **(Plate 14)** prior to initiating the PRK retreatment. (See Chap. 5.)

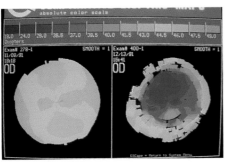 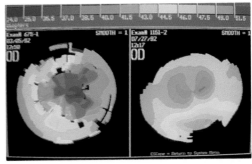

Plates 15 *(left)* **and 16** *(right)*. Videokeratography showing preoperative and postoperative topography at 1, 3, and 6 months following excimer laser PRK for high myopia. Myopic regression is apparent topographically, with the 6-month postoperative image being nearly similar to that of the preoperative image. (See Chap. 5.)

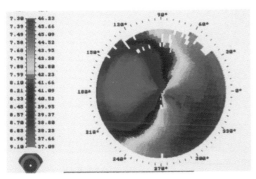 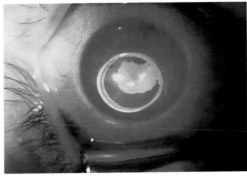

Plate 17. Videokeratography demonstrating marked decentration following excimer laser PRK. (See Chap. 5.)

Plate 18. Excimer laser retreatment for decentration showing an asymmetric area of peripheral epithelial breakthrough (decreased fluorescence) in area of previously untreated cornea. (See Chap. 5.)

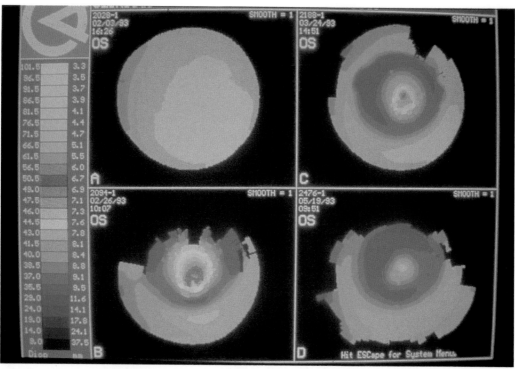

Plate 19. Videokeratography of a steep central island and its partial resolution over time, demonstrated by a preoperative image *(top left)* and postoperative images at 1 week *(bottom left)*, 1 month *(top right)*, and 3 months *(bottom right)*. The topographic size and magnitude of a steep central island appears to diminish at both 1 and 3 months postoperatively. (From RR Krueger et al. Clinical analysis of steep central islands after excimer laser photorefractive keratectomy. *Arch Ophthalamol* April. Copyright 1996, American Medical Association.) (See Chap. 5.)

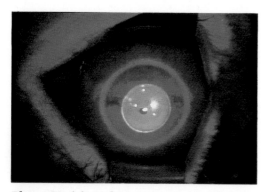 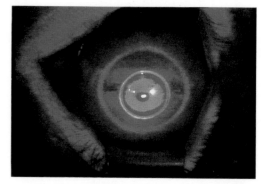

Plates 20 *(left)* **and 21** *(right)*. Excimer laser retreatment for a persistent steep central island 1 year following excimer laser PRK. The retreatment begins with a transepithelial PTK performed until a central **(Plate 20)** and peripheral **(Plate 21)** breakthrough of the epithelium (decreased fluorescence) is seen. (See Chap. 5.)

Corneal Haze and Scarring

Superficial stromal opacification following excimer PRK is an extremely common finding that depends on the biologic healing response of the cornea. Corneal stromal wound healing following excimer PRK has been studied in considerable depth in animal models in association with new collagen formation, cellular infiltration, and the presence of glycosaminoglycans. Studies of corneal histology and immunofluorescence in nonhuman primate eyes have demonstrated a deposition of type III collagen, early absence with later increase of sulfated keratan sulfate, and increased levels of hyaluronic acid [71–73]. These findings have been seen in eyes demonstrating haze following excimer PRK, with the quantity of deposition in some cases in direct correlation with the magnitude of haze [74].

Typically, stromal haze after excimer laser PRK takes on a reticular appearance. It appears during the first postoperative month, peaks at somewhere between 1 and 3 months, and gradually decreases thereafter. Objective assessment of the magnitude of haze can be difficult. Lohmann and colleagues have developed a continuous color display (CCD) camera system mounted to a slit lamp for objective assessment of back-scattered light [75, 76]. Because this technology is not widely available and practical for routine measurement, subjective measurement criteria developed by Fantes [74] and later Seiler [54] have been routinely employed. The most widely used scale of haze utilizes the following criteria for grade of haze.

> 0 = clear cornea
> 0.5 = barely detectable or trace haze
> 1.0 = mild haze that does not interfere with refraction
> 2.0 = moderate haze that does interfere with refraction
> 3.0 = marked haze that obscures iris detail
> 4.0 = severe haze that precludes a view of iris detail

Because haze is part of the normal healing process after excimer PRK, lower levels of haze are clinically insignificant. Loss of best corrected acuity, glare acuity, and contrast sensitivity have not been correlated to most levels of haze but rather to irregular astigmatism and spherical aberration [36, 77, 78]. Nevertheless, there is a certain level of haze that can contribute to clinical symptoms.

Most investigators consider a haze grade of 2.0 or greater clinically significant and reportable as a complication [9, 56, 77]. Corneas with grade 2.0 haze or higher are often referred to as having a scar due to the increased density of the haze. The incidence of 2.0 haze, or scarring, after excimer PRK is shown in Table 5-6 [40, 41, 55, 56,

Table 5-6. Incidence of grade 2.0 haze and greater (scarring) after excimer PRK

Reference	Optical zone	Attempted correction	Postoperative examination	Corticosteroids	Grade 2+ haze
Seiler et al. [41, 56] (Summit)	5.0 mm	−1.25 to −3.0	1–6 mo	Dexamethasone 1% 4 mo taper	0% (0/48)
	5.0 mm	−3.1 to −6.0			1.1% (1/93)
	4.0–5.0 mm	−6.1 to −9.0			15.0% (6/40)
	4.0 mm	−9.1 to −17.5			16.7% (2/12)
Ficker et al. [80] (Summit)	4.5–5.0 mm	−1.0 to −10.0	3 mo	Dexamethasone 0.1% for 1 mo	7.4% (6/81)
Kim et al. [40] (Summit)	N/A	−2.0 to −7.0	1 yr	Prednisone acetate 0.25%	0% (0/135)
		−7.25 to −13.5			3% (2/67)
Ehlers [81] (Meditec)	5.0 mm	−5.0 to −8.0	6 mo	Dexamethasone 1% or prednisone acetate 1% 1–5 mo bid	9% (2/22)
		−9.0 to −12.0			17% (3/18)
VISX [82] (Phase III)	5.0–6.0 mm	−1.0 to −6.0	1 mo	Fluorometholone 0.1% taper 4 mo	1.3% ( )
			3 mo		2.3% ( )
			6 mo		0.8% ( )
			1 yr		0.4% ( )
Maguen [55] (VISX)	5.0–5.5	−1.25 to −7.5	1–6 mo	Fluorometholone 0.1% taper 4 mo	4.9% (10/206)
Pop [83] (VISX)	Multizone pass (6 mm)	−1.0 to −27.0	6 mo	Fluorometholone 0.1% bid	0%(0/315)
	Single pass (6 mm)				2.2% (3/138)

80–83]. It is readily apparent that increased levels of myopia result in higher levels of corneal scarring, ranging from 0–5% for low myopia less than 6.0 D, to 3–17% for higher myopia greater than 10.0 D.

Overall, the mean level of haze seen at various points within the first year after excimer PRK for low myopia (< 6.0 D) varies from a mean score of grade 0.1 to slightly greater than grade 1.0 [32, 41, 84]. The mean maximum level peaks at 1–3 months and decreases with time, often to a level of clinical insignificance or even complete resolution. During VISX trials in the United States, the level of haze in eyes treated with nitrogen gas blowing was significantly higher than in eyes treated without nitrogen gas blowing [32]. Similarly, the level of haze in eyes with greater than 4.0 D of myopia was significantly higher than in those with less than 2.0 D [32].

Management. For patients who have marked haze or scarring at the first postoperative month, topical corticosteroids can be helpful in reducing the level of haze as well as any refractive regression. Patients who are being treated with topical fluorometholone as part of the routine postoperative management can be switched to topical dexamethasone. This more potent inhibitor of keratocyte activation can be helpful in minimizing the aggressive wound-healing response of some patients.

For patients in whom corneal scarring persists beyond 6 months, excimer laser retreatment can be performed. Because nearly all these patients will have concomitant regression and myopic undercorrection, a simple myopic ablation profile is the best choice. Some investigators, however, warn that these patients will redevelop haze and scarring after retreatment and suggest waiting until the magnitude of the haze resolves. There is no evidence that haze and regression after retreatment will be any less if the procedure is performed later. Others report that these patients do well after excimer retreatment, and suggest the following strategy: Transepithelial ablation (i.e., PTK) can be performed until a substantial area of decreased fluorescence is observed. Thereafter, a myopic PRK can be performed according to the level of residual myopia [13].

Delayed Epithelial Healing

In most cases, the epithelium heals promptly after excimer PRK, but occasionally healing delayed beyond 4–5 days can occur. When the epithelium takes longer than 1 week to close (Fig. 5-5), a cause for concern arises because delayed healing can result in worsening of corneal haze and scarring. Additionally, delayed epithelial closure increases the risk of infection. Consequently, conditions that predispose to poor epithelial healing should be sought out and prevented prior to surgery.

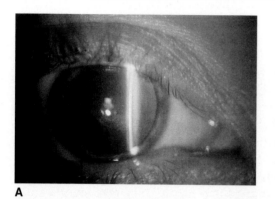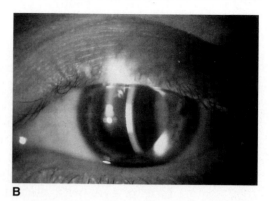

A   B

Fig. 5-5. Corneal epithelial defect persisting beyond the first postoperative week in a patient following excimer laser PRK (**A**). The other eye of this patient has a corneal scar at the 6-month visit, in an area where the epithelium did not heal for 18 days after surgery (**B**). (Courtesy of Andrew Garfinkle, M.D., Ph.D., Cornwall, Ontario.)

One relatively common condition that can result in poor epithelial healing is keratoconjunctivitis sicca. Patients with a tear deficiency may be motivated to seek refractive surgery because it often complicates soft contact lens wear. Preliminary results with the VISX excimer laser suggest that a decreased Schirmer's test consistent with a tear deficiency state is associated with increased corneal haze and epitheliopathy after excimer PRK. Thus, it is important to prescreen all patients for a tear deficiency and to pretreat them with artificial tear supplements or punctal occlusion, if appropriate.

The incidence of delayed epithelial healing with closure times longer than 4 days has been reported in several large studies (Table 5-7), with the incidence ranging from 0–38% of cases [41, 51, 57, 85, 86]. Some of the differences in closure rate may not be entirely due to preoperative conditions but to intraoperative and postoperative conditions as well. Excessively large corneal epithelial debridement can unnecessarily delay epithelial closure, as can nitrogen gas blowing during the procedure [30, 32]. Although mechanical epithelial debridement is employed by most surgeons, transepithelial laser ablation has been advocated by some. Ronald Jans from Calgary, Alberta, Canada, has suggested that transepithelial ablation not only reduces the time for epithelial closure but slightly decreases the level of postoperative corneal haze [6a]. These results, however, were not statistically substantiated, and prospective clinical studies are needed.

The possible factors in postoperative management associated with delayed epithelial healing include the use and abuse of topical anti-inflammatory agents (corticosteroids and nonsteroidal anti-inflammatory drugs), prophylactic antibiotics, and therapeutic soft contact

Table 5-7. Incidence of epithelial healing delayed beyond 4 days after PRK

Reference	Optical zone	Attempted correction	Contact lens/patch	Early steroids	Delayed re-epithelialization
Seiler et al. [41] (Summit)	4.5–5.0 mm	−1.25 to −17.5 D	Patch	None	1.5% (4/255)
Dutt et al. [85] (Summit)	5.0 mm	−1.5 to −6.0 D	Patch	Dexamethasone ung	0% (0/47)
Talley et al. [57] (VISX)	6.0–7.0 mm	−1.0 to −7.5 D	SCL	Fluorometholone q2h	0% (0/91)
Brancato et al. [51] (Summit)	3.5–5.0 mm	−0.8 to −25.0 D	N/A	Dexamethasone or fluorometholone	9.4% (106/113)
Pallikaris et al. [86] (Autonomous)	6 mm	−1.0 to −6.0 D	SCL	Tobradex	38% (16/42)

N/A = not available; SCL = soft contact lens.

lenses. Epithelial toxicity secondary to these medications and lenses may limit the speed of re-epithelialization. Superficial keratopathy related to preservatives or the medications themselves can also occur, even after re-epithelialization. All these factors may contribute to an increased level of postoperative corneal haze. Therapeutic soft contact lenses can be fit too tightly or become dislocated, resulting in ocular redness and irritation, again contributing to diminished epithelial healing.

Undiagnosed autoimmune conditions can also impede re-epithelialization and even result in stromal ulceration. A persistent epithelial defect associated with stromal ulceration may warrant a system autoimmune workup.

Management. When epithelial healing is delayed, every effort should be made to understand the cause for delayed re-epithelialization and appropriate measures taken. If corticosteroids or nonsteroidal anti-inflammatory agents are being used, they should be discontinued. The use of pressure patching, nonpreservative ophthalmic lubrication and ointments, and topical antibiotics with a different type of preservative should be considered. By paying careful attention to delays in re-epithelialization, one should be able to diagnose and correct unexpected postoperative conditions and minimize side effects that influence the visual and refractive outcome.

Epithelial Erosions

Epithelial erosions or predisposing basement membrane abnormalities can be seen infrequently following excimer PRK. Seiler [87] has observed only one case in 600 of a patient describing symptoms of an erosion, although no erosion was seen. Gartry [26, 37], on the other hand, reported 22 cases in 120 (18%) of foreign body sensation on waking and tenderness with eye rubbing. No erosions were noted in these patients, and all resolved within a 6-month period.

Both symptomatic and asymptomatic epithelial erosions and basement membrane changes have been observed in 5 eyes of 4 patients in the Cedar-Sinai series, in an incidence of 2.1% [32]. This incidence is close to that reported in the general population. In this series, the epithelial abnormalities were seen both within and away from the ablation zone, suggesting that an epithelial dystrophy pre-existed in these eyes. On the other hand, epithelial dots have also been reported within the ablation zone following excimer PRK. These persisted after repeat epithelial debridement, demonstrating abnormal regeneration of the epithelial basement membrane [88].

Figure 5-6 shows an example of a basement membrane redundancy leading to erosive symptoms in an area outside the actual treatment zone but within the zone of epithelial debridement. Whether epi-

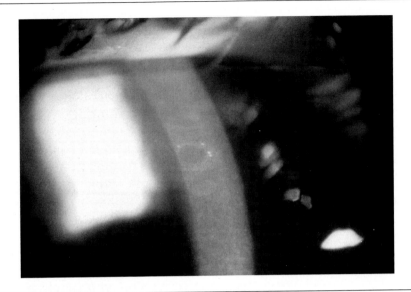

Fig. 5-6. Anterior basement membrane redundancy seen following excimer laser PRK outside the actual treatment zone but within the zone of epithelial debridement. No erosions were seen or experienced in this patient. (Courtesy of Neal Sher, M.D., Minneapolis.)

thelial debridement or the laser ablation itself compromises the reformation of hemidesmosomal attachments is unknown. But factors such as long-standing contact lens wear and even prior excimer laser treatment have been found to be associated with more difficult epithelial debridement, suggesting that the attachments are even stronger in these cases. In fact, in cases of recurrent epithelial erosions unrelated to excimer laser surgery, excimer PTK has been successfully used in treatment of refractory cases [32].

Management. The treatment of symptomatic epithelial erosions after PRK is similar to their treatment when not associated with laser therapy. The use of hypertonic saline 3% solution and ointment should be effective in most patients. In those refractory to topical medications, excimer laser PTK can be used. One case of excimer laser retreatment (PTK) for an epithelial erosion has been reported [32].

Elevated Intraocular Pressure

The routine use of topical corticosteroids in the management of excimer PRK is a topic of ongoing discussion. The earliest treatments with excimer laser PRK utilized high doses of potent corticosteroids, such as prednisolone acetate and dexamethasone, in an effort to prevent scarring and titrate refraction [9, 26, 54]. Later, because of steroid response and other concerns, fluorometholone was adopted by many investigators, with subsequent reduction in the incidence of intraocular pressure (IOP) spikes.

The mechanism of IOP elevation in response to corticosteroids is believed to be due to the influence of glycosaminoglycans [62]. As mentioned earlier, corticosteroids decrease the consumption of glycosaminoglycans by endothelial cells in the trabecular meshwork, allowing the trabecular meshwork to thicken with outflow obstruction in some patients (steroid responders) [62, 63]. In other patients, corticosteroids decrease the production of hyaluronic acid (glycosaminoglycan) by keratocytes in the corneal stroma, thereby reducing the regression associated with glycosaminoglycan deposition [61]. In general, patients who have an inadequate wound-healing response are also those who tend to be steroid responders [56]. This is a favorable association because the discontinuation of corticosteroids due to an early pressure rise happens to be the same management recommended for an inadequate wound healer who is overcorrected. To avoid overcorrection in correlation with steroid response, some have advocated testing patients for corticosteroid-induced IOP elevation prior to surgery [13].

The incidence of IOP elevation at 1 month following excimer PRK is outlined in Table 5-8 for both dexamethasone and fluorometholone, as reported by various centers [9, 15, 37, 38, 40, 51, 56–58, 82, 85]. Table 5-8 clearly demonstrates a much higher incidence of pressure rise in the dexamethasone-treated eyes over those treated with fluorometholone. Also, the incidence of IOP elevation is significantly higher in higher myopes with refraction greater than −9.0 D. With the dexamethasone-treated eyes, some patients had severe and symptomatic IOP elevation. Three patients reported transient loss of vision on rising rapidly from a chair and were found to have IOP in excess of 45 mm Hg [37]. Anecdotal reports of visual field loss have been reported in some patients with prolonged IOP elevation following excimer laser PRK.

Management. If a significant IOP rise is detected at 1 month after surgery, cessation or at least reduction of the topical steroid should be made, with the concurrent administration of a topical β-blocker. The IOP usually returns to normal within 1 or 2 weeks, and no reports of persistent pressure elevation can be found in the literature.

Reactivation of Herpes Simplex Keratitis

Although no known cases of primary herpes simplex keratitis have been observed after excimer laser PRK, several cases of reactivation of herpes keratitis in eyes with corneal scarring have been observed following PTK [89–94]. In two of these cases, PTK was performed to remove the corneal scar, with reactivation being seen 3 months later

Table 5-8. Incidence of intraocular pressure elevation at 1 month following excimer PRK

Reference	Number of eyes	Attempted correction	Steroid	Postoperative examination	Increased IOP
Salz et al. [15]	146	−1.25 to −7.5 D	Fluorometholone 0.1%	N/A	3% > 24 mm Hg
Piebenga et al. [58]	129	−1.0 to −6.0 D	Fluorometholone 0.1%	< 3 mo	2.3% > 21 mm Hg
Talley et al. [57]	85	−1.0 to −7.5 D	Fluorometholone 0.1%	3 mo	2.3% > 21 mm Hg
VISX FDA study [82]	691	−1.0 to −6.0 D	Fluorometholone 0.1%	N/A	3% > 5 mm Hg rise
Dutt et al. [85]	47	−1.5 to −6.1 D	Fluorometholone 0.25%	< 3 mo	10% > 22 mm Hg
Kim et al. [40]	135	−2.0 to −7.0 D	Prednisolone acetate 0.25%	N/A	14%
	67	−7.25 to −13.5 D			24%
Brancato et al. [51]	1236	−0.8 to −25.0 D	Dexamethasone or fluorometholone 0.1%	< 1 mo	25% > 26 mm Hg
Tengroth et al. [38]	420	−1.5 to −7.5 D	Dexamethasone 0.1%	N/A	13% > 24 mm Hg
Garty et al. [37]	120	−1.5 to −7.0 D	Dexamethasone 0.1%	2–6 wk	12% > 25 mm Hg
Seiler et al. [9]	26	−1.0 to −7.5 D	Dexamethasone 0.1%	1 mo	24% > 5 mm Hg rise
					3% > 30 mm Hg
Seiler et al. [56]	181	−1.25 to −9.0 D	Dexamethasone 0.1%	1 mo	28% > 5 mm Hg rise
	12	−9.0 to −17.5 D			50% > 5 mm Hg rise

N/A = not available; IOP = intraocular pressure.

while topical corticosteroids were being used concurrently [89]. Another case demonstrated recurrence 1 month after astigmatic PRK in a corneal graft of a former herpetic patient, again while topical steroids were being used [87, 91]. Due to the latency of reactivation, these cases strongly suggest the influence of topical steroids rather than the ultraviolet laser energy as the stimulus for recurrence. In another study of PTK, the incidence of recurrence was not different from other previously infected eyes [93].

In an experimental animal study of herpes reactivation following excimer PTK, viral shedding was observed in a percentage of both excimer-treated eyes and those treated with chemical scraping of the epithelial surface [94]. Although corticosteroids did not play a role in this experimental model, mechanical factors, rather than the ultraviolet laser light, were a likely contributor.

In a clinical case of herpes virus reactivation, keratitis was seen 8 days after an excimer PTK in which the topical steroids were discontinued 2 days prior to treatment [92]. Despite the initiation of topical and oral acyclovir, the herpetic keratitis did not resolve until topical steroids were reinitiated 2 weeks later. In this case, topical steroids had a beneficial effect.

All these reports indicate that multiple factors may contribute to the reactivation of herpes simplex keratitis following excimer laser corneal surgery. Although the ultraviolet light of the excimer laser might be suspect, it is more likely that immunologic, mechanical, and chemical factors are responsible.

Management. Oral acyclovir for several weeks after surgery should be considered as a prophylaxis in all patients with a history of ocular herpetic disease. The management of patients developing active viral keratitis following the procedure should include acyclovir 200 mg PO 5 times daily, trifluorothymidine eye drops 9 times per day, and discontinuation of topical steroids. Treatment should be continued until the acute keratitis has subsided.

Posterior Subcapsular Cataracts

Several cases of posterior subcapsular cataracts have been observed with the use of dexamethasone phosphate 0.1% within the first year following excimer laser PRK. In a series of 3 patients, reported by Maguen and Machat [32], the duration and frequency of topical steroid use varied from 4 times daily for 3 months to every 2 hours for 8 months. In no reported cases was the use of topical fluorometholone drops associated with the formation of a posterior subcapsular cataract.

Excimer laser stress waves have also been recorded intraocularly with an intensity maximum at a distance of approximately 6 to 7 mm posterior to the corneal surface [94a]. Although these stress waves peak just behind the posterior lens capsule, no sign of posterior subcapsular cataracts have been observed except for those explained by the frequent use of potent corticosteroid drops.

Management. Patients developing visually significant posterior subcapsular cataracts following excimer laser PRK may be considered for cataract extraction with intraocular lens implantation at a point at least 6 months to 1 year following the keratectomy. Keratometry values used in calculating the power of the implant may best be determined by subtracting the spherical equivalent change in refractive error (corrected by the vertex distance to the corneal plane) from the keratometry reading recorded before excimer laser PRK [95]. In eyes where the preoperative keratometry readings are unavailable, a computer program estimating the effective keratometric values following excimer laser PRK has been reported, utilizing videokeratography data weighted with the Stiles-Crawford effect. [96]. Both simple keratometry and nonweighted videokeratography data tend to underestimate the effective topographic change [96].

Infectious and Ulcerative Keratitis

Few cases of infectious keratitis following excimer laser PRK have been reported. One of the first was in the VISX U.S. national blind eye study in a patient treated postoperatively with a pressure patch rather than a soft bandage contact lens [97]. Since that time, every other report of a corneal infection following excimer PRK has been associated with the use of therapeutic soft contact lenses, with the exception of one [98]. The most significant report is by Faschinger and colleagues [7] of four patients who developed fungal keratitis with *Aspergillus* in reasonably close proximity to each other. All four patients wore a disposable contact lens after the surgery during a period of hospital renovation in the hot, humid summer months. Three of the four developed severe ulceration, which resulted in grade 3.0–4.0 haze and scarring after treatment with antifungal agents (Fig. 5-7). One patient developed culture-negative endophthalmitis, which was effectively treated with antifungal agents. The incidence of infectious keratitis in this series was as high as 1.4% (4/297), whereas in other series with larger numbers of patients (> 3000) it is less common (0.1–0.2%) [32]. Other than the cases of fungal keratitis, a culture-positive result is most commonly seen as staphylococcal epidermitis [32, 97], whereas some reports indicate a culture-negative result [98] or no culture results at all [99].

Ulcerative keratitis and nonhealing epithelial defects can also be due to an undiagnosed systemic autoimmune condition or collagen vascular disease. One case has been reported of progressive ulceration

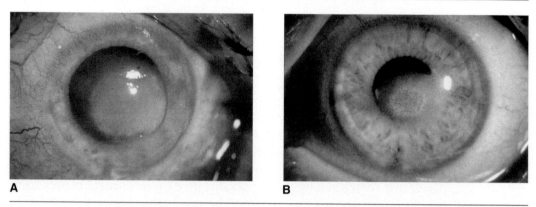

A   B

Fig. 5-7. **A.** Severe *Aspergillus* infectious keratitis noted several days following excimer laser PRK with the use of a bandage soft contact lens. **B.** Following effective
treatment with antifungal agents, a large, grade 3.0–4.0 zone of haze and scarring
was observed. (Courtesy of Christoph Faschinger, M.D., Graz, Austria.)

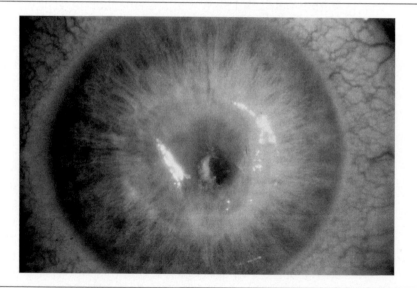

Fig. 5-8. Noninfectious ulcerative keratitis leading to corneal perforation 1 month
after excimer laser PRK in a patient with systemic lupus erythematosus. (From
T Seiler et al, Complications After Myopic PRK, Primarily with the Summit
Excimer Laser. In JJ Salz [ed], *Corneal Laser Surgery.* Mosby–Year Book, 1995.)

leading to corneal perforation 1 month after excimer PRK in a patient
with undiagnosed systemic lupus erythematosus (Fig. 5-8) [56]. Another patient experienced corneal ulceration leading to perforation in
a yet undiagnosed allergic or autoimmune condition. Her ulceration
led to perforation within days, and histopathology of the transplanted
corneal button demonstrated an unusually high number of eosino-
phils [David Silver, personal communication, November 1995].

Management. At the first sign of infection or infiltration, contact lens use should be discontinued and cultures of the cornea and contact lens performed. Broad-spectrum topical antibiotics should be initiated immediately, with antifungals if appropriate. Gram's stain and culture results will verify the proper selection of antibiotics. Corticosteroids can usually be added after several days of treatment or when a culture-negative result is reported (see Sterile Corneal Infiltrates below).

Topical or systemic corticosteroids or immunosuppressants can also be used when an autoimmune-related ulceration is suspected. Accordingly, knowledge of a systemic autoimmune condition is a contraindication to excimer laser treatment.

When stability of an infectious or ulcerative condition is achieved, residual opacity or irregular astigmatism can be treated with a therapeutic rigid contact lens, excimer laser phototherapeutic retreatment, or corneal transplantation if needed. One of the four patients with *Aspergillus* keratitis had a successful excimer PTK of the residual scar, with a corrected visual acuity of 15/20. Successful corneal transplantation was performed in both patients with autoimmune ulcerative keratitis and perforation, leading to a good visual outcome with no further tendency toward ulceration.

Sterile Corneal Infiltrates

With the widespread use of soft contact lenses with diclofenac sodium after excimer laser PRK, an additional complication of sterile corneal infiltrates has been reported [6]. Sterile subepithelial infiltrates are a well-recognized complication of soft contact lens wear in the absence of surgery, but typically they are peripheral, not central or paracentral, as they are after excimer laser PRK. Diclofenac sodium also appears to contribute to the formation of these infiltrates. Diclofenac sodium, when used without corticosteroids, is associated with a statistically significant increase in the number of polymorphonuclear cells entering the anterior stroma following experimental excimer surgery in rabbit eyes [1]. As a nonsteroidal anti-inflammatory agent, diclofenac sodium or ketorolac effectively blocks the cyclooxygenase pathway to reduce the level of prostaglandins in tissue. The chemotactic effect of leukotrienes, however, is not blocked, presumably contributing to leukocyte infiltration and the formation of sterile corneal infiltrates.

A photograph of a patient with a paracentral subepithelial infiltrate 48 hours after PRK is shown in Fig. 5-9. The incidence of sterile corneal infiltrates after excimer PRK is approximately 0.4%, being seen in as many as 28 patients who were retrospectively analyzed by 17 Canadian surgeons [6]. The lesions are unlike infectious keratitis

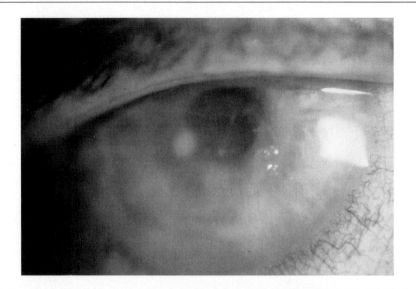

Fig. 5-9. Sterile corneal infiltrates 48 hours following excimer PRK in a patient using topical diclofenac sodium and a bandage soft contact lens as postoperative management. (From N Sher et al, Role of topical corticosteroids and nonsteroidal antiinflammatory drugs in the etiology of stromal infiltrates after excimer PRK. *J Refract Corneal Surg* Sept/Oct 1994.)

in that they are usually subepithelial, multiple, and repeatedly culture negative with an absence of organisms on Gram's stain. They usually appear between 24 and 48 hours after surgery and can be associated with immune rings or stromal melting. All the patients reported in this series received a soft contact lens with topical diclofenac sodium or ketorolac prior, during, and 4 times a day following excimer laser PRK. None of the patients received concurrent topical steroids. All patients responded similarly, with 90% of eyes experiencing stromal scarring and a line or two of loss of BSCVA [6]. Current incidence of sterile infiltrates with the concurrent postoperative use of topical steroids is dramatically decreased.

Management. As with infectious keratitis, a presumed subepithelial sterile infiltrate should be first cultured with a Gram's stain and then started on a topical antibiotic, with discontinuation of the contact lens and topical diclofenac. Topical corticosteroids should also be started as soon as possible when the presence of a sterile infiltrate is suspected. As mentioned above, scarring and loss of BSCVA are associated with most cases, regardless of the management.

Although long-term management of these cases has not been reported, excimer PTK retreatment may be effective in patients with dense superficial scarring that precludes good vision.

Subretinal Hemorrhages

Patients with high myopia may at times develop subretinal neovascularization, which can lead to bleeding, resulting in a Fuchs' spot, or subretinal hemorrhage. Several reports of subretinal hemorrhage following excimer laser PRK have been cited [13, 51, 100], leading to the question of whether their occurrence is due to the laser-induced shock wave or subject to the natural history of the disease. In an Italian series of 1236 patients treated with the Summit excimer laser, three patients had severe visual loss due to subretinal hemorrhage at an unspecified time interval following excimer PRK [51]. Two other patients developed a subretinal hemorrhage 2 months after surgery in a German series of several thousand patients [13, 87], and another developed a hemorrhage in a Korean series of 1821 patients [100]. Angiographic evidence of subretinal neovascularization was found in one of the fellow eyes of the German patients, which did not progress to bleeding [13, 87].

Studies of excimer laser stress waves in the eye have recorded focused amplitudes of at least several orders of magnitude within the anterior vitreous. Although these were first believed to be the cause of subretinal Fuchs' spot, they are not of sufficient magnitude to be referred to as shock waves, and they attenuate significantly before reaching the retinal surface [94a].

Although subretinal hemorrhage is not a major risk factor of excimer PRK, it does result in severe visual loss and warrants a careful preoperative examination of the fundus with attention to the macula as well as the retinal periphery. A patient should be counseled regarding the possibility of subretinal hemorrhage as a complication of PRK.

Additionally, one case of presumed cystoid macular edema has been reported after PRK [101], and this should also be considered when counseling the patient.

Management. Unfortunately, the management of subretinal hemorrhage is observation with no therapy leading to its resolution. The management of cystoid macula edema is discussed elsewhere.

Ptosis, Anisocoria, and Iritis

Unilateral blepharoptosis has been reported in a small percentage of cases after excimer PRK. In the Berlin experience, blepharoptosis of more than 1 mm was found in 1% of cases at 1 month after surgery [13, 56]. By 6 months, the ptosis had significantly improved. In the Cedar-Sinai series, only one case occurred, requiring surgical correction [32]. The exact cause of the ptosis is unknown, but some suggest it is due to steroid use or stretching of Müller's muscle with the lid speculum. Whatever the pathogenesis, it is not something unique to excimer PRK because cases have also been reported after RK [102].

Anisocoria has been reported after excimer PRK, with pupil enlargement in up to 9% (97/1165) of eyes, beginning within the first postoperative month and disappearing within 1 year [51]. In the Berlin series, 5% of unilaterally treated patients developed anisocoria that persisted beyond 1 year [13]. The mechanism for the anisocoria is unknown, but it is presumed to be due to a uniquely prolonged postoperative response of pupillary dilation by homatropine.

Iritis has been reported in a few rare instances after excimer PRK. Only one patient in the VISX phase III clinical trials [82] and two in a series from the Laser Center (TLC) [32] have developed iritis after excimer PRK. Only one patient in the latter series was positive for HLA-B27, and the rest had no history or risk factor for iritis. All had resolution within several days with topical steroid treatment.

Management. The management of these conditions is mostly observation, with resolution often occurring in time or with mild intervention. In only one case of ptosis was a surgical procedure necessary (Müller's muscle-conjunctival resection) [32]. In all the remaining cases mentioned above, improvement was seen without any further intervention and without any adverse sequelae.

References

1. Phillips AF, et al. Arachidonic acid metabolites after excimer laser corneal surgery. *Arch Ophthalmol* 11:1273–1278, 1993.
2. Wu WCS, Stark WJ, Green WR. Corneal wound healing after 193-nm excimer laser keratectomy. *Arch Ophthalmol* 109:1426–1432, 1991.
3. Sher NA, et al. Excimer laser photorefractive keratectomy in high myopia. *Arch Ophthalmol* 110:935–943,1992.
4. Eiferman RA, Hoffman RS, Sher NA. Topical diclofenac reduces pain following photorefractive keratectomy. *Arch Ophthalmol* 111:1022, 1993.
5. Sher NA, et al. Topical diclofenac in the treatment of ocular pain after excimer photorefractive keratectomy. *Refract Corneal Surg* 9:425–436, 1993.
6. Sher NA, et al. The role of topical steroidal and nonsteroidal anti-inflammatory drugs in the etiology of stromal infiltrates after excimer photorefractive keratectomy. *J Refract Corneal Surg* 10: 587–588, 1994.
6a. Jans R. Preventing and managing excimer PRK complications. Presented at Meeting of the American Society of Cataract and Refractive Surgery, San Diego, April 1995.
7. Faschinger C, Grasl M, Ganser K. Infectious corneal ulcerations and endophthalmitis after photorefractive keratectomy with use of disposable contact lenses. *Eur J Implant Ref Surg* 7:1–8, 1995.

8. Verma S, Corbett MC, Marshall J. A prospective, randomized, double-masked trial to evaluate the role of topical anesthetics in controlling pain after photorefractive keratectomy. *Ophthalmol* 102:1918–1924, 1995.

9. Seiler T, Wollensak J. Myopic photorefractive keratectomy with the excimer laser. **One-year** follow-up. *Ophthalmology* 98:1156–1163, 1991.

10. McDonald MB, et al. Central photorefractive keratectomy for myopia. Partially sighted and normally sighted eyes. *Ophthalmology* 98: 1327–1337, 1991.

11. Sher NA, et al. The use of the 193-nm excimer laser for myopic photorefractive keratectomy in sighted eyes. A multicenter study. *Arch Ophthalmol* 109:1525–1530, 1991.

12. Gauthier CA, et al. Epithelial alterations following photorefractive keratectomy for myopia. *J Refract Surg* 11:113–118, 1995.

13. Seiler T, Schmidt-Petersen H, Wollensak J. Complications after Myopic Photorefractive Keratectomy, Primarily with the Summit Excimer Laser. In JJ Salz (ed.). *Corneal Laser Surgery*. St. Louis: Mosby, 1995.

14. Thompson KP, et al. Photorefractive Keratectomy with the Summit Excimer Laser: The Phase III U.S. Results. In JJ Salz (ed.). *Corneal Laser Surgery*. St. Louis: Mosby, 1995.

15. Salz JJ, et al. A two-year experience with excimer laser photorefractive keratectomy for myopia. *Ophthalmology* 100:873–882, 1993.

16. Durrie DS, Sanders DR, Schumer DJ. Computerized Corneal Topography of Surface Ablations with the EyeSys System. In JJ Salz (ed.). *Corneal Laser Surgery*. St. Louis: Mosby, 1995.

17. Gartry DS, Kerr Muir MG, Marshall J. The effect of topical corticosteroids on refraction and corneal haze following excimer laser treatment of myopia: An update. A prospective, randomized double-blind study. *Eye* 7:584–590, 1993.

18. O'Brart DPS, et al. The effects of topical corticosteroids and plasmin inhibitors on refractive outcome, haze and visual performance after photorefractive keratectomy. A prospective, randomized, observer-masked study. *Ophthalmology* 101:1565–1574, 1994.

19. Brancato R, et al. Corticosteroids vs diclofenac in the treatment of delayed regression after myopic photorefractive keratectomy. *Refract Corneal Surg* 9:376–378, 1993.

20. Nassaralla BA, et al. Effect of diclofenac on corneal haze after photorefractive keratectomy in rabbits. *Ophthalmology* 102:469–474, 1995.

21. Talamo JH, et al. Modulation of corneal wound healing after excimer laser keratomileusis using topical mitomycin C and steroids. *Arch Ophthalmol* 109:1141–1146, 1991.

22. Morlet N, et al. Effect of topical interferon-alpha 2b on corneal haze after excimer laser photorefractive keratectomy in rabbits. *Refract Corneal Surg* 9:443–451, 1993.

23. Wilson SE. Excimer laser (193 nm) myopic keratomileusis: Differential stability in lower and higher myopes. *Refract Corneal Surg* 6:383–385, 1990.

24. Seiler T, Derse M, Pham T. Repeated excimer laser treatment after photorefractive keratectomy. *Arch Ophthalmol* 110:1230–1233, 1992.

25. Uozato H, Guyton DL. Centering corneal surgical procedures. *Am J Ophthalmol* 103:264–275, 1987.

26. Gartry DS, Kerr Muir MG, Marshall J. Photorefractive keratectomy with an argon fluoride excimer laser: A clinical study. *Refract Corneal Surg* 7:420–435, 1991.

27. Dougherty PJ, Wellish KL, Maloney RK. Excimer laser ablation rate and corneal hydration. *Am J Ophthalmol* 118:169–176, 1994.

28. Campos M, et al. Corneal wound healing after excimer laser ablation: Effects of nitrogen gas blower. *Ophthalmology* 99:893–897, 1992.

29. Krueger RR, et al. Corneal surface morphology following excimer laser ablation with humidified gases. *Arch Ophthalmol* 111:1131–1137, 1993.

30. Maguen E, et al. Effect of nitrogen flow on recovery of vision after excimer laser photorefractive keratectomy without nitrogen flow. *J Refract Corneal Surg* 10:321–326, 1994.

31. Krueger RR, et al. Clinical analysis of excimer laser photorefractive keratectomy using a multiple zone technique for severe myopia. *Am J Ophthalmol* 119:263–274, 1995.

32. Maguen E, Machat JJ. Complications of Photorefractive Keratectomy, Primarily with the VisX Excimer Laser. In JJ Salz (ed.). *Corneal Laser Surgery*. St. Louis: Mosby, 1995.

33. Pallikaris IG, et al. Rotating brush for fast removal of corneal epithelium. *J Refract Corneal Surg* 10:239–442, 1994.

34. Sher NA, et al. The use of the 193-nm excimer laser for myopic photorefractive keratectomy in sighted eyes: A multicenter study. *Arch Ophthalmol* 109:1525–1530, 1991.

35. Krueger RR. The excimer laser: A step-up in complexity and responsibility for the ophthalmic laser surgeon. *J Refract Corneal Surg* 10: 83–86, 1994.

36. Seiler T, Reckmann W, Maloney RK. Effective spherical aberration of the cornea as a quantitative descriptor in corneal topography. *J Cataract Refract Surg* 19(Suppl.):155–165, 1993.

37. Gartry DS, Kerr Muir MG, Marshall J. Excimer laser photorefractive keratectomy. 18-month follow-up. *Ophthalmology* 99:1209–1219, 1992.

38. Tengroth B, et al. Excimer laser photorefractive keratectomy for myopia. Clinical results in sighted eyes. *Ophthalmology* 100:739–745, 1993.

39. Gimbel HV, et al. Visual, refractive and patient satisfaction results following bilateral photorefractive keratectomy for myopia. *Refract Corneal Surg* 9(Suppl.):S5–S10, 1993.

40. Kim JH, et al. Photorefractive keratectomy in 202 myopic eyes: One year results. *Refract Corneal Surg* 9(Suppl.):S11–S16, 1993.

41. Seiler T, Wollensak J. Results of a prospective evaluation of photorefractive keratectomy at 1 year after surgery. *German J Ophthalmol* 2: 135–142, 1993.

42. O'Brart DPS, et al. The effects of ablation diameter on the outcome of excimer laser photorefractive keratectomy: A prospective, randomized, double-blind study. *Arch Ophthalmol* 113:438–443, 1995.

43. Dello Russo J. Night glare and excimer laser ablation diameter. *J Cataract Refract Surg* 19:565, 1993.

44. Roberts CW, Koester CJ. Optical zone diameters for photorefractive corneal surgery. *Invest Ophthalmol Vis Sci* 34:2275–2281, 1993.

45. Seiler T, Hell K, Wollensak J. Diurnal variation in refraction after excimer laser refractive keratectomy. *German J Ophthalmol* 1:19–21, 1992.

46. Schanzlin DJ, et al. Diurnal change in refraction, corneal curvature, visual acuity, and intraocular pressure after radial keratotomy in the PERK study. *Ophthalmology* 93:167–175, 1986.

47. Lynn MJ, et al. Stability of refraction after radial keratotomy compared with unoperated eyes in the PERK study. *Invest Ophthalmol Vis Sci* 28(Suppl.):223, 1987.

48. Nizam A, et al. Stability of refraction and visual acuity during 5 years with simple myopia. *Refract Corneal Surg* 8:439–477, 1992.

49. Krueger RR, McDonnell PJ. Progressive hyperopia following excimer laser refractive keratectomy. *Am J Ophthalmol* 117:668–670, 1994.

50. O'Brart DPS, et al. An investigation to determine the effects of ablation diameter, depth and profile on the outcome of excimer laser photorefractive keratectomy (PRK). *Invest Ophthalmol Vis Sci* 36(4):S1063, 1995.

51. Brancato R, et al. Excimer laser photorefractive keratectomy for myopia: Results in 1165 eyes. *Refract Corneal Surg* 9:95–104, 1993.

52. Sher NA, et al. 193 nm excimer photorefractive keratectomy in high myopia. *Ophthalmology* 101:1575–1582, 1994.

53. Heitzmann J, et al. The correction of high myopia using the excimer laser. *Arch Ophthalmol* 111:1627–1634, 1993.

54. Seiler T, Kahle G, Kriegerowski M. Excimer laser (193 nm) myopic keratomileusis in sighted and blind human eyes. *Refract Corneal Surg* 6: 165–173, 1990.

55. Maguen E, et al. Results of excimer laser photorefractive keratectomy for the correction of myopia. *Ophthalmology* 101:1548–1556, 1994.

56. Seiler T, et al. Complications of myopic photorefractive keratectomy with the excimer laser. *Ophthalmology* 101:153–160, 1994.

57. Talley AR, et al. Results one year after using the 193-nm excimer laser for photorefractive keratectomy in mild to moderate myopia. *Am J Ophthalmol* 118:304–311, 1994.

58. Piebenga LW, et al. Excimer photorefractive keratectomy for myopia. *Ophthalmology* 100:1335–1345, 1993.

59. Carones F, et al. Efficacy of corticosteroids in reversing regression after myopic photorefractive keratectomy. *Refract Corneal Surg* 9(Suppl.): S52–S60, 1993.

60. Brancato R, et al. Corticosteroids vs. diclofenac in the treatment of delayed regression after myopic photorefractive keratectomy. *Refract Corneal Surg* 9:376–378, 1993.

61. Fitzsimmons TD, Fagerholm P, Tengroth B. Steroid treatment of myopic regression: Acute refractive and topographic changes in excimer photorefractive keratectomy patients. *Cornea* 12:358–361, 1993.

62. Segawa K. Ultrastructural changes of the trabecular tissue in the primary open angle glaucoma. *Jpn J Ophthalmol* 19:317, 1975.

63. Seiler T. The resistance of the trabecular meshwork to aqueous humor outflow. *Graefe's Arch Ophthalmol* 223:88–91, 1985.

64. Schwartz-Goldstein BH, et al. Corneal topography of Phase III excimer laser photorefractive keratectomy. Optical zone centration analysis. *Ophthalmology* 102:951–962, 1995.

65. Lin DTC. Corneal topographic analysis after excimer photorefractive keratectomy. *Ophthalmology* 101:1432–1439, 1994.

66. Colin J, Cochener B, Gallinaro C. Central steep islands immediately following excimer photorefractive keratectomy for myopia. *Refract Corneal Surg* 9:395–396, 1993.

67. Krueger RR, Saedy NF, McDonnell PJ. Clinical analysis of topographic steep central islands following excimer laser photorefractive keratectomy (PRK). *Arch Ophthalmol* 114:377–381, 1996.

68. Parker PJ, et al. Central topographic islands following photorefractive keratectomy. *Invest Ophthalmol Vis Sci* 34(Suppl.):803, 1993.

69. Hersh PS, et al. Corneal topography of phase III excimer laser photorefractive keratectomy. Characterization and clinical effects. *Ophthalmology* 102:963–978, 1995.

70. Schmidt-Petersen H, et al. Central islands detected by two different devices of corneal topography. Presented at Meeting of the American Society of Cataract and Refractive Surgery, San Diego, April 3, 1995.

71. Malley DS, et al. Immunofluorescence study of corneal wound healing after excimer laser anterior keratectomy in the monkey eye. *Arch Ophthalmol* 108:1316–1322, 1990.

72. SundarRaj N, et al. Healing of excimer laser ablated monkey corneas: An immunohistochemical evaluation. *Arch Ophthalmol* 108:1604–1610, 1990.

73. Fitzsimmons TD, et al. Hyaluronic acid in the rabbit corneal after excimer laser superficial keratectomy. *Invest Ophthalmol Vis Sci* 33:3011–3016, 1992.

74. Fantes F, et al. Wound healing after excimer laser keratomileusis (photorefractive keratectomy) in monkeys. *Arch Ophthalmol* 108:665–675, 1990.

75. Lohmann CP, et al. Corneal light scattering after excimer laser photorefractive keratectomy: The objective measurement of haze. *Refract Corneal Surg* 8:114–121, 1992.

76. Lohmann CP, et al. Corneal light scattering and visual performance in myopic individuals with spectacles, contact lenses, or excimer laser photorefractive keratectomy. *Am J Ophthalmol* 115:444–453, 1993.

77. Seiler T, et al. Aspheric photorefractive keratectomy with excimer laser. *Refract Corneal Surg* 9:166–172, 1993.

78. Harrison JM, et al. Forward light scatter at one month after photo-refractive keratectomy. *J Refract Surg* 11:83–88, 1995.
79. Lin JC, et al. Myopic excimer laser photorefractive keratectomy: An analysis of clinical correlations. *Refract Corneal Surg* 6:321–328, 1990.
80. Ficker LA, et al. Excimer laser photorefractive keratectomy for myopia: 12 month follow-up. *Eye* 7:617–624, 1993.
81. Ehlers N, Hjortdal JO. Excimer laser refractive keratectomy for high myopia: 6-month follow-up of patients treated bilaterally. *Acta Ophthalmol* 70:578–586, 1992.
82. VISX FDA data. Transcript of Proceedings, Ophthalmic Devices Panel Meeting, Gaithersburg, MD, October 1995.
83. Pop M, Aras M. Multizone/multipass photorefractive keratectomy: six months. *J Cataract Refract Surg* 21:633–643, 1995.
84. Caubert E. Cause of subepithelial corneal haze over 18 months after photorefractive keratectomy for myopia. *Refract Corneal Surg* 9(Suppl.): S65–S70, 1993.
85. Dutt S, et al. One-year results of excimer laser photorefractive keratectomy for low to moderate myopia. *Arch Ophthalmol* 112:1427–1436, 1994.
86. Pallikaris I, et al. T-PRK for low myopia: 6 month clinical results. *J Refract Surg* 12:240–247, 1996.
87. Seiler T, McDonnell PJ. Excimer laser photorefractive keratectomy. *Survey Ophthalmol* 40:89–118, 1995.
88. Busin M, Meller D. Corneal epithelial dots following excimer laser photorefractive keratectomy. *J Refract Corneal Surg* 10:357–359, 1994.
89. Vrabec MP, Durrie DS, Chase DS. Recurrence of herpes simplex after excimer laser keratectomy. *Am J Ophthalmol* 116:101–102, 1992.
90. Vrabec MP, et al. Electron microscopic findings in a cornea with recurrence of herpes simplex keratitis after excimer laser photo-therapeutic keratectomy. *CLAO J* 20:41–44, 1994.
91. McDonnell PJ, et al. Photorefractive keratectomy for astigmatism. Initial clinical results. *Arch Ophthalmol* 109:1370, 1991.
92. Tervo T, Tuunanen T. Excimer laser and reactivation of herpes simplex keratitis. *CLAO J* 20:152–157, 1994.
93. Fagerholm P, Ohman L, Orndahl M. Phototherapeutic keratectomy in herpes simplex keratitis. Clinical results in 20 patients. *Acta Ophthalmol* 72:457–460, 1994.
94. Pepose JS, et al. Reactivation of latent herpes simplex virus by excimer laser photokeratectomy. *Am J Ophthalmol* 114:45–50, 1992.
94a. Seiler T, et al. Stress wave amplitude after laser surgery of the cornea. *Invest Ophthalmol Vis Sci* (in press).
95. Hoffer KJ. Intraocular lens power calculation for eyes after refractive keratotomy. *J Refract Surg* 116:490–493, 1995.
96. Young JA, Talamo JH. A new parameter substitutes for keratometry after photorefractive keratectomy. *Ophthalmology* (in press).
97. McDonald MB, et al. Central photorefractive keratectomy for myopia. The blind eye study. *Arch Ophthalmol* 108:799–808, 1990.

98. Waked NE, Ojeimi GK. Excimer laser photorefractive keratectomy in Lebanon. *J Refract Surg* 11(Suppl.):S270–S273, 1995.

99. Lavery FL. Photorefractive keratectomy in 472 eyes. *Refract Corneal Surg* 9(Suppl.):598, 1993.

100. Kim JH, et al. Some problems after photorefractive keratectomy. *J Refract Corneal Surg* 10(Suppl.):S226–S230, 1994.

101. JanKnecht P, Soriano JM, Hansen LL. Cystoid macular oedema after excimer laser photorefractive keratectomy. *Br J Ophthalmol* 77:681, 1993.

102. Caroll RP, Lindstrom RL. Blepharoptosis after radial keratotomy. *Am J Ophthalmol* 102:800–801, 1986.

Phototherapeutic Keratectomy (PTK)

6 PTK: Indications, Surgical Techniques, Postoperative Care, and Complications Management

Dimitri T. Azar, Jonathan H. Talamo, Marco C. Helena,
Walter J. Stark, Shu-Wen Chang, and Sandeep Jain

PTK: General Considerations

Excimer laser phototherapeutic keratectomy (PTK) has great potential to treat visually significant corneal opacities and to smooth corneal surface irregularities. The excimer laser provides corneal surgeons with an excellent cutting instrument for the management of anterior stromal opacities [1], as the depth and shape of tissue removal can be accurately controlled [1–4], facilitating exact removal of the stroma and providing a relatively smooth base for better re-epithelialization [1, 3, 5].

As opposed to manual keratectomy surgery, there is a very clear boundary between the treated and untreated area following PTK at the histologic level [6]. With PTK, re-epithelialization and wound healing begin shortly after surgery and are associated with a small degree of tissue reorganization [6, 7]. Compared to the 193-nm argon fluoride (ArF) excimer laser [6], incisions made with diamond and steel blades produce relatively irregular and more diffuse tissue damage. The 193-nm ArF laser improves on the 248-nm krypton excimer laser, which produces irregular and scattered areas of tissue damage. With PTK, patients may potentially postpone or avoid more invasive surgical procedures, such as penetrating or lamellar keratoplasty [5].

Although excimer photoablation offers significant theoretical and technical advantages, limitations also exist. Many ocular surface disorders are easily and effectively treated with more conventional, time-honored, and less expensive medical and surgical therapies. These include bandage contact lenses and anterior stromal micropuncture for recurrent erosion syndrome or manual superficial keratectomy for corneal nodules such as encountered in keratoconus

Table 6-1. Management of ocular surface disorders

Lubrication
Bandage contact lenses
Epithelial debridement
Anterior stromal micropuncture
Manual superficial keratectomy
Excimer phototherapeutic keratectomy

or Salzmann's nodular degeneration (Table 6-1). Such techniques are, and continue to be, an integral part of the corneal surgeon's therapeutic armamentarium. PTK should be viewed as an adjunct to, not an expensive replacement for, these procedures.

Indications and Contraindications

Indications for PTK differ from those of photorefractive keratectomy (PRK) utilized for the treatment of myopia and astigmatism (Table 6-2). Indications for PTK include opacities resulting from surgical or nonsurgical trauma, corneal inflammations, dystrophies, and degenerations limited to the anterior one-third of the cornea. Of 271 consecutive PTK cases at 17 VISX (Santa Clara, CA) centers in the United States reviewed by Sanders [8], 55% of patients had corneal scars or leukomas, 39% had corneal dystrophies, and 5% had corneal surface irregularities.

Surface irregularities resulting from epithelial dystrophies, Reis-Bückler's dystrophy, band keratopathy, and corneal surgical procedures can be improved with PTK, particularly if the surface irregularities are associated with significant visual impairment. PTK is less effective in treating deep scars, nodules, and band keratopathy. Calculated posttreatment corneal thickness should not be less than 250 mm. The use of PTK to treat microbial keratitis, including infectious crystalline keratopathy [9–12] is also very limited because of the risk of spreading microorganisms during treatment [13].

Keratoconjunctivitis sicca, uncontrolled uveitis, severe blepharitis, lagophthalmos, and systemic immunosuppression may constitute contraindications to PTK under many circumstances. Hyperopia is a relative contraindication because PTK often results in further flattening of the cornea. Following PTK in human corneas, hyperopic shifts have frequently been observed [5, 14–19]. In a series of 35 PTKs, Sher at al. [15] observed hyperopic shift in 50%. Campos et al. [17] detected hyperopic shift in 56% of 18 consecutive cases.

Deep ablation in the central cornea associated with treatment of central pathology causes central flattening and a hyperopic shift. This may be desirable if the eye is myopic but not hyperopic preopera-

Table 6-2. PTK indications

Corneal opacities
  Dystrophies
    Anterior basement membrane
    Reis-Bückler's
    Granular
    Lattice
    Schnyder's crystalline
  Scars
    Posttraumatic
    Postsurgical
    Postinfectious
  Other
    Band keratopathy
    Climatic droplet keratopathy
    Active infectious processes
Irregular surfaces
  Anterior basement membrane and other dystrophies
  Post-pterygium removal
  Salzmann's nodular degeneration
  Band keratopathy
  Climatic droplet keratopathy
Epithelial breakdown
  Recurrent erosion
  Band keratopathy
Irregular astigmatism

tively. In contrast, relatively greater ablation in the paracentral cornea is associated with relative central steepening and a myopic change and is more desirable if the eye is hyperopic preoperatively (Plate 22). Excessive PTK in the paracentral cornea, however, can induce unwanted astigmatism, especially at the edge of the ablation zone.

Preoperative Evaluation

Preoperative evaluation typically includes visual acuity, visual potential (evaluated with pinhole, hard contact lens, or potential acuity meter), pupil size, slit-lamp biomicroscopy, and dilated fundus examination. It should also include the type and depth of pathology, proximity to the center of the pupil, and refractive error. Preoperative determination of the type of pathology and the ablation characteristics are important to plan the most effective procedure. The excimer laser is effective for removal of pathology in Bowman's layer or in the anterior stroma. Disorders such as map-dot-fingerprint dystrophy and

Salzmann's nodular degeneration can usually be scraped mechanically off Bowman's layer. Excimer laser can remove residual nodules and smooth the surface if mechanical removal is incomplete. The depth of the intended treatment can be determined using optical pachymetry. The clinical outcome is best if the treatment is limited to pathology in the anterior 100 μm of the stroma. Central corneal surface irregularities and anterior stromal opacities are good indications for PTK, unlike lesions in the periphery, because the latter are generally not visually significant. An important principle to remember when examining patients is that it is often possible to achieve a satisfactory visual result without ablating the opacity completely. This is particularly true for cases of stromal dystrophy, where partial removal of tissue opacities may dramatically improve visual function but still leave easily visible dystrophic material behind.

Surgical Technique: Diagnosis-Specific Considerations

Corneal Opacities and Dystrophies

Treatment of anterior corneal opacities has been shown to produce significant improvement of visual function [5]. However, with deeper postinfectious and posttraumatic scars, visual improvement is less likely to occur [15, 17]. The scar may ablate at a different rate than the adjacent normal stroma, resulting in an irregular corneal surface if masking agents are not used. Peripheral elevated nodules may be treated with laser ablation after truncation with sharp blades. Central elevated nodules remain a major operative challenge.

Corneal scars that have been successfully treated with PTK to improve visual function include postinfectious, posttraumatic, herpetic, trachomatous climatic droplet keratopathy and pterygium-related scars. Greater success has been achieved with superficial corneal scars, such as those following pterygium surgery (Fig. 6-1) than with deeper postinfectious and posttraumatic scars. Despite the reported success in treating herpetic scars (Fig. 6-2), several investigators caution against using the excimer laser in herpetic disease because of the risk of recurrence [5, 17, 20, 21].

Recurrence of the primary pathology in penetrating keratoplasty for corneal dystrophies is not uncommon. Patients with superficial stromal and epithelial basement membrane dystrophies (Schnyder's, Reis-Bückler, granular, and Lattice) may respond well to PTK, thus obviating the need for conventional penetrating keratoplasty (Fig. 6-3). Patients with recurrent granular or lattice dystrophy in a graft have relatively superficial lesions. The success rate in these cases is very high and is similar to that for primary Reis-Bückler's dystrophy,

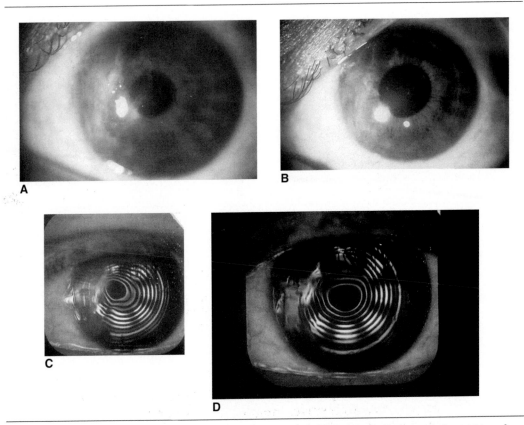

Fig. 6-1. PTK for post-pterygium scarring. Appearance of cornea before (**A**) and 1 week after (**B**) excimer PTK. BCVA with spectacles was 20/80 before surgery and 20/25 with +1.00–2.75 × 175 1 week after surgery. Photokeratoscopy demonstrates improved regularity of the central mire (Preop **C**, Postop **D**). (From JH Talamo, RF Steinert, CA Puliafito. Clinical strategies for excimer laser phototherapeutic keratectomy. *Refract Corneal Surg* 8:319–324, 1992.)

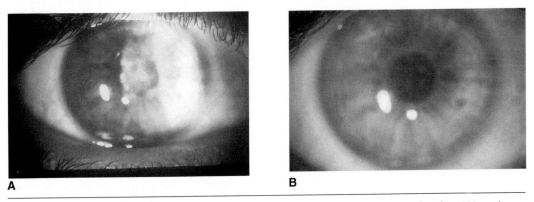

Fig. 6-2. Herpetic anterior stromal scar before (**A**) and 6 months after (**B**) excimer PTK. (From JH Talamo, RF Steinert, CA Puliafito. Clinical strategies for excimer laser phototherapeutic keratectomy. *Refract Corneal Surg* 8:319–324, 1992.)

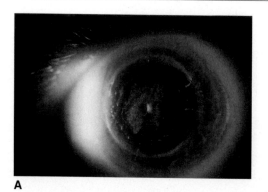 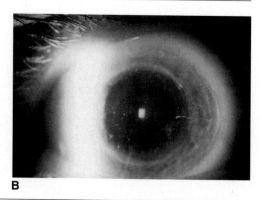

A   B

Fig. 6-3. PTK for recurrent granular dystrophy. This 56-year-old female patient
developed recurrent granular corneal dystrophy 12 years following penetrating
keratoplasty. Best corrected visual acuity (BCVA) was 20/100 corrected with −0.25
+ 2.75 × 157 (**A**). One year following excimer PTK (45 microns central depth with
an edge modification using a 2.0 mm spot diameter delivering 200 microns of
treatment at the periphery for 360 degrees), the cornea is smooth and free of
haze (**B**). BCVA was 20/30 with −1.5–2.25 × 45 of spectacle correction.

in which the deposits are limited to Bowman's layer [5]. Most patients achieve a relatively smooth ablation bed when treated through
the epithelium. For patients with granular dystrophy, the objective is
to ablate most of the areas of diffuse haze between the granular
deposits and not necessarily all the granular hyaline deposits. In
treating these anterior corneal pathologies in which the surface is
smooth, it may be advisable to leave the epithelium intact and ablate
through it, taking advantage of the epithelium's capacity to act as a
smoothing agent that fills in small irregularities. Once the pathology
is encountered, however, the treatment should be halted and masking fluid applied as needed to provide for a smoother ablation of the
now uneven surface.

Infectious Keratitis

Although the treatment of active infectious keratitis with PTK has
been reported, this practice has not met with widespread acceptance
[9–12] and should be discouraged. Stromal involvement in most
corneal infections extends deeper than the clinically evident lesion.
Given that tissue penetration depth of 193-nm radiation is at most 1
micron, it is unlikely that PTK could be used to treat mid- or deep
stromal infiltrates. In addition, dissemination of microorganisms as a
result of PTK treatment is also of great concern [13].

Surface Irregularities

Following epithelial removal, whether manually or by laser, a masking fluid (0.3% carboxymethylcellulose [Refresh Plus], 1% carboxymethylcellulose [Celluvisc], or 0.3% hydroxypropyl methylcellulose and 0.1% dextran [Tears Naturale]) is usually applied to improve the smoothness of the stromal surface. The fluid in valleys prevents ablation of underlying tissue, leaving the exposed peaks to be ablated. Comparing the smoothing effects on irregular corneal surfaces of Tears Naturale II, 1% carboxymethylcellulose sodium (Celluvisc), and 0.9% saline (Unisol), Kornmehl et al. [22] obtained better results in the Tears II treatment group. More recently, synthetic human collagen gels have been used with promising results. This material has an ablation rate similar to stroma and can be used to make a mold of an irregular corneal surface, which is placed on the cornea during PTK.

Corneal scars causing surface irregularity that have been successfully treated with PTK to improve visual function include those due to pterygium removal (see Fig. 6-1) (smooth and rough) and apical scars or nodules in keratoconus (Fig. 6-4). Removal of apical nodules in keratoconus by excimer PTK may result in a smoother surface than that resulting from manual techniques, and dramatically improved contact lens tolerance has been reported [23]. Treatment of band keratopathy has proven difficult. The use of ethylenediaminetetraacetic acid (EDTA) combined with manual debridement is still the standard treatment for this condition, with PTK employed as a last resort [5, 15, 17, 20]. Anecdotal reports have suggested that PTK may

Fig. 6-4. Apical corneal nodule. Appearance before (**A**) and immediately after (**B**) excimer PTK. Methylcellulose 1% was used to shield adjacent normal corneal tissue during photoablation with 242 pulses using a 1 mm spot diameter. (From JH Talamo, RF Steinert, CA Puliafito. Clinical strategies for excimer laser phototherapeutic keratectomy. *Refract Corneal Surg* 8:319–324, 1992.)

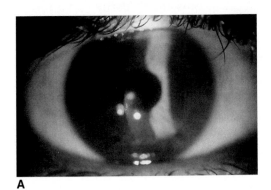

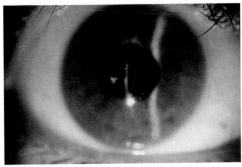

A   B

help delay the need for penetrating keratoplasty or conjuctival flap procedures in cases of painful bullous keratopathy.

Recurrent Corneal Erosions

Conventional surgical methods of treating recurrent corneal erosions include manual epithelial debridement and anterior stromal puncture. Patients with recalcitrant recurrent corneal erosions (not relieved by conventional surgery) may benefit from excimer PTK. In the treatment of recurrent epithelial erosion, it is important to draw an accurate corneal map showing where the recurrent epithelial breakdown occurs. All loose epithelium should be meticulously removed with a microsponge or blade, or both. This usually encompasses a larger area than the area of recurrent epithelial breakdown itself. In most cases, the use of surface modulators before laser ablation is not necessary. After epithelial debridement, a cellulose sponge can be used to sweep any residual deposits. The laser is then centered over the area of recurrent breakdown and fired. The treatment depth is relatively minimal (3–8 microns) and is usually limited to Bowman's layer. Accordingly, significant postoperative hyperopic shift is not observed, and corneal wound healing is less prolonged.

Irregular Astigmatism

Irregular astigmatism is a refractive error that cannot be corrected with spherocylindrical spectacle lenses. Corneal surface abnormalities often cause irregular astigmatism. These surface changes need not be extensive and often arise from small, focal abnormalities within visually significant portions of the cornea. Irregular astigmatism is common after lamellar keratoplasty, penetrating keratoplasty, or corneal trauma, though, and focal surface elevations or depressions are often not visible by slit-lamp examination. In such cases, corneal topography prior to surgery is essential because it allows the surgeon to perform at least a rough calculation of how much tissue elevation to remove in a specific area of cornea with respect to a particular reference point, such as the pupil center. Stepwise techniques for the treatment of irregular astigmatism are discussed in greater detail below (see Treating Irregular Astigmatism).

Surgical Technique: Specific Intraoperative Considerations

Surgical technique and judgment is perhaps more critical in PTK than in PRK because the individual treatment may require customization.

Deciding when to terminate the laser treatment, in particular, is a matter of experienced judgment. During laser ablation, the cornea becomes opaque from drying, making the intraoperative evaluation of the amount of residual scar difficult. To accomplish this, slit-lamp examination may need to be performed after the initial ablation to determine whether further treatment is required. In addition to serial slit-lamp examinations, identification of corneal abnormalities at a level consistent with maximal treatment can be a useful tool in judging treatment depth. If necessary, the patient should be repositioned under the laser and additional laser pulses administered until a satisfactory result is achieved. Because repeating PTK is simpler than restoring excised tissue, it is much better to err on the conservative side and initially undertreat patients.

PTK Technique Algorithm

To avoid the complications of unintended refractive changes, decentered ablations, and incomplete excision of corneal lesions, it is useful to have in mind some type of treatment algorithm or mental flowchart when approaching each patient. With careful attention not only to the type of pathology but also its horizontal and vertical configuration within the cornea and with respect to the central optical zone overlying the pupil, more consistent results should be achievable. A proposed algorithm for an approach to PTK technique is given in Figure 6-5.

Laser Calibration and Operation

The laser is calibrated before each treatment session to ensure optimal performance, as it would be for PRK procedures. The operation of the laser is confirmed by ablating a standard treatment into a calibration plate made of polymethylmethacrylate (PMMA) test block or other material, depending on the laser used. The appropriate corneal ablation rate is generally determined using nomograms and is entered into the laser computer program in a manner similar to that previously described for PRK. Nitrogen gas flow, used during the PMMA calibration in some lasers, is rarely used today [14].

Epithelial and Stromal Ablation: Basic Approaches

The decision whether to ablate using the laser or to remove the epithelium manually is based on the smoothness of the epithelium relative to the expected smoothness of Bowman's layer. The ultimate goal is to achieve as smooth a surface as possible after photoablation, thus minimizing irregular astigmatism. The epithelium is ablated with the laser if the epithelial surface is smooth and the anterior stromal

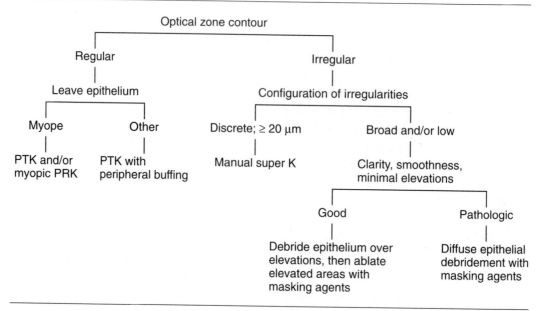

Fig. 6-5. PTK technique algorithm. (Adapted from JH Talamo, RF Steinert, CA Puliafito. Clinical strategies for excimer laser phototherapeutic keratectomy. *J Refract Corneal Surg* 8:319–324, 1992.)

surface is judged to be irregular and, in this manner, acts as a built-in masking agent (Fig. 6-6). If the anterior stromal surface is judged to be smooth, the epithelium may be removed manually with a Bard-Parker blade or a blunt spatula. In some cases, however, the epithelium is strongly attached to the underlying corneal layers, and it is difficult to remove. Adjunctive chemical de-epithelialization techniques (e.g., EDTA in band keratopathy or dilute ethanol solutions 10–18%) may occasionally be helpful.

A transition zone is usually created during stromal ablation to allow for better re-epithelialization over the ablation bed. Sher et al. [15] used a smoothing technique in their early cases, wherein the eye was moved in a circular manner under the laser beam. A similar polishing technique was used in the Summit (Waltham, MA) excimer laser clinical trials [24, 25]. The surgeon moved the patient's head in a brisk controlled circular manner under the laser beam to "polish" the corneal surface. Stark et al. [5] later described a modified taper technique, wherein the surgeon attempts to decrease central flattening by moving the eye under the laser in a circular fashion and treating the circumference of the ablation zone with a 200-micron deep, 2-mm diameter spot. This edge modification creates a ring-shaped ablation pattern at the periphery of the PTK to reduce the hyperopic shift that

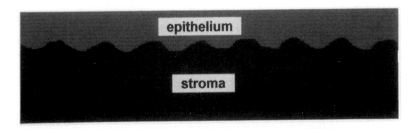

Fig. 6-6. Smoothing effect of the corneal epithelium on underlying stromal irregularities.

is commonly seen after PTK. It is important and worth stressing that the objective of PTK should be to reduce the pathology to a point where nature's own smoothing agent, the epithelium, can take over and create a smooth tear-air interface. Excessive treatment increases the risk of inducing large refractive changes and stromal scarring.

Varying Ablation Rates Among Tissues

The ablation rates of different corneal tissue constituents by the excimer laser have been extensively studied [26–29]. When the energy density (fluence) of 193-nm excimer laser light exceeds a critical value, individual molecular bonds are irreversibly broken, leading to tissue ablation. Different molecular structures have different ablation rates, and, consequently, so do different tissue components. The ablation rate of the epithelium is the highest, followed in descending order by stroma, Bowman's layer, corneal scar, and calcium deposit. If laser energy is applied directly to a surface where tissues of variable ablation rates coexist, such as calcium deposits in band keratopathy or stromal scars of any etiology, the resulting treatment surface may be irregular (Fig. 6-7A). In these cases, masking fluids are indicated during ablation. Depending on their viscosity and surface tension, masking fluids are able to fill in depressions and expose elevations of an irregular corneal surface. These substances absorb laser energy, shielding tissue components with higher ablation rates while over-exposing tissues with lower ablation rates (Fig. 6-7B).

A variety of substances can be used for masking purposes. The most important principle of technique is to use just enough fluid to coat the "valleys," or tissue depressions, while leaving "peaks" or elevations exposed, otherwise excessive ablation may be required. A highly viscous fluid (1–2% hydroxymethylcellulose or sodium hyaluronate [Healon]) does not cover an irregular surface uniformly and tends to

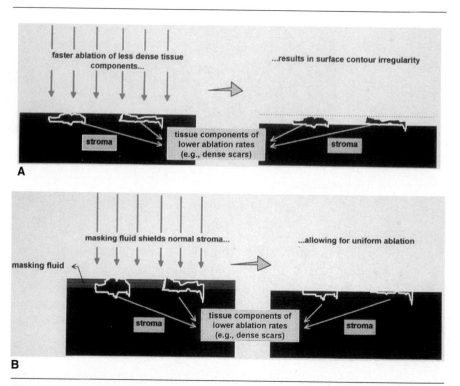

Fig. 6-7. **A.** Variable ablation rate of different tissue contstituents. **B.** Shielding effect of masking fluids. (Adapted from J Marshall et al. Photoablative reprofiling of the cornea using an excimer laser: Photorefractive keractectomy. *Laser Ophthalmol* 1:23–44, 1986.)

partially cover peaks as well as valleys. A fluid of low viscosity (hydroxypropyl-methylcellulose 0.1% with dextran [Tears Naturale II]) may expose both peaks and valleys. In our experience, carboxymethylcellulose 0.5% (Refresh Plus) offers the appropriate viscosity to efficiently shield most superficial focal elevated pathology. It is often necessary to have both types of masking agent present and to determine by trial and error which substance is most appropriate. In addition to creating a smooth corneal surface, masking agents may reduce the amount of induced hyperopia. When rather large peaks or "chunks" of pathology are present, a surgical blade and 0.12-mm forceps are used to debride as much abnormal material as possible, followed by laser treatment using a masking agent. Use of the laser alone to ablate the large bulky lesions would require such a large number of pulses that there would be a significant risk of ablating deeply into the surrounding tissue or inducing excessive refractive changes.

Selection of Ablation Zone Size Parameters

Paracentral anterior stromal lesions are common indications for PTK as they may decrease visual acuity by blocking the entrance of light rays (opacity) and/or by causing irregular astigmatism as well as glare and light scattering. Although treating each lesion with an appropriately sized ablation zone diameter set according to the size of the lesion can potentially decrease the total amount of tissue ablation, asymmetric paracentral ablations may induce significant irregular astigmatism. Glare and monocular diplopia may result if the margins of paracentral ablations are too close to the center of the entrance pupil. As such, small, elevated paracentral lesions are often best treated with manual superficial keratectomy alone or in combination with PTK. Alternatively, paracentral lesions may be treated with large optical zones centered over the entrance pupil, using masking agents to shield areas of normal corneal tissue as necessary.

Minimizing Hyperopic Shift

The PTK mode of photoablation was designed to ablate corneal tissue uniformly without altering surface refractive power. Thus, the surface profile of a standard PMMA test block is preserved after applying excimer laser with a PTK beam profile, but this is not the case for corneal tissue, where a hyperopic refractive shift often occurs. Possible mechanisms for the hyperopic shift after PTK are as follows: (1) ablation products may provide greater shielding toward the edge of the ablation zone if deposited in a centrifugal fashion (Fig. 6-8A); (2) the decreasing angle of incidence of the laser beam on more peripheral cornea may reduce laser efficacy as the edge of the ablation zone is approached (Fig. 6-8B); and (3) the abrupt margins of the ablation zone following PTK may result in peripheral epithelial and stromal hyperplasia, thus creating a myopic lens effect (Fig. 6-8C).

As mentioned previously, strategies to reduce hyperopic shift have been developed. Sher et al. [15] initially described a smoothing technique in which the eye was moved via head rotation in a circular manner under a laser beam of varying aperture size. This has been termed the *buff-and-polish technique*, and it is still useful in some situations. Later, the same authors decided to perform a hyperopic ablation immediately following an initial therapeutic ablation. Stark et al. [5] attempted to decrease or even reverse central flattening by setting the laser depth at 200 μm and the diameter at 2 mm and firmly grasping the patient's head to move the eye under the laser beam, treating the margins of the ablation zone with a 20-μm deep, 2-mm diameter annulus. A case successfully treated in this manner is illustrated in Plates 22 through 24.

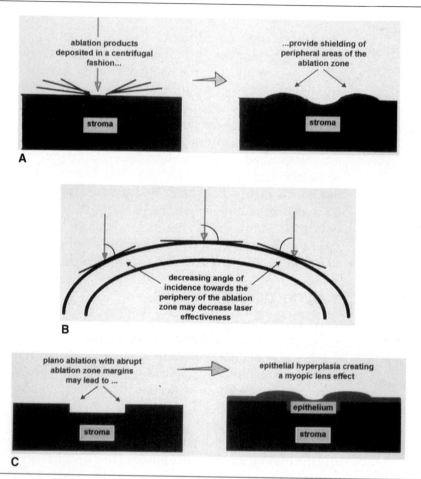

Fig. 6-8. **A–C.** Possible mechanisms of hyperopic shift after PTK.

A positive correlation between depth of PTK ablation and hyperopic shift has been detected [16, 18]. Therefore, monitoring the depth of ablation required in each case is extremely important to avoid unnecessary tissue removal. When removing stromal opacities, it is often difficult to assess ablation depth with the patient supine under the operating microscope. Tissue should be excised conservatively, frequently returning the patient to an upright position to allow for intraoperative slit-lamp examination. It is wiser to proceed in a stepwise fashion, adding more treatment as needed, than to irreversibly overtreat a patient.

Inducing Myopic Shift

To induce a myopic shift, the cornea must be more deeply ablated in the periphery than at the center. Although less common than induced hyperopia, myopic shifts can occur following PTK, as illustrated in Plates 22 through 24. Sher et al. [15] observed myopic shift in 3% of PTK-treated patients, and Campos et al. [17] observed myopic shift in 16.6%. The exact mechanism of induced myopia is not always clear, but if the treatment is directed to paracentral areas with the central cornea protected by masking agents, such an effect can be achieved [20].

Minimizing Decentration

Centration of PTK is variable because it depends heavily on the distribution of surgical pathology. In cases where extensive treatment is required, the ablation zone should be large and centered, as in PRK. Treatment of small lesions, however, is generally centered over the lesions themselves, with the laser spot diameter adjusted according to the size of the lesion. When such lesions are peripheral or paracentral, surgeons should proceed with caution, utilizing adjunctive manual superficial keratectomy whenever possible because treatment can result in irregular astigmatism or myopic shift.

Technical factors that may induce decentration include (1) inappropriate patient fixation, (2) misalignment of the laser beam and the microscope, and (3) use of miotics before the surgery, which may nasally displace the center of the physiologic entrance pupil in a small subpopulation of individuals. Treatment should be interrupted as soon as poor centration is noted. Once adequate centration is obtained, ablation should be resumed after ensuring an appropriate degree of corneal stromal hydration and reapplication of a masking agent, if indicated.

Treating Irregular Astigmatism

Correction of irregular astigmatism in the absence of focal pathology has not been possible using previously available keratorefractive surgical technology, and photoablative techniques for this indication are in their infancy. Using a topographic map as a guide, Gibralter et al. [30] created a custom excimer ablation program designed to treat irregular astigmatism after penetrating keratoplasty (see Fig. 6-6). The program consisted of a combination of phototherapeutic and photorefractive ablation patterns. After identifying high, steep areas of cornea, the authors ablated them by local, focal treatment using small-diameter ablations (≤ 4 mm). This technique neutralized the irregular astigmatism by minimizing the differences between steeper and flatter geographic areas within the optical zone. The 4-mm laser treatments were placed over the steeper corneal zones and then residual myopia was corrected by treating directly over the entrance pupil, as in PRK for myopia. Based on the preoperative corneal topographic analysis, the amount of tissue to be removed was calculated on the basis of the diameter and steepness of the irregular areas of the corneal surface.

Using a similar approach, Talamo et al. [31] corrected irregular astigmatism in conjunction with residual myopia and ablation decentration after PRK. Plates 25 and 26 illustrate computerized video-keratography (CVK) maps before and after successful retreatment.

Improvements in analysis and treatment, especially those which combine topographical analysis of actual corneal elevation (rather than reflected ring images) with control of the pattern of photoablation with scanning-slit or flying-spot lasers (see Chaps. 14 and 15 and Chaps. 16–18, respectively), may be helpful in treating irregular astigmatism. In this way, a more regular surface might be achieved, as evidenced by smooth topography, reduced refractive astigmatism, and a more rapid progression to improved uncorrected visual acuity.

Routine Postoperative Management

Postoperative medications include prophylactic antibiotics and anti-inflammatory agents. Injection of corticosteroid and antibiotic beneath Tenon's capsule at the conclusion of surgery is optional. After topical application of antibiotic ointment (bacitracin and erythromycin) and instillation of a cycloplegic agent (homatropine), the eye is patched. Alternatively, a therapeutic soft contact lens is applied with frequent application of topical antibiotic drugs. Because the patient may experience severe pain in the first 24 hours, topical nonsteroidal anti-inflammatory drugs (NSAIDs) and systemic sedative-analgesics may be needed for the first few days. One percent (1%) prednisolone acetate or 0.1% dexamethasone phosphate drops are used 4 times daily for 1 week, then tapered to once daily for 1 month. In many compromised corneas undergoing PTK, the benefits of continued steroid drops may be outweighed by the potential side effects of steroid-responsive intraocular pressure (IOP), cataract, and risk of microbial infection or recurrent herpetic disease.

Patients are generally examined every 24–48 hours until re-epithelialization is complete, and then at 1 month, 3 months, 6 months, 12 months, and 24 months. Re-epithelialization occurs within 1 week in most patients. Following re-epithelialization, the postoperative examination at each visit includes symptomatic evaluation, CVK, manifest refraction, and a detailed anterior segment examination.

Corneal haze is graded subjectively using slit-lamp biomicroscopic examination, as suggested by many investigators:

0 = clear
0.5 = barely detectable
1.0 = mild, not affecting refraction
1.5 = mildly affecting refraction
2.0 = moderate, refraction possible but difficult
3.0 = opacity preventing refraction, anterior chamber easily viewed
4.0 = impaired view of anterior chamber
5.0 = anterior chamber not visible

For examples of corneal haze grading after PRK, please see Figure 5-5 and Plates 10–12.

Postoperative Complications

Postoperative complications of PTK are summarized in Table 6-3. Because many of these problems are not unique to PTK and are addressed in Chapter 5, here we focus on the issues unique or most relevant to PTK.

Postoperative Optical Complications

A smooth and regular anterior corneal surface following PTK results in a better visual outcome. The corneal epithelium plays a critical role

Table 6-3. Postoperative PTK complications

Optical
  Hyperopic shift
  Myopic shift
  Irregular astigmatism
  Decentration
  Glare, halos, polyopia
  Residual opacity
Medical
  Pain
  Persistent epithelial defect
  Infection
  Incomplete treatment (opacity, irregularity)
  Recurrent dystrophy or degeneration
  Excessive stromal scarring
  HSV keratitis reactivation
  Endothelial decompensation
  Graft rejection

HSV = herpes simplex virus.

in modulating such smoothnes by compensating for certain degrees of stromal irregularity, as illustrated in Fig. 6-6. However, even seemingly small changes in the anterior stromal profile may significantly alter the refractive characteristics of the corneal surface, resulting in myopic or hyperopic shifts as well as irregular astigmatism and its attendant symptomatology (glare, halos, polyopia). As with almost any keratorefractive surgical procedure, careful surgical planning and meticulous attention to detail intraoperatively to prevent unwanted refractive shifts is the best therapy for such problems.

If the patient experiences significant optical aberrations following PTK, retreatment may or may not be indicated because PTK is often used as a final attempt to avoid more invasive surgery, such as lamellar or penetrating keratoplasty. Although there is often little risk to performing repeat PTK, one should carefully assess the potential for additional visual or symptomatic benefit.

Postoperative Medical Complications

Pain

The human cornea is innervated by the ciliary nerves, which originate from the nasociliary branch of the trigeminal nerve. Sensory impulses are mediated by A delta fibers and C fibers that course from the periphery to the center of the cornea by way of the epithelium and stroma. Following excimer laser ablation, a large number of corneal nerve fibers are severed, which often results in significant pain. Generally, pain begins 30–60 minutes after the procedure and may become severe within 4–6 hours, diminishing steadily over 24–48 hours as re-epithelialization progresses. Because PTK is often performed in corneas that are already medically compromised, postoperative inflammation may occur in excess of that observed after PRK procedures in otherwise healthy eyes. As such, postoperative pain may be a significant problem after PTK, and thus the pathophysiology of this phenomenon warrants detailed discussion.

Arachidonic acid metabolites, such as prostaglandins and leukotrienes, are important biologic mediators of inflammation and pain after excimer photoablation. Arachidonic acid is released into the intracellular space from cell plasma membranes by phospholipases. Prostaglandins and thromboxanes are generated via the cyclooxygenase pathway, whereas leukotrienes arise through the lipoxygenase pathway. Prostaglandins may increase nerve ending sensitivity and produce hyperalgesia. Leukotrienes may increase pain by promoting inflammatory cell chemotaxis.

Initially, management of pain after excimer laser corneal ablation was not satisfactory for a majority of patients. It consisted of counseling and treatment with pressure patching or bandage contact lenses, cycloplegics, ice packing, and oral analgesics, including narcotics. The introduction of topical NSAIDs has greatly improved this situation. In general, these drugs reduce the production of prostaglandins and thromboxanes by inhibiting the cyclooxygenase pathway. Because of lipoxygenase pathway overload, however, some of these drugs can enhance leukotriene production, leading to increased inflammatory cell infiltration, which may appear clinically as corneal infiltrates [32].

Although topical NSAIDs, such as ketorolac tromethamine and flurbiprofen sodium, have been shown to be effective in reducing pain after PRK [33], diclofenac sodium is the agent most extensively studied for corneal excimer laser procedures. Diclofenac has been shown to reduce pain and light sensitivity significantly following PRK [33, 34]. Phillips et al. [32] observed significant reduction of prostaglandin E_2 but increased leukocyte infiltration using diclofenac in PRK-treated rabbit corneas. Interestingly, no detectable changes in the leukotriene B_4 levels (potent chemotactic agents) were found. It has been shown that high doses of diclofenac not only inhibit the cyclooxygenase pathway but also decrease the bioavailability of intracellular arachidonic acid [35].

Szerenyi et al. [36] demonstrated that diclofenac acutely decreases corneal sensitivity when 1 drop is applied every 5 minutes to normal, unoperated human eyes. Sensitivity returns to normal within less than 1 hour after discontinuation of the drug. The mechanism involved is unclear. Although transient hypoesthesia occurs from topical NSAID administration as well as the PRK procedure itself, within 3 months following PRK corneal sensitivity generally returns to preoperative levels, although this return to normal sensitivity may be more delayed after deeper ablations.

Despite claims that diclofenac may delay re-epithelialization, Sher et al. [34] found no significant difference in the re-epithelialization rate between post-PRK patients receiving topical diclofenac qid and controls. In a survey of Canadian surgeons performing PRK, 28 reports (approximately 1 in 250 treated eyes) of subepithelial corneal infiltrates were found in association with pre- and postoperative use of topical NSAIDs (diclofenac or ketorolac) and contact lens fitting [36a]. No patient in this series received topical steroids. Sher et al. [37] reported 1 patient with similar corneal infiltrates and 1 patient with an immune ring among 16 patients treated with topical diclofenac qid, and 1 patient with a corneal infiltrate among 16 patients treated with placebo. However, in a review of 700 consecutive cases of PRK in which either ketorolac or diclofenac were used postoperatively in conjunction with 0.1% fluorometholone and a bandage contact lens, no complications (including corneal infiltrates) were observed in association with this regimen.

Topical steroids are potent anti-inflammatory drugs, stabilizing lysosomal membranes, inhibiting arachidonic acid pathways and decreasing inflammatory cell margination and migration. Fluorometholone has decreased intraocular penetration and may be preferable to prednisolone or dexamethasone preparations so as to minimize topical steroid–induced complications, such as glaucoma, cataract, and ptosis. Campos et al. [38] demonstrated that fluorometholone significantly reduces leukocyte infiltration in rabbit corneas 24 hours after PRK. Based on these data, it is conceivable that fluorometholone may decrease the incidence of corneal infiltrates associated with topical NSAIDs by reducing the influx of inflammatory cells. Because steroids and NSAIDs have synergistic effects, topical regimens combining both drugs are commonly used following excimer laser procedures to control pain and inflammation, supplemented by systemic analgesics as appropriate.

Persistent Epithelial Defects

Rapid and stable re-epithelialization after PTK is desirable for a number of reasons, including the reduction of pain, discomfort, inflammation, and risk of infection as well as the promotion of more rapid improvement of visual acuity. In most cases, the epithelium heals completely within 1 week. However, because corneas undergoing PTK are more often medically compromised than corneas undergoing PRK, cases of persistent epithelial defect [14, 18] or recurrent epithelial erosions [39] are more likely.

The absence of or damage to the remaining Bowman's layer, the toxicity of topical postoperative medications, and the presence of active ocular surface and eyelid inflammatory processes are possible etiologies. Corneal anesthesia may impede epithelial healing, as may abnormalities of eyelid anatomy and globe apposition. Particularly in older patients, consideration should be given to the possibility of a previously undiagnosed or overlooked systemic condition or medication that might compromise epithelial wound healing. Prevention and management of impaired epithelial healing consists of (1) meticulous preoperative control of ocular surface and adnexal disease; (2) patching or bandage contact lens fitting, followed by tarsorrhaphy if needed; (3) proper corneal lubrication; and (4) suspension or substitution of potentially toxic topical medications.

Bacterial Keratitis

The risk of infection after PTK has not been assessed in large-scale prospective clinical trials. However, many indications for PTK are disorders associated with significant ocular surface pathology that may impede healing and potentially allow organisms access to stroma via iatrogenic postoperative epithelial defects.

No reports of bacterial keratitis following manual superficial keratectomy have been published, but the numbers of cases surveyed are small. In the single published report of bacterial infection after PTK, Al-Rajhi et al. [40] encountered bacterial keratitis in 3 of 258 eyes undergoing PTK [40]. The visual outcome was poor in all cases, and all three patients had climatic droplet keratopathy and were infected with gram-positive organisms. No infections were observed in 75 other eyes undergoing PTK for other anterior corneal disorders. The authors concluded that infection after PTK for climatic droplet keratopathy still has a lower incidence than that associated with the natural history of the disease.

As with PRK, the risk of bacterial keratitis is most likely increased by the use of bandage soft contact lenses, but the risk is still considered low and probably worth the increased comfort and decreased epithelial healing time accompanying their use. Appropriate antibiotic prophylaxis and management of the postoperative epithelial defect are advised. Patients with bandage contact lenses should be monitored daily for signs of infection or delayed closure of the epithelial defect.

Incomplete Treatment

Dense corneal scar tissue and calcium deposits are difficult to photoablate. As a result, large numbers of pulses are needed to achieve a given ablation depth. Meticulous use of masking fluids is required to avoid extensive ablation of adjacent normal corneal tissue in the ablation zone. Slit-lamp examination at regular intervals during PTK may ensure adequate treatment.

Unsuccessful treatment of stromal scarring due to its low ablation rate has been reported [41]. Although some surgeons prefer not to treat band keratopathy by PTK for the same reason, O'Brart et al. [39] obtained good results in a series of 122 eyes. In cases of rough band keratopathy, mechanical keratectomy to remove calcific plaques was performed, followed by a PTK to remove focal remnants and to smooth the stromal surface. The same approach has been suggested for treating other pathologies, such as Salzmann's nodular degeneration, where, again, mechanical removal of the lesion should be performed prior to PTK. Such manual debulking procedures minimize the need for excessive photoablation of these areas of abnormal corneal tissue, where tissue ablation rate may fluctuate greatly, even within lesions that have a uniform clinical appearance. Because it is difficult to evaluate the depth of treatment through the operating microscope, careful slit-lamp examination during surgery is instrumental in the intraoperative planning and performance of PTK.

Recurrent Disease or Stromal Scarring

Dystrophic processes often recur following PTK. If the location of the disease process and corneal thickness are appropriate, PTK retreatment can be applied, although never in the setting of active infection or inflammation. It is important to be mindful of the patient's refractive error in the fellow eye; however, the combination of induced anisometropia and contact lens intolerance can be problematic in some situations, even if visual acuity is substantially improved. If appropriate, it may be prudent to reconsider manual superficial keratectomy techniques, which minimize refractive shifts.

As with PRK, visually significant stromal scarring can ensue after PTK. Retreatment is possible in select cases, but watchful waiting for at least 12 months is advised, as many cases of ablation-related haze improve spontaneously. If rapid visual rehabilitation for significant stromal disease is the primary goal, keratoplasty is often a sensible option at this juncture.

Herpes Simplex Virus Reactivation

Herpes simplex virus (HSV) is the most common infectious cause of corneal blindness in the developed world, and herpetic keratitis is the third most common preoperative diagnosis in patients undergoing penetrating keratoplasty. Within 48 hours of primary infection, virions may travel via any of the major divisions of the trigeminal nerve to the trigeminal, ciliary, and sympathetic ganglia, as well as to mesencephalic nuclei of the brainstem, wherein it enters a latent state. There is also evidence that the cornea may serve as a site of latency. Viral shedding and reactivation may occur and may cause infectious blepharoconjunctivitis, keratitis, and keratouveitis. Among the many factors that may trigger HSV reactivation, of special concern for corneal laser surgeons are ultraviolet (UV) light, acoustomechanical trauma, and local immunosuppression.

The most common surgical treatments for herpetic corneal scars are penetrating keratoplasty (PK) and lamellar keratoplasty (LK). Drawbacks of these techniques include (1) risks of major intraocular surgery, (2) increased risk of graft rejection in inflamed and highly vascularized corneas, (3) the frequent need for intensive topical steroid therapy after surgery, and (4) the high cost of donor tissue and operating room time.

PTK is a potential alternative for treatment of superficial herpetic scars and offers a decreased cost. It is possible, however, that HSV reactivation may be induced by excimer laser. McDonnell et al. [42] described one case of herpes epithelial keratitis recurrence 4 weeks following astigmatic PRK in a patient who had undergone penetrating keratoplasty for herpetic stromal scar. Vrabec et al. [21] reported recurrence of herpetic dendritic keratitis 3 months (2 cases) and 18 months (1 case) following PTK to treat stromal scar secondary to recurrent herpetic keratitis. Pepose et al. [43] demonstrated that excimer laser photoablation can reactivate HSV epithelial keratitis in latently infected mice. In addition, one case of disciform keratitis recurred 3 times in a 28-month period following PTK [16]. Therefore, pre- and postoperative prophylaxis with oral acyclovir and perhaps low doses of topical antiviral agents seem appropriate when performing PTK on patients with previous history of HSV blepharoconjunctivitis or keratitis. Topical corticosteroids should be used sparingly in these patients.

Endothelial Cell Damage

The 193-nm excimer laser produces precise etching of corneal tissue with minimal damage to adjacent areas. The laser energy is almost completely absorbed by the ablated corneal tissue without transmission to deeper layers. As such, direct damage to endothelial cells by the excimer laser radiation should not be expected. Endothelial damage can result, however, from indirect effects. Photoablative procedures modify corneal anatomy and physiology: The corneal stroma is reduced in thickness and Bowman's layer is frequently removed [44]. Theoretically, these modifications could affect endothelial metabolism [45]. In addition, the shock waves produced by the impact of each laser pulse can lead to acute mechanical cell trauma [46].

Endothelial injury has been demonstrated in animal models following excimer laser ablation, and it may be of greater theoretical concern with PTK because treatments are often performed on compromised corneas. Marshall et al. [4] performed deep excimer laser incisions in rabbit corneas and found endothelial cell loss when the ablation depth was within 40 μm of Descemet's membrane. Dehm et al. [46] performed excimer laser and diamond knife incisions to 90% of corneal depth in rabbits and observed similar endothelial alterations with both methods.

These experiments do not represent photoablative procedures currently performed in humans. Excimer PRK and PTK involve much more superficial layers of the cornea. Recent clinical trials of PRK have failed to demonstrate endothelial damage or loss. Fantes et al. [47] did not detect any endothelial abnormalities by light and electron transmission microscopy following PRK in monkeys. Amano et al. [48] performed endothelial specular microscopy in a series of 26 eyes undergoing PRK and observed no statistically significant difference in mean cell density or coefficient of variation of mean cell area among preoperative and 1-month and 1-year postoperative measurements. In a series of 14 human eyes, Perez-Santonja et al. [49] observed no change in endothelial cell density and hexagonality 1 year following PRK but significant improvement from preoperative readings of the coefficient of endothelial cell area variation (polymegathism). Carones et al. [44] performed a similar study in 76 eyes undergoing PRK, and after 1 year, not only did the coefficient of cell area variation improve but so did the percentage of hexagonal cells without significant change in cell density. The authors postulated that the postoperative improvement in endothelial cell parameters resulted from discontinuation of contact lens wear and an attendant decrease in chronic corneal hypoxia.

Endothelial damage is a serious concern following new corneal surgical techniques. Currently, there is no indication of clinically significant endothelial damage following PRK or PTK. Nevertheless, corneal surgeons should remain mindful of this possibility because longer-term follow-up is not yet available.

Graft Rejection

The main cause of corneal transplant failure is immune-mediated graft rejection, occurring in 16–30% of recipients. Cellular immune mechanisms appear to play a key role, but humoral components have also been detected. Risk factors include (1) corneal vascularization, (2) graft size and proximity to the limbus, (3) infections, (4) persistent epithelial defects, and (5) other disorders associated with inflammation, including surgical trauma.

Graft rejection has been reported in two cases following excimer photoablation. One patient underwent PTK to treat recurrent lattice dystrophy in a corneal graft [50], and another underwent PRK to reduce postkeratoplasty astigmatism [51]. In both cases, rejection was successfully treated medically. Epstein et al. [51] have altered their protocol to include the use of 1% prednisolone every 2 hours as opposed to 0.1% fluorometholone following excimer photoablation of corneal grafts.

Summary

Excimer PTK is not and should not be a rigidly standardized procedure. Strategies and techniques vary depending on the characteristics of the individual corneal disorder for a specific patient. Although a number of different complications may occur, they are rarely sight threatening. Given the existing alternatives, PTK seems to be a safe and useful technique for the treatment of anterior corneal pathology.

References

1. Marshall J, et al. Photoablative reprofiling of the cornea using an excimer laser: Photorefractive keratectomy. *Laser Ophthalmol* 1:23–44, 1986.
2. Gaster RN, et al. Corneal Surface ablation by 193-nm excimer laser and wound healing in rabbits. *Invest Ophthalmol Vis Sci* 30:90–97, 1989.
3. Trokel SL, Srinivasan R, Braren B. Excimer laser surgery of the cornea. *Am J Ophthalmol* 96:710–715, 1983.
4. Tuft SJ, Zabel RW, Marshall J. Corneal repair following keratectomy. *Invest Ophthalmol Vis Sci* 30:1769–1777, 1989.
5. Stark WJ, et al. Clinical follow-up of 193-nm ArF excimer laser photo-keratectomy. *Ophthalmology* 99:805–811, 1992.
6. Marshall J, et al. A comparative study of corneal incisions induced by diamond and steel knives and two ultraviolet radiations from an excimer laser. *Br J Ophthalmol* 70:482–500, 1986.
7. van Setten GB, et al. Expression of tenascin and fibronectin in the rabbit cornea after excimer laser surgery. *Graefe's Arch Clin Exp Ophthalmol* 230:178–182, 1992.
8. Sanders D. Clinical evaluation of phototherapeutic keratectomy: VISX twenty/twenty excimer laser. FDA submission—written communication February 7, 1994.
9. Keates RH, Drago PC, Rothchild EJ. Effect of excimer laser on micro-biological organisms. *Ophthalmic Surg* 19:715–718, 1988.
10. Gottsch JD, et al. Excimer laser ablative treatment of microbial keratitis. *Ophthalmology* 98:146–149, 1991.
11. Serdarevic O, et al. Excimer laser therapy for experimental *Candida* keratitis. *Am J Ophthalmol* 99:534–538, 1985.
12. Eiferman RA, Forgey DR, Cook YD. Excimer laser ablation of infectious crystalline keratopathy. *Arch Ophthalmol* 110:18, 1992.
13. Krueger RR, et al. Corneal surface morphology following excimer laser ablation with humidified gases. *Arch Ophthalmol* 111:1131, 1993.
14. Hersh PS, et al. Phototherapeutic keratectomy: Strategies and results in 12 eyes. *J Refract Corneal Surg* 9(Suppl.):90–95, 1993.
15. Sher NA, et al. Clinical use of 193-nm excimer laser in the treatment of corneal scars. *Arch Ophthalmol* 109:491–498, 1991.
16. Fagerholm P, et al. Phototherapeutic keratectomy: Long-term results in 166 eyes. *J Refract Corneal Surg* 9(Suppl.):76–81, 1993.
17. Campos M, et al. Clinical follow-up of phototherapeutic keratectomy for treatment of corneal opacities. *Am J Ophthalmol* 115:433–440, 1993.

18. Chamon W, et al. Phototherapeutic keratectomy. *Ophthalmol Clin North Am* 6:399–412, 1993.

19. Rapuano CJ, Laibson PR. Excimer laser phototherapeutic keratectomy. *CLAO J* 19:235–240, 1993.

20. Azar DT, et al. Phototherapeutic keratectomy: The VISX experience. In JJ Salz, PJ McDonnell, MB McDonald (eds.). *Corneal Laser Surgery*. St. Louis: Mosby, 1995. Pp 213–226.

21. Vrabec MP, et al. Electron microscopic findings in a cornea with recurrence of herpes simplex keratitis after excimer laser phototherapeutic keratectomy. *CLAO J* 20:41, 1994.

22. Kornmehl EW, Steinert RF, Puliafito CA. A comparative study of masking fluids for excimer laser phototherapeutic keratectomy. *Arch Ophthalmol* 109:860–863, 1991.

23. Talamo JH, Steinert RF, Puliafito CA. Clinical strategies for excimer laser phototherapeutic keratectomy. *Refract Corneal Surg* 8:319–324, 1992.

24. Thompson V, Durrie DS, Cavanaugh TB. Philosophy and technique for excimer laser phototherapeutic keratectomy. [Review]. *Refract Corneal Surg* 9(Suppl. 2):81–85, 1993.

25. Durrie DS, Schumer JD, Cavanaugh T. Phototherapeutic keratectomy: The VISX experience. In JJ Salz, PJ McDonnell, MB McDonald (eds.). *Corneal Laser Surgery*. St. Louis: Mosby, 1995. Pp 227–235.

26. Krueger SL, Trokel SL. Quantitation of corneal ablation by ultraviolet laser light. *Arch Ophthalmol* 103:1741–1742, 1985.

27. Puliafito CA, Wong K, Steinert RF. Quantitative and ultrastructural studies of excimer laser ablation of the cornea at 193 and 248 nanometers. *Laser Surg Med* 7:155–159, 1987.

28. Van Saarlos PP, Constable IJ. Bovine corneal stroma ablation rate with 193-nm excimer laser radiation: Quantitative measurement. *J Refract Corneal Surg* 6:424–429, 1990.

29. Seiler T, et al. Ablation rate of human corneal epithelium and Bowman's layer with the excimer laser (193 nm). *J Refract Corneal Surg* 6: 99–102, 1990.

30. Gibralter R, Trokel SL. Correction of irregular astigmatism with the excimer laser. *Ophthalmol* 101:1310–1315, 1994.

31. Talamo JH, Wagoner MD, Lee SL. Management of ablation decentration following excimer photorefractive keratectomy. *Arch Ophthalmol* 113: 706–707, 1995.

32. Phillips AF, et al. Arachidonic acid metabolites after excimer laser corneal surgery. *Arch Ophthalmol* 111:1273–1278, 1993.

33. Arshinoff S, et al. Use of topical nonsteroidal anti-inflammatory drugs in excimer laser photorefractive keratectomy. *J Cataract Refract Surg* 20: 216–222, 1994.

34. Sher NA, et al. Topical diclofenac in the treatment of ocular pain after excimer photorefractive keratectomy. *J Refract Corneal Surg* 9:425–436, 1993.

35. Ku EC, et al. Effect of diclofenac sodium on the arachidonic acid cascade. *Am J Med* 80(Suppl. 4B):18–23, 1986.

36. Szerenyi K, et al. Decrease in normal human corneal sensitivity with topical diclofenac sodium. *Am J Ophthalmol* 118:312–315, 1994.

36a. Sher NA, et al. The role of topical steroidal and non-steroidal anti-inflammatory drugs in the etiology of stromal infiltrates after excimer PRK. *J Refract Surg* 10:587–588, 1994.

37. Sher NA, et al. Role of topical corticosteroids and nonsteroidal anti-inflammatory drugs in the etiology of stromal infiltrates after excimer photorefractive keratectomy. *J Refract Corneal Surg* 10:587–588, 1994.

38. Campos M, Abed HM, McDonnell PJ. Topical fluorometholone reduces stromal inflammation after photorefractive keratectomy. *Ophthalmic Surg* 24:654–657, 1993.

39. O'Brart DPS, et al. Treatment of band keratopathy by excimer laser phototherapeutic keratectomy: Surgical techniques and long term follow-up. *Br J Ophthalmol* 7:702–708, 1993.

40. Al-Rajhi AA, et al. Bacterial keratitis following phototherapeutic keratectomy. *J Refract Surg* 12:123–127, 1996.

41. McDonnell JM, Garbus JJ, McDonnell PJ. Unsuccessful excimer laser phototherapeutic keratectomy. *Arch Ophthalmol* 110:977–979, 1992.

42. McDonnell PJ, et al. Photorefractive keratectomy for astigmatism. *Arch Ophthalmol* 109:1370–1373, 1991.

43. Pepose JS, et al. Reactivation of latent herpes simplex virus by excimer laser photokeratectomy. *Am J Ophthalmol* 114:45–50, 1992.

44. Carones F, et al. The corneal endothelium after myopic excimer laser photorefractive keratectomy. *Arch Ophthalmol* 112:920–924, 1994.

45. Kermani O, Lubatschowski H. Struktur und dynamik photoakustischer shockwellen bei der 193 nm excimerlaserphotoablation der hornhaut. *Fortschr Ophthalmol* 88:748–753, 1991.

46. Dehm EJ, et al. Corneal endothelial injury in rabbits following excimer laser ablation at 193 and 248 nm. *Arch Ophthalmol* 104:1364–1368, 1986.

47. Fantes FE, et al. Wound healing after excimer laser keratomileusis (photorefractive keratectomy) in monkeys. *Arch Ophthalmol* 108:665–675, 1990.

48. Amano S, Shimizu K. Corneal endothelial changes after excimer laser photorefractive keratectomy. *Am J Ophthalmol* 116:692–694, 1993.

49. Perez-Santonja JJ, et al. Short-term corneal endothelial changes after photorefractive keratectomy. *J Refract Corneal Surg* 10(Suppl.):194–198, 1994.

50. Hersh PS, Jordan AJ, Mayers M. Corneal graft rejection episode after excimer laser phototherapeutic keratectomy. *Arch Ophthalmol* 111:735–736, 1993.

51. Epstein RJ, Robin JB. Corneal graft rejection episode after excimer laser phototherapeutic keratectomy. *Arch Ophthalmol* 112:157, 1994.

Laser In-Situ Keratomileusis (LASIK)

7 LASIK Surgical Techniques

Maria Clara Arbelaez, Peter A. Rapoza, and Jesus Vidaurri-Leal

History

Laser-assisted in-situ keratomileusis (LASIK) is a keratorefractive surgical technique that combines the precision of excimer laser photoablation with the theoretical advantages of an intrastromal procedure that maintains the integrity of Bowman's layer and the overlying corneal epithelium. The technique is a descendant of myopic keratomileusis as originally performed in 1949 by Jose Barraquer, in his pioneering work in Bogota, Colombia. Dr. Barraquer's initial technique required the freehand dissection of a half-thickness corneal disc, which was subsequently shaped with a modified contact lens lathe and then sutured to the recipient bed. Advances in instrumentation allowed the procedure to become more reproducible and accurate in the hands of other surgeons. The development of a cryolathe in the 1950s improved the method for shaping of the corneal disc. A modified, miniaturized dermatome was designed that eased the removal of the corneal disc.

The work described above culminated in the development of the automated corneal shaper by Luis A. Ruiz during the 1980s in collaboration with the Steinway Instrument Company and HANSA Research and Development (Miami, FL). The automated corneal shaper was used not only to remove a corneal cap but to perform a refractive cut, removing a second corneal disc from the corneal bed (automatic lamellar keratoplasty [ALK] or keratomileusis in situ). The corneal cap was then replaced with or without suturing; after this technique was refined to create a hinged flap, no suturing was necessary. The next logical step was the application of excimer laser photoablation to replace the microkeratome in creating the refractive cut, with the potential advantages of (1) increased accuracy and decreased risk of complications, (2) the ability to create a lenticular rather than a planar lamellar resection, and (3) the ability to correct astigmatism. Two principal techniques are now in use to perform laser keratomileusis: the Buratto technique and LASIK. Only LASIK will be discussed here.

For LASIK, the procedure is conducted in a fashion similar to ALK, but once the hinged flap is created, the laser ablation is performed in the stromal bed. The LASIK technique using a hinged flap is most widely accepted and is currently used for the correction of myopia, hyperopia, and astigmatism.

Microkeratome Instrumentation

LASIK is performed with the automated corneal shaper (designed by Luis A. Ruiz, Chiron Ophthalmics, Irvine, CA) or another, similar instrument. Technology is advancing rapidly, and other acceptable automated and hand-driven microkeratomes are now available. Companies currently producing microkeratomes available for purchase include SCMD (Phoenix, AZ), Eye Technology (St. Paul, MN), Phoenix Instruments (San Diego, CA) and Herbert Schwind (Kleinostheim, Germany).

The Chiron Automated Corneal Shaper

The authors use the automated corneal shaper, which is currently the most widely distributed instrument. The apparatus consists of the corneal shaper head, shaper motor, and pneumatic fixation ring (Fig. 7-1) and is powered by a control unit, containing the electrical source and a suction pump. Each component is described below in detail.

Shaper Head

The shaper head consists of upper and lower parts hinged together to ease insertion of the blade and to prevent the parts from being maladjusted. The upper portion of the shaper head contains the *blade holder*, in which coupling occurs between the blade and the motor. The lower portion of the shaper serves as a plane that accepts a preset thickness of corneal tissue for incision by the oscillating blade, as presented by the *suction apparatus*. A *stainless steel blade* is placed inside the blade holder in the lower surface of the upper portion of the corneal shaper. Blades must be of the highest quality, and great care must be exercised to ensure that the edge is not damaged during assembly or operation of the automatic corneal shaper. Blade length, thickness, and bevel should be checked before insertion into the blade

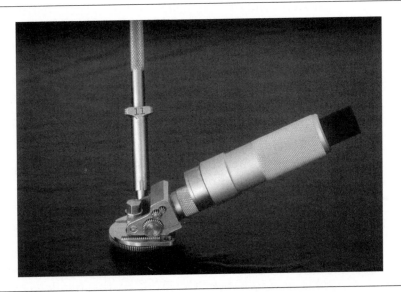

Fig. 7-1. Automated corneal shaper consisting of the shaper head, motor, and pneumatic fixation ring.

holder. The blade holder is designed to allow only the proper placement of the blade. The blade angle in the automatic corneal shaper is fixed at 25 degrees. After the blade is placed in the blade holder, the corneal shaper is closed and secured in place with a nut. A *probing shank,* identical in shape to the motor shaft that drives the blade, is inserted into the shaper head and gyrated while the blade is inspected for normal oscillation. If oscillation is normal, the shaper head is then coupled to the motor. On coupling the shaper head to the motor shaft, the *eccentric* (a cylindrical body at the end of the motor) enters a groove in the blade holder. When the power is activated, the motor spins at 7500 rpm, thereby driving the blade holder with the attached blade at a constant oscillation speed.

Inspection of the shaper head from the front reveals a recess designed for the placement of a plate that is selected by the surgeon to define the thickness of the resected tissue. The thickness of a given plate defines the distance between the external surface of the plate and the cutting edge of the blade, thereby determining the thickness of the tissue to be resected. Each plate is marked with a plate number, which corresponds to a given desired resection calibrated to be within a 5-micron range of accuracy. Although numerous plate sizes are needed to perform two-pass ALK, only the 130- and 160-micron plates are needed for LASIK.

The plate is shaped to allow its attachment to the shaper head in the desired fashion. A cylindrical boss accepts a screw, which is secured firmly to the plate with a wrench, leaving no play between the shaper and the plate. An accessory called a *stopper* has been developed for making hinged, or flap, cuts. Newer microkeratomes have a stopper in the shaper head, whereas in older models the stopper is installed over the knurled nut of the shaper head. A two-part foot pedal switch activates the forward motion of the microkeratome. The lower lip of the stopper is placed under the flat surface of the head. The stopper causes the shaper to cease forward motion at a precisely defined point to create a flap resection. When the stopper has been reached, the motor's direction is reversed by stepping on the opposite side of the two-position foot switch.

Shaper Motor

The motor for the automated corneal shaper is contained in a cylindrical handpiece by which the instrument is held. The 12-volt motor spins at 7500 rpm. The front of the handpiece has a pinion that couples with pinions in the shaper head. An electrical cable exits the proximal end, connecting to the power source.

Pneumatic Fixation Ring

A pneumatic fixation ring is an integral part of the microkeratome. It is a circular chamber that fixates the eye by means of a vacuum. Because the diameter of the flap created for LASIK is constant, it is not necessary to vary the height of the ring. Fixation of the eye is imperative in this procedure; usually it is carried out under topical anesthesia. The underside of the fixation range has a vacuum chamber that seals against the globe. A suction handle is provided that communicates with a pump for evacuating the chamber and providing the vacuum for fixation. The intraocular pressure (IOP) must exceed 65 mm Hg to obtain a resection that is both uniform and regular and the appropriate diameter.

Control Unit

The control unit of the automated corneal shaper serves as the power source for controlling the oscillation of the blade and the forward or reverse motion of the corneal shaper. As mentioned above, a dual-position foot pedal initiates forward or reverse motion of the keratome. A voltmeter indicates by inclination to the left or right whether the shaper is moving forward or backward. The control unit also contains a suction pump that delivers vacuum to the fixation ring at 22 inches Hg. A separate foot pedal is depressed once to initiate suction and again to break the vacuum.

*The SCMD Turbokeratome**

The Turbokeratome, manufactured by SCMD, Inc., and distributed by VisionAerie, Inc. (Wilmington, DE) is another widely used keratome that is specifically designed for single-cut LASIK procedures. This hand-driven keratome consists of the shaper head, the turbine hand-piece, the pneumatic fixation ring, and a control unit that provides a suction pump and control of the nitrogen gas input used to drive the turbine (Fig. 7-2).

Shaper Head and Pneumatic Fixation Ring

The shaper head is a three-piece unit; the main body splits into upper and lower portions, and a blade holder slots into the upper portion. The lower portion of the shaper head has dovetail tracks at the base that correspond to similar tracks on the surface of the fixation ring. This lower portion is engineered to allow the blade holder to rest in a shaped groove, and to allow the blade to emerge through a horizontal slit when the upper and lower portions of the unit are connected. The thickness of corneal tissue presented for incision by the oscillating blade, which emerges from the base of the shaper head, is fixed at 150 microns for LASIK procedures without the use of any further plates or adjustments. A single blade is used for each procedure. These blades are stainless steel with a symmetrical (i.e., center-cutting, non-bevel) edge and are clipped onto the blade holder after

Fig. 7-2. SCMD Turbokeratome control unit.

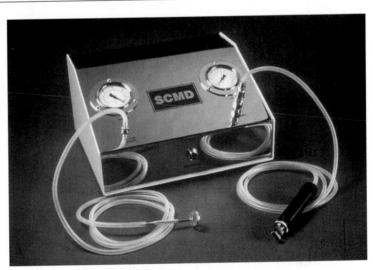

*Turbokeratome information courtesy of Steven Verity, M.D.

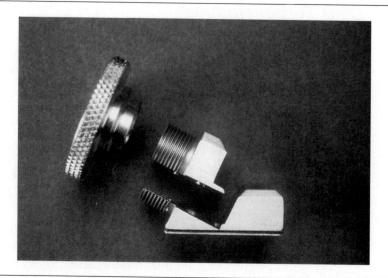

Fig. 7-3. Turbokeratome blade holder.

the holder is placed in the upper portion of the shaper head (Fig. 7-3). Once the blade is placed, the shaper head can be assembled upside down by carefully sliding the two portions together until the locating pins in the upper portion fit into corresponding holes in the lower portion. This assembly must be performed with care to ensure no damage to the blade edge. When the shaper head is assembled, a stop ring is screwed onto the rear of the head to secure the unit. In this unit, the blade angle is fixed at 22.5 degrees. There is a choice between four stop rings when assembling the unit, with different rings being used to control the forward motion of the shaper head to allow more precise control of the excursion of the head within the suction handpiece. In this manner, the hinge size for a LASIK procedure can thus be varied by using different combinations of fixation ring and stop ring: The fixation ring controls the height and diameter of corneal tissue presented to the shaper head for lamellar incision for a given eye, while the stop ring limits the horizontal excursion of the blade/shaper head complex. Instead of the plates utilized with the Chiron shaper, several sizes of fixation ring are available so that the surgeon can vary the corneal flap thickness.

Control Unit

The Control unit of the Turbokeratome provides control for both the nitrogen gas supply to the turbine and the suction pump for the fixation ring (see Fig. 7-2). The suction pump provides 20–25 inches

Hg vacuum to the fixation ring and is controlled by a foot pedal. The pump is driven by a battery inside the control unit that is independent from the external power supply, allowing procedures to be completed even in the case of power loss. The unit is connected to an external source of nitrogen gas through a regulator adjusted to give running pressure at the turbine of 42 psi as indicated on the control unit pressure gauge. The turbine rotation is controlled by a second foot pedal.

Using Microkeratome with an Excimer Laser

All microkeratomes can be used in conjunction with any excimer laser as long as the optics of the laser's operating microscope provide an adequate working distance (5 inches or more is optimal). We currently use the Keracor 117 (Chiron, Inc.; Irvine, CA) and the Coherent-Schwind Keratom I (Kleinostheim, Germany).

Preoperative Evaluation

It is imperative that all patients considering surgical correction of refractive error be well informed as to the risks and benefits of any procedure they might undergo. Especially important is the matching of motivations and expectations so that patient and surgeon can be more assured of a satisfactory outcome. Currently, myopia of −1.00 to −30.00 D and astigmatism of 0.50 to 10.00 D is amenable to correction with LASIK. Clinical trials are now under way to evaluate the technique for the treatment of hyperopia up to +8.00 D and presbyopia. Several preoperative considerations are unique to the LASIK procedure. These are outlined in Table 7-1 and discussed in detail below.

Examination of the patient usually includes measurement of visual acuity without correction for distance and near. Contact lens wearers should discontinue the use of soft contact lenses for 2 weeks and rigid contact lenses for 3 weeks before evaluation. A refraction should be performed with and without cycloplegia. The best corrected visual acuity (BCVA) is recorded for distance and near. Surgery should only be considered if the refractive error has been stable (0.5 D change in sphere or cylinder of ≤ 0.5 D) for 1 year or longer. Keratometry and corneal topography are routinely performed. Glare testing and contrast sensitivity testing may be obtained. All patients should undergo a detailed ophthalmologic evaluation before surgery, including careful slit-lamp examination and IOP determination. The fundus should be evaluated through a dilated pupil.

Table 7-1. Special preoperative considerations for LASIK

Exposure of globe

   If exposure is not adequate, suction ring application and microkeratome pass may be complicated

   Consider omitting lid speculum

Corneal thickness

   After flap and ablation, avoid being closer than 250 microns to the endothelium

   Pachymetry of < 530 microns may dictate need for a thinner flap (130 vs. 160 microns) or shallower ablation, or both

   Do not operate on corneas with central thickness < 450 microns

History of glaucoma or vascular disease

   Eye must tolerate IOP > 65 mm Hg during flap resection

IOP = intraocular pressure

Ultrasonic pachymetry of the central cornea is an essential ancillary test. LASIK is not recommended for corneas with central thickness measurements less than 450 microns. For corneas thinner than 530 microns or where an extremely high myopic ablation is planned (> −15 D), consideration should be given to using a thinner flap (130 microns) combined with multiple and smaller ablation zone diameters to minimize the excision depth at the center of the laser keratectomy. In no case should residual corneal bed thickness after laser ablation measure less than 250 microns because this may result in progressive central corneal ectasia.

The eyelids and adnexa should be scrutinized for potential sources of infection or conditions that might lead to wound healing problems, such as dry eyes or exposure keratopathy. Deeply set globes may be more difficult to approach due to the size of the pneumatic fixation ring. In such cases, it may be useful to omit the lid speculum during surgery. If one is in doubt as to the ability to adequately couple the microkeratome suction ring to the globe, it is not unreasonable to test this before surgery.

Exclusion criteria for LASIK are similar to those for photorefractive keratectomy (PRK). Patients with keratoconus should not undergo the procedure. Monocular patients and pregnant women are excluded. Surgeons should be mindful that the patient must tolerate an intraoperative IOP of at least 65 mm Hg for up to several minutes during the LASIK procedure. Thus, patients with glaucoma, retinal vascular disease, and systemic vascular disease should be excluded.

Before surgery, the procedure is explained in detail to the patient, and written informed consent is obtained. Remember that inappropriate expectations also constitute a contraindication to surgery.

Surgical Procedure

Anesthesia and Other Preoperative Medications

LASIK is usually performed under topical anesthesia with mild systemic sedation. Patients receive diazepam (Valium) 10 mg PO 30–60 minutes before the procedure. A topical anesthetic agent (either proparacaine 0.5%, tetracaine 0.5%, or mucous membrane lidocaine [Xylocaine] 4%) is instilled 4 times at 5-minutes intervals, beginning 20 minutes prior to surgery. Many surgeons also use preoperative broad-spectrum antibiotic drops and pilocarpine 1%, which helps maintain pupillary miosis to assist with centration.

Surgical Calculations

Either the manifest or cycloplegic refraction is utilized for planning the surgical procedure. In cases where a great discrepancy exists between the manifest and cycloplegic refraction, the former should be retested once the cycloplegic effect has ended. Parameters are entered into the excimer laser's terminal before surgery. Protocols continue to vary and are beyond the scope of this text. The reader should be aware that ablation algorithms for intrastromal ablation during LASIK may differ substantially from those for surface PRK, generally employing fewer pulses to achieve a given correction (i.e., assume a higher ablation rate per pulse). A standard conversion formula should not be assumed, and the surgeon should consult the appropriate individual(s) at each manufacturer or someone familiar with the particular use of the machine in question before proceeding.

Preparation of Instruments

The microkeratome is prepared by inserting a new blade into the shaper head for each procedure. In older models, the stopper is firmly attached to the keratome. For the Chiron units, the probing shank is used to check the blade holder and blade assembly. The gears should turn freely when the shank is rotated between the thumb and forefinger. The 160-micron plate is attached to the shaper head. In the near future, optional calibration microscopes may be available to verify the gap distance between the blade and the lower portion of the shaper head. For patients with greater than −15.00 D of myopia or corneal thickness less than 530 microns, a 130-micron plate (Chiron) or different suction ring (SCMD) is utilized. The motor is attached to the corneal shaper, and the shaper is attached to the pneumatic fixation ring, where forward and reverse motion are assessed. The Turbokeratome is prepared by inserting a blade onto the blade holder

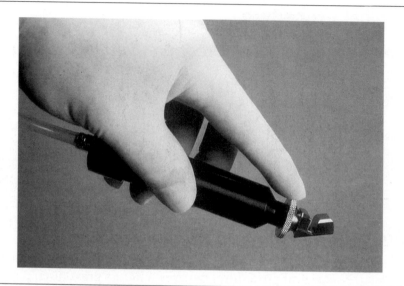

Fig. 7-4. Turbokeratome turbine handpiece.

for each procedure. The head is then assembled and the chosen stop ring attached. The tip of the drive shaft is lightly lubricated and the head is then attached to the turbine handpiece (Fig. 7-4). The turbine should be activated to ensure that the head is correctly attached to the handpiece and that the blade moves freely. Suction may be checked on the fixation ring for both units by occluding the ring with the thumb.

When using the Turbokeratome, the keratome head is engaged in the dovetails of the fixation ring and manually advanced until the blade edge is about 2 mm away from engaging corneal tissue (Fig. 7-5). At this point, the turbine is activated and the blade begins to oscillate. The keratome is then advanced smoothly across the fixation ring until the stop ring is encountered, making the lamellar incision in a 1- to 2-second pass. The turbine then stops and the keratome is withdrawn from the fixation ring until it disengages. Suction is then removed. The pressure obtained should be more than 25 inches Hg for the Chiron unit and more than 22 inches for the SCMD.

The laser system is activated and a fluence test performed as recommended by the manufacturer. The patient's demographic and refractive data are entered at the excimer laser's terminal. Before commencing the procedure, it is useful to test the patient's ability to fixate the blinking fixation light, as this will aid both marking for the procedure and the laser ablation itself.

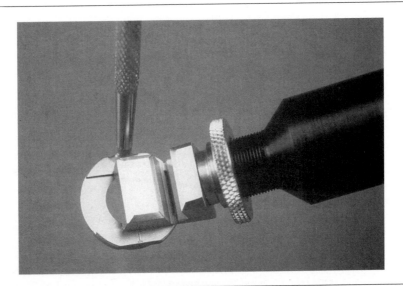

Fig. 7-5. Turbokeratome head engaged in the dovetails of the fixation ring.

Surgical Technique

The anesthetized eye is irrigated with saline solution. The eye and face are prepped and draped in the usual fashion for intraocular surgery. A plastic drape or tape is applied to keep the lashes outside the surgical field. One drop of 0.5% povidone-iodine (Betadine) is instilled in the surgical eye. A blepharostat is placed. A specially designed marker, consisting of an internal circle 3.0 mm in diameter joined by paired pararadial lines to an external circle of 10.5 mm, is prepared for imprinting by dipping in gentian violet or application of a marking ink (Fig. 7-6). The inner circle is placed concentrically with the pupil to aid with centration. The outer circle aids the concentric placement of the pneumatic fixation ring. The pararadial line serves to reorient the disc to correctly denote the appropriate orientation of the epithelial surface and the axis in cases where a complete cap is dissected. If a marker of this type is not available, the crucial reference points to mark are (1) the pupil center and (2) a radial mark on the peripheral corneal epithelium to allow correct reapposition of the hinged corneal flap.

Maximal exposure of the globe is obtained via the blepharostat. The pneumatic fixation ring is applied to the globe. To ease exposure and avoid resting the instrument against the patient's nose, the handle of the ring should be directed inferiorly for the right eye and superiorly for the left eye for the Chiron unit, but may be oriented in either

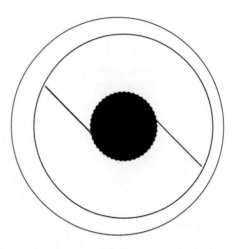

Fig. 7-6. Marking the cornea for LASIK. Specialized LASIK markers have concentric 3-mm and 10.5-mm circular marks connected by a pair of radial lines. The concentric marks aid positioning of the suction ring with respect to the pupil (3 mm) and the limbus (10.5 mm). The radial lines assist with reapposition of the hinged flap.

direction for the SCMD unit. Centering movements can be performed by the surgeon by moving the cornea with a fingertip or the pneumatic fixation ring prior to engaging suction. The suction is then activated. The IOP should be elevated to 65 mm Hg or higher, which is the IOP necessary to obtain a resection of appropriate diameter and thickness with the corneal shaper. A Barraquer tonometer is utilized to measure the IOP before resection. This conical plastic instrument has a convex dome that magnifies the flat lower surface and its inscribed applanation ring. The tonometer, held by a plastic ring, is applied to the dry cornea inside the pneumatic fixation ring. If the IOP is 65 mm Hg, the applanation created by the cornea in contact with the tonometer will be exactly equal to the diameter of the inscribed circle. Too high a pressure is indicated by a smaller applanation, and too low a pressure is detected by an applanation larger than the inscribed circle. The IOP may be varied by altering the pressure applied to the eyeball via the pneumatic fixation ring and how it is held.

The eye is now ready for the lamellar resection of the cornea. The microkeratome is inspected to be certain that the shaper head components are still in position. Patients with −15.00 D or greater of myopia or those with central pachymetry of 530 microns may benefit from a flap resection thickness in the 130-micron range rather than 150–160 microns. A single drop of balanced salt solution is placed on the underside of the shaper head as a lubricant for the advancing, oscillating microkeratome blade. Some surgeons prefer more aggressive irrigation, but the important principle to remember is "Cut wet, ablate dry."

The Chiron microkeratome head is placed on the pneumatic fixation ring by inserting the dovetail into the dovetail groove, lowering to the horizontal position, then inserting the shaper into the fixation ring notch until a tooth of the largest pinion is engaged into the dented rack. The forward pedal is depressed, and the microkeratome moves forward and performs the lamellar incision (Fig. 7-7). The shaper stops when the stopper is reached. The reverse pedal is then depressed to move the microkeratome backward on the pneumatic fixation ring.

A similar set of maneuvers is employed for the SCMD Turbokeratome (described above), with the principal difference being that a dovetailed groove without a gear track is utilized and the shaper head is passed manually along the dovetail track of the suction ring (see Fig. 7-5). The shaper head is then carefully withdrawn backwards out of the dovetailed groove. The suction to the pneumatic fixation ring is interrupted by depressing the suction foot pedal. The pneumatic fixation ring may be maintained in position to stabilize inadvertent eye movements. An irrigation cannula can be utilized to fold the hinged corneal flap to the nasal side of the eye (Plate 27). The flap should be carefully inspected before proceeding with laser ablation of the stromal bed. If the flap is too thin or the microkeratome becomes stuck during advancement, it is best to abort the procedure and reattempt after at least 3 months. The same resection depth can be utilized. If

Fig. 7-7. Chiron Automated Corneal Shaper performs the lamellar resection of the cornea.

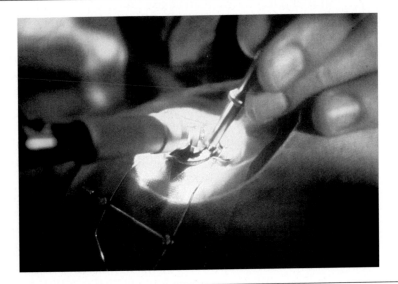

the flap appears thick (a very rare occurrence), it is prudent to measure the thickness of the stromal bed by ultrasonic pachymetry prior to proceeding. If a total cap is resected, the cap can be left inside the microkeratome head to preserve its orientation during laser ablation.

The excimer laser is focused on the center of the bed, and ideally there is a delay of no more than 30 seconds before the laser is activated to perform the keratectomy. During excimer photoablation, great care should be taken to ensure that the ablation is centered. Patient fixation is poor during LASIK ablations, as the stromal bed surface possesses less optical regularity than during surface PRK, and the transient retinal hypoperfusion induced during flap resection creates additional difficulty with fixation. Eye-tracking devices seem to work less well during LASIK than PRK, and retention of the suction ring to manipulate the eye is quite helpful. It is also important to avoid ablation of the flap hinge. This complication can create postoperative topographic and refractive abnormalities, and in rare instances it may actually result in perforation of the flap by the laser. One means of minimizing the chance of this complication is to assist visualization of the laser ablation in progress by applying a single drop of dilute fluorescein solution to the stromal bed just before laser activation, as described by Jesus Vidaurri-Leal, M.D. Excess fluid is removed with a dry cellulose sponge, and the ablation can then be elegantly localized with respect to the pupil center while it is in progress (Plates 28 and 29). This is particularly useful during astigmatic and hyperopic ablations because the outer diameter of laser energy delivery may measure 8–9 mm and can easily ablate the underside of the hinged flap. For this reason, it is advantageous to use as large a flap as possible when performing such treatments. For astigmatic ablation, another option is to align the meridian of the flap hinge as much as possible with the steep axis, where the shorter chord diameter of elliptical astigmatic ablations is present.

Variations in stromal hydration are an issue during LASIK ablations as the appearance of a central "spot" of surface wetting seems to be more common during LASIK than during PRK. For this reason, many surgeons will routinely interrupt the laser treatment every 150–200 pulses to allow drying of the bed with a cellulose sponge. Whether this intervention decreases the incidence of central islands and other postoperative topographic abnormalities awaits further clarification through clinical experience.

Following laser ablation, the stromal bed and the underside of the corneal flap are cleaned of cells and foreign debris by irrigation with a stream of filtered balanced salt solution while these surfaces are brushed with a wet cellulose sponge and excess fluid is suctioned out of the fornices. Additional irrigation is then performed with the irrigation cannula to completely clean the interface and reposition the flap. The flap is then gently recentered over the resected bed using either a wet cellulose sponge or a curved tying forceps. If a complete cap has been resected, the cap can now be carefully removed from the microkeratome head and replaced, taking care to align the radial orientation marks in the epithelium. Only rarely is it necessary to place sutures in this situation. The edge of the circular incision is dried with a stream of filtered air or simply allowed to air dry for 5 minutes with the blepharostat in place. It is imperative that the pararadial mark from the centration instrument be aligned across the edge of the lamellar incision to prevent wrinkling of the flap and other tissue alignment abnormalities, which may result in irregular astigmatism. The pneumatic fixation ring is removed without disturbing the flap. Forceps are used to indent the peripheral cornea to assess for the presence of striae passing from the periphery into the flap, which confirms adequate adhesion across the interface. The lid speculum is then removed and 1 drop of broad-spectrum antibiotic instilled. An eye shield is placed to prevent the patient from rubbing the globe and dislodging the flap during the first postoperative night.

Postoperatively, the patient is instructed to use acetaminophen, aspirin, or a nonsteroidal anti-inflammatory agent orally for any discomfort. The first postoperative visit is scheduled for the day after surgery. The eye shield is removed and visual acuity assessed. The eye is examined at the slit lamp to ensure that the flap is in its expected position and without evidence of significant interface opacities (Plate 30). Postoperative medications include fluorometholone 0.1% (FML) and a topical broad-spectrum antibiotic agent, 1 drop tid to the operated eye for 1 week. Artificial tears may be instilled as needed. Some surgeons use topical steroids for at least 1 month because they feel this may decrease the incidence of refractive regression over time. The patient is reexamined 1, 3, 6, and 12 months after surgery. A refraction is performed at these visits. If the expected refractive outcome is not achieved (uncorrected visual acuity ≤ 20/40 with ≤ 1 D of residual refractive error), adjunctive corneal topography and pachymetry are obtained and a repeat procedure can be performed if appropriate within 3 months after the initial surgery by simply re-elevating the lamellar flap. A more detailed discussion of postoperative management is given in Chapters 8 and 9.

Retreatments

If an enhancement procedure is performed within 1 year of the initial procedure, blunt dissection with spatula or Suarez spreader can often be used to open the interface. If more than 1 year has passed since the initial procedure or the interface cannot be opened without difficulty, the enhancement is approached as if the eye had not been previously operated on using the same microkeratome settings employed during the initial surgery but using the current subjective refraction as a guide to re-ablation. Retreatments are discussed in greater detail in Chapters 8 and 9.

Bibliography

Barraquer JI. Method for cutting lamellar grafts in frozen corneas. *Arch So Am Ophthalmol* 1:237, 1958.

Barraquer JI. Queratoplastia refractiva. *Estudios Inform Oftal Inst Barraquer* 10:2–10, 1949.

Barraquer JI. Querato mileusis para la correccian de la myopia. *Arch Soc Am Optom* 5:27–48, 1964.

Bas AM, Onnis R. Excimer laser in situ keratomileusis for myopia. *J Refract Corneal Surg* 11(3):S229–S233, 1995.

Buratto L, Ferrari M, Rama P. Excimer laser intrastromal keratomileusis. *Am J Ophthalmol* 113(3):291–295, 1992.

Fiander DC, Tayfour F. Excimer laser in situ keratomileusis in 124 myopic eyes. *J Refract Corneal Surg* 11(3):S234–S238, 1995.

Krawicz T. Lamellar corneal stromectomy. *Am J Ophthalmol* 57:828–833, 1964.

Kremer FB, Dufek M. Excimer laser in situ keratomileusis. *J Refract Corneal Surg* 11(3):S244–S247, 1995.

Leal JV. Meeting of the American Society of Cataract and Refractive Surgery, Seattle, WA, June 1996.

Pallikaris IG, et al. Laser in situ keratomileusis. *Laser Surg Med* 10:463–468, 1990.

Pureskin N. Weakening ocular refraction by means of partial stromectomy of cornea under experimental conditions. *Vestnik Oftalmologii* 80:19–24,1967.

Rozakis GW. Keratomes. In GW Rozakis (ed.). *Refractive Lamellar Keratoplasty.* Thorofare, NJ: Slack, 1994.

Ruiz LA, Rowsey J. In situ keratomileusis *Invest Ophthalmol Vis Sci* 29(Suppl.):392, 1988.

Salah T, Waring GO, El-Magrhaby A. Excimer Laser Keratomileusis. In JJ Salz (ed.). *Corneal Laser Surgery.* St. Louis: Mosby, 1994. Pp. 187–195.

Salah T, et al. Excimer laser in situ keratomileusis under a corneal flap for myopia of 2 to 20 diopters. *Am J Ophthalmol* 121:143–155, 1996.

Slade SG, Berkeley RG. History of Keratomileusis. In GW Rozakis (ed.). *Refractive Lamellar Keratoplasty.* Thorofare, NJ: Slack, 1994. Pp. 1–16.

Slade SG, Brint SF. Excimer Laser Myopic Keratomileusis. In GW Rozakis (ed.). *Refractive Lamellar Keratoplasty.* Thorofare, NJ: Slack, 1994. Pp. 125–137.

8 LASIK Routine Postoperative Management

Arturo S. Chayet

LASIK is a new laser refractive surgical procedure. Although it was conceived for the surgical correction of high myopia (because more complications are seen when performing surface photorefractive keratectomy [PRK] at this level), in some parts of the world it is rapidly becoming the standard refractive procedure for the correction of all levels of myopia as well as hyperopia. The reason LASIK has been so well accepted by some is that the epithelium and Bowman's layer are preserved, resulting in more rapid visual rehabilitation and a more comfortable postoperative course. Although the procedure itself is more complicated than PRK, the postoperative follow-up appears to be simpler, with a lower incidence of pain, infection, and poor healing, manifested haze, and scarring. The ease of follow-up and speed of recovery make LASIK a popular alternative for the laser refractive surgeon. Nevertheless, several factors in postoperative care are important to consider, and these are the subject of this chapter.

Immediate Postoperative Period

First Day

At the conclusion of the surgical procedure, the corneal flap should be folded back to its original position and carefully inspected, making sure all reference marks are well aligned. The cornea should be allowed to air dry for 5 minutes so the flap will adhere firmly without sutures. Topical steroids and antibiotics are then instilled over the cornea.

Some surgeons retire the eyelid speculum and have the patient blink a few times to verify that the flap is still in place before discharging the patient. Other surgeons close the eyelids with an adhesive strip to prevent blinking and to decrease the potential for subsequent flap displacement. Others use a bandage contact lens for the first 16–24 hours, a practice we have adopted as our standard of care. The reason for this approach is to prevent flap displacement due to contact with the eyelid and to allow for a more comfortable postoperative period, in case an epithelial defect was created. Some surgeons believe that a bandage contact lens induces more corneal edema and, therefore, delayed visual rehabilitation; it is our impression that the visual acuity the next day is not affected by the use of the contact lens (Fig. 8-1). Before the flap technique was adopted, patching the eye was the preferred method to prevent loss of the cap. Now that generation of a free corneal cap is a rare occurrence, patching can be reserved for such instances.

Topical antibiotics and steroids are prescribed four times per day for the first 24 hours, after which no further medications are usually needed. Most patients are comfortable within 1 day or show no visible signs of ocular surface inflammation. Artificial tears, however, are quite helpful and should be prescribed at least 4 times daily for several weeks after LASIK.

First Week

Epithelial Margin Healing

On the first postoperative day, the cornea is clear, and the epithelial margins of the flap are generally healed and sometimes difficult to

Fig. 8-1. Slit-lamp photograph of an eye revealing an uneventful postoperative course 1 day after LASIK following use of a bandage contact lens.

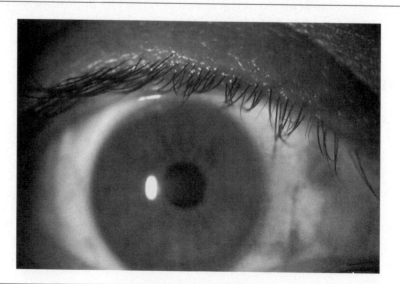

see. Very rarely, an epithelial defect may be present in the area of the flap. In such cases, it is important to patch the eye for 24 hours or until full re-epithelialization occurs. It is our impression that bad cases of epithelial ingrowth into the flap interface are more common in the presence of a postoperative epithelial defect. In such instances, the epithelial ingrowth is secondary to early exposure and gaping of the flap margin, which may be a strong stimulus for epithelial regeneration to cover the defect. We have encountered one case of epithelial ingrowth after lamellar surgery, in which the patient had a large epithelial defect that extended over the margins of the flap. Epithelial ingrowth was not seen until the third postoperative day and appeared patchy and localized to the inferior part of the flap interface in the region of the epithelial defect. On the seventh postoperative day, the epithelial ingrowth was better organized and had migrated centrally into the center of the flap (Fig. 8-2). After 2 weeks, the flap was lifted and the epithelium cleared from the interface with a spatula, leaving a mild central opacity. Some surgeons advocate the use of absolute alcohol when removing interface epithelial ingrowth, but this is probably unnecessary if the stromal bed is cleaned promptly and meticulously.

Interface Clarity

After our first few cases, we found more interface debris following LASIK than subsequently (Fig. 8-3). Our recommendations for avoiding interface debris are the following:

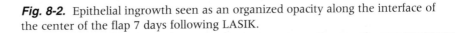

Fig. 8-2. Epithelial ingrowth seen as an organized opacity along the interface of the center of the flap 7 days following LASIK.

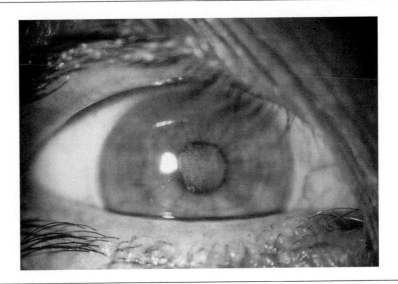

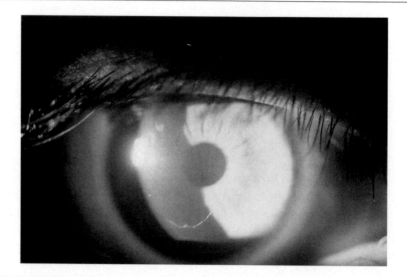

Fig. 8-3. Interface debris consisting of linen on the first postoperative day following LASIK; debris resulted from a sterile cloth used for instrument placement.

1. Do not use powdered gloves.
2. Do not place any instrument or material to be used during the procedure in contact with fibers, such as cloth or linen. (We place all our instruments on plastic surfaces.)
3. Make sure the instruments are clean and in perfect condition.
4. Irrigate vigorously only the posterior surface of the flap. (We have found it unnecessary to irrigate the bed unless it shows particles or debris.)
5. Avoid epithelial defects.
6. Make sure the instruments are free of chemical solutions.
7. Avoid excessive use of topical anesthetics because they promote epithelial defects.
8. Do not touch the posterior face of the flap or the bed with any instrument or material that has been in contact with the epithelium.

Flap Smoothness and Stability

In almost every case, the flap adheres to its bed immediately after surgery and remains in this configuration. During the first postoperative week, corneal topography and keratometry mires are not as regular as those seen in later weeks. This is likely due to mild edema of the flap in conjunction with epithelial roughness. As the cornea thins and the epithelium smooths over the flap margins, the regularity of the keratometric and topographic mires improves.

Wound Healing Phase

First Month

During the first postoperative month, the cornea stays clear and quiet. Other than artificial tears, no further medications are needed. The main focus of attention at this time and thereafter is on optical and visual rehabilitation. Although it is important to remain vigilant, by this time epithelial ingrowth or flap dislocation should have been identified and properly managed.

The role of topical steroids in the postoperative management of LASIK is uncertain, although generally steroids are not used as extensively as they are after PRK. Most surgeons believe that because no haze is seen after LASIK, there is no need for topical steroids postoperatively. Nevertheless, we utilized topical steroids empirically in an attempt to assess their potential role in preventing regression after LASIK. So far, no conclusive evidence of their benefit has been observed, but we have observed adverse side effects from steroids. One patient experienced a sudden loss of uncorrected visual acuity 10 days after LASIK. At her sixth postoperative day, she had an uncorrected visual acuity of 20/30, with a clear cornea and uneventful postoperative course. On the tenth postoperative day, her uncorrected vision dropped to 20/70, corrected to 20/25 with a −2.00 D lens. On slit-lamp examination, the cornea showed an unusual diffuse haze localized to the interface (Plate 31). Corneal thickness changed dramatically from 0.430 mm to 0.495 mm. We suspected corneal edema secondary to increased intraocular pressure (IOP) and verified this assumption with an IOP measurement of 48 mm Hg. The diagnosis of topical steroid–induced glaucoma was made, and immediate medical treatment was started, including the discontinuation of the topical steroid. Seven days later, the cornea was clear, IOP returned to normal, and the patient's uncorrected visual acuity improved to 20/25 with a refraction of −0.50 D. Following this incident, and because there is as yet no scientific support for the use of topical steroids after LASIK, we have abandoned the use of topical steroids until controlled clinical trials demonstrate their utility.

Subsequent Months

Most serious complications of LASIK become evident within the first postoperative month. Thereafter, continued observation is warranted to monitor for refractive regression or persistent irregular astigmatism. The technique and timing of LASIK retreatments are discussed in detail in Chapter 9.

When we started to perform LASIK, all our cases were more than −10.00 D of myopia. The mean spherical equivalent of our first 35 cases was −14.5 D with a range of −10.00 to −22.00 D. Each case showed some degree of regression, depending on the amount of the intended correction. In general, the higher the preoperative myopia, the larger the regression, being on average about 20% of the preoperative spherical equivalent.

One example of refractive regression after LASIK was a patient who had a preoperative spherical equivalent of −19.00 D. Following treatment at 1 week, he was plano, but at 6 months the refraction was −6.00 D (almost 30% regression). Another example is a patient with −11.50 D of preoperative myopia; at 7 days after treatment the refraction was −0.50 D. Over the following months, he had a slow regression, leading to a refraction of −2.00 D (a 15% regression) (Plates 32–34).

Another case was a patient for whom, due to a large hinge, we chose a smaller ablation zone but the same laser correction as that intended for the larger optical zone. The patient's preoperative spherical equivalent was −16.00 D, and 1 month after treatment the manifest spherical equivalent was + 3.00 D. Regression occurred over the next several months, and at 6 months, her refraction was plano with an uncorrected visual acuity that was one line better than her best corrected visual acuity preoperatively. Her vision and refraction remained the same at 1 year.

With increasing acceptance of the procedure, LASIK can be done for lower myopic corrections as well. We have found that when a low or moderate myopic correction is attempted, regression of the effect is minimal. Our experience correlates favorably with the results of other reported studies [1, 2]. When calculating a LASIK algorithm, as with PRK, one must take regression into account and look for ways to minimize its effect. The use of a multizone pattern ablation with a very smooth transition zone is one new approach, and preliminary results suggest less regression with this approach than after single-zone treatments.

The pathogenesis of myopic regression after LASIK remains somewhat uncertain. In the higher myopes, deeper stromal ablations are required and produce a 20–30% thinner cornea. Initial concern was that as the cornea becomes thinner, it can become ectatic. Nevertheless, our early experience has shown the opposite; that is, the cornea progressively thickens over the first 6 postoperative months.

From this observation, we decided to conduct a prospective study to analyze cornea thickness and curvature after LASIK. Our study included refraction, central pachymetry, and corneal topography before surgery and at follow-up visits at 1 week, 1 month, 3 months, 6 months, and 1 year. At this writing, 6-month data are available for 52 highly myopic eyes that underwent LASIK, with a mean preoperative spherical equivalent of −13.4 D. A mean myopic shift of 11.3%, increased corneal thickness of 3.2%, and increased corneal power of 2.2% occurred between the 1-week and 6-month follow-up visits. Regression was proportional to the amount of intended correction.

In another group of patients who underwent LASIK for more moderate myopia (mean spherical equivalent of −7.8 D), a mean myopic shift of 5.2% was found at the 3-month follow-up visit, in contrast to 11.3% of high myopes and 12.3% in an extreme myopic group (mean preoperative refraction of −21.7 D). Furthermore, an average additional 3.2% of regression was seen between the 3- and 6-month follow-up visits for the high myopic group (mean preoperative refraction of −13.1 D). Although not analyzed yet, our initial impression is that our low myopic correction group (−1.00 to −6.00 D) has a much smaller overall myopic shift that is between 2–5% of the initial attempted correction. These observations are similar to those made from early experiences with myopic keratomileusis (MKM). Professor Barraquer, in his masterly report 30 years ago, noted that an early overcorrection of 20% was desired to compensate for future regression of the effect [3].

Because deposition of new collagen material over the ablated bed is unlikely, it has been theorized that the pathogenesis of increased corneal thickness after LASIK and other types of keratomileusis is due to epithelial hyperplasia. Using high-frequency ultrasound (50 MHz), Francis Roy [personal communication, 1996] was able to measure epithelial thickness after LASIK and found a pattern of increasing epithelial thickness over the first postoperative months. It is our impression that there is a limit for the process of epithelial hyperplasia after LASIK with a consequent stabilization of the refractive effect at 6 months; conclusive proof awaits results of prospective, controlled studies. Longer follow-up time and closer observation of regression will help us better understand the natural course of the refractive effect of LASIK and, consequently, will improve the predictability and decrease the percentage of re-operations through generation of better treatment algorithms.

References

1. Fiander DC, Tayfour F. Excimer laser in situ keratomileusis in 124 myopic eyes. *J Refract Surg* 11(Suppl.):S234–S238, 1995.
2. Salah T, et al. Excimer laser in-situ keratomileusis (LASIK) under a corneal flap for myopia of 2 to 20 D. *Am J Ophthalmol* 121:143–155, 1996.
3. Barraquer JI. Keratomileusis. *Int. Surg.* 48:103–117, 1967.

9 LASIK Complications Management

Ioannis Pallikaris and Dimitrios Siganos

The vast majority of LASIK complications are intraoperative. Postoperative complications are almost always related to events that occurred during surgery. Most complications unique to LASIK are microkeratome related. With improvement in microkeratome technology, many of the complications encountered with older generations of microkeratomes should eventually become historic.

New technological advances have improved the safety and efficacy of automated lamellar corneal surgery using microkeratome instrumentation. An impressive example is the intraoperative use of ultrasonic pachometry, which allows measurement of flap thickness directly or indirectly by subtracting the bed thickness from the preoperative corneal thickness. If this instrument had been available in the early days of our practice, perforation into the anterior chamber during ablation (a complication encountered in our first series of 10 eyes) could have been avoided.

Computerized videokeratography (CVK), whose evolution has closely paralleled that of laser keratorefractive surgery, is another advance that has proved an invaluable tool, not only for performing LASIK and guiding modification of surgical results but also for its ability to help solve many of the optical enigmas of refractive surgery, often while eliciting new questions to be solved. Although intraoperative modulation of corneal curvature is currently in its infancy, this new capability will undoubtedly lay the groundwork for the next leap forward in LASIK-related technology development.

Intraoperative Complications

Microkeratome-Related Complications

Suction

When the suction ring handpiece is applied to the conjuctiva, variable chemosis may result. If this occurs, the suction may not work properly because conjunctival tissue can occlude the pneumatic ring suction port(s). If minimal chemosis is encountered, a spatula or muscle hook can be used to massage the excess fluid posteriorly so that the ring seats properly. When severe chemosis is present, excess fluid can be drawn into an insulin syringe. In this case, the conjuctiva should be entered with a 27- to 30-gauge needle posterior to the suction ring position.

When the suction ring is fully engaged, intraocular pressure (IOP) should be 65 mm Hg or greater. The pressure is checked by applanation using a surgical tonometer. If tonometry indicates an IOP of less than 65 mm Hg, do not proceed with surgery unless the IOP can be corrected; otherwise the flap created will have a variable and suboptimal thickness because an inadequate amount of tissue will have been introduced through the suction ring opening. For the same reason, the flap diameter will be smaller, allowing only for a smaller and thus, more likely, a poorly centered laser ablation. Flap thickness may also influence refractive outcome: If a laser nomogram is used that is based on the ablation rate of corneal tissue starting at an assumed specific depth in the stromal bed, predictability of the refractive result is affected.

Gear Mechanism

Foreign material, debris, and salt crystals from saline solutions that are used during surgery can become caught between the microkeratome gear mechanisms, resulting in malfunction of the system during passage of the instrument across the cornea.

In such instances, the gears do not advance, or they do so for a distance and then stop, resulting in an incomplete flap, often with an irregular bed (Fig. 9-1 and Plate 35). Proper assembly, cleaning, and checking of the gears and dovetail track, as well as proper alignment and lubrication of the drive gears in the dovetail, ensure free advancement of the microkeratome.

Blade

Always use a new blade for each case. Compared to new blades, used blades are poor quality, often having a thicker and more irregular

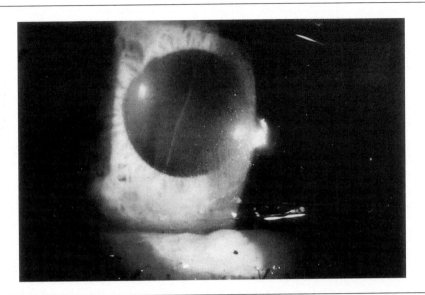

Fig. 9-1. Mild striae and intrastromal undulations due to arrest of keratome.

cutting edge, which may result in thin flaps or uneven flap thickness, or both.

Only blades that are made expressly for the brand of microkeratome being used should be selected. By doing so, the surgeon can ensure appropriate sharpness and edge quality. In addition, the blades will fit precisely into the microkeratome head—a sharp blade does not produce good results if its orientation inside the microkeratome is askew.

Depth Calibration

We consider a 130- to 160-micron thick flap to be of optimal thickness. When a flap is too thin, it cannot be handled easily and ultimately may adhere to underlying stroma in an irregular or rotated position (see Flap-Related Complications below). Moreover, a very thick flap results in a deeper ablation. If the intended correction is too high, especially with larger ablation zones, there is a postsurgical risk of progressive corneal ectasia, endothelial decompensation, or perforation of the anterior chamber.

Perforation of Anterior Chamber

During Microkeratome Use. At least two cases of microkeratome-related globe perforation with consequent severe visual loss have been verbally reported at major ophthalmic meetings. In both instances, it seems that insertion of an inappropriately sized steel plate into the microkeratome head was the cause. As emerging instrument designs eliminate this potential source of human error, this devastating complication should be eliminated.

Theoretically, perforation might also occur after prolonged application of the suction ring at high vacuum levels. Under such conditions, excess corneal tissue could be drawn up above the advancing microkeratome blade. Fortunately, no such occurrence has been reported, and such an event seems highly unlikely with current techniques and instrumentation.

During Laser Ablation

Perforation of the anterior chamber is a complication that we hope will never again be reported. This occurred through the cornea of a 28-year-old male with a preoperative central thickness of 480 microns, which was measured both optically and ultrasonically.

Although mobilization of the hinged flap appeared uneventful, aqueous humor was encountered at the center of the ablated area after 18 D were ablated of a planned 20-D correction.

The ablation was stopped immediately and the flap secured back to its original position with three 10.0 nylon sutures at 3, 1, and 5 o'clock. One milliliter of subconjunctival gentamicin 20 mg and dexamethasone 1 mg were injected into the lower fornix. Atropine sulfate was also instilled topically, and the eye was pressure-patched.

The next day the eye appeared quiet, but the cornea displayed marked central stromal edema. Patching, subconjuctival injection, and atropine sulfate eye drops were repeated for the first 3 postoperative days, after which the patch was removed. Combined tobramycin-dexamethasone and atropine sulfate eye drops were prescribed for the next week. At 1 month, slit-lamp examination revealed that the hinged lamellar flap had been extremely thick, leaving behind only a thin stromal bed to be ablated at the time of surgery. The cornea became ectatic after surgery, but over time CVK maps showed an initially central, localized keratoconus that decreased in magnitude. At the last recorded follow-up visit in October 1995 (4 years after surgery), the topographic appearance of central ectasia was still prominent (Fig. 9-2), and manifest refraction with $-2.00 - 4.00 \times 180$ yielded best spectacle-corrected visual acuity of 20/40.

Flap-Related Complications

Total Cap Instead of a Flap

This is a relatively common complication, and in our experience it has accounted for 4% of all complications. Total cap generation can occur via three mechanisms: (1) intraoperative IOP lower than 65 mm Hg

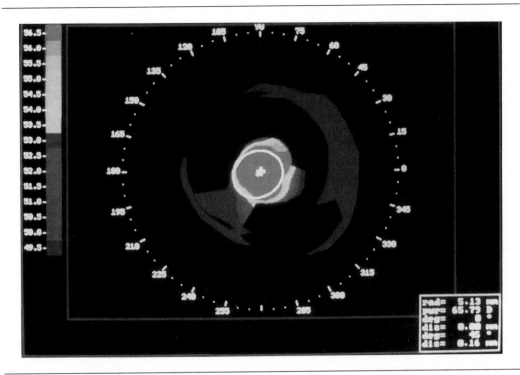

Fig. 9-2. Corneal topography of an iatrogenically induced keratoconus. The eye sustained perforation into the anterior chamber during excimer laser ablation for LASIK.

during suction fixation; (2) a small cornea (< 10.5 mm in diameter); the microkeratome, calibrated to produce a hinged flap in a cornea of 11 mm or more, stops farther peripherally than is required for a small cornea; (3) the keratome stopper was not fixed.

By itself, a cap is not a serious complication and can be managed easily. Ablation may proceed as usual and the cap replaced. In most cases, air drying is enough to promote adherence of the cap to the bed. If there is any doubt regarding cap adhesion, anchor sutures can be placed.

Reapposition of the corneal cap should be as exact as possible. To best manage this complication, the cornea should be marked out at one or more points at its edge preoperatively with a radial keratotomy (RK) marker or similar device especially designed for this purpose so that reference marks are present on both sides of the lamellar resection (see Chap. 7, LASIK Surgical Techniques).

Excessive handling of the cap (or flap) should be avoided. In addition to the defects that excessive handling could produce and the potential for overhydration or dehydration, differentiation of the epithelial and stromal surfaces can become extremely difficult. This problem is best prevented by leaving the cap undisturbed in the microkeratome head slit while performing the laser ablation. In this way, the cap is handled less and the position of the flap in the microkeratome head dictates the proper alignment for later placement and adherence to the stromal bed.

Once the epithelial surface of the cap has been identified, the corneal bed is flooded with balanced salt solution (BSS), the cap is gently reposited, aligned with fine movements, and dried using humidified air. A wet cellulose sponge works quite well for this maneuver; however, some surgeons prefer to use tying forceps or a fine (27 or 30) gauge cannula. Under no circumstances should a toothed forceps be used as the corneal disc tears easily.

Some surgeons believe that retraction of the flap edges, caused by excessive air drying, might lead to irregular astigmatism. In our experience, air drying does not appear to be problematic. An alternative is to apply air from a greater distance, at a lower flow rate, or to simply wait a longer period of time for the cap to adhere without forced air-drying. The *striae sign,* in which striae are seen in the cap when pressing gently with a Merocel sponge on the peripheral cornea, is an excellent indicator that cap adherence to underlying stroma is sufficient.

Incomplete Flap

Occasionally, despite meticulous, systematic preoperative inspection and cleaning of the microkeratome, mechanical problems may arise during microkeratome operation. We have encountered three cases in which the microkeratome, after mobilizing half the flap, ceased forward movement and did not respond to any attempts to free it (see Plate 35). In such cases, the suction is released and the suction ring–microkeratome complex is gently removed from the eye as one piece, taking great care not to induce any damage to the flap. Following removal of the microkeratome, the flap interface is irrigated with BSS solution using an air cannula to remove any epithelial cells, and the flap is reposited and dried. Combined antibiotic-steroid drops, a cycloplegic agent, and topical nonsteroidal anti-inflammatory drug (NSAID) are placed onto the eye, and a bandage contact lens is applied for 1–2 days to help maintain the orientation of the partial flap as it heals; the steroid-antibiotic drops are continued 4 times per day for 1 week. If there is concern that a bandage contact lens may not be tolerated acutely, the eye can be pressure-patched and lens fitting attempted the next day.

LASIK can be repeated after 3–6 months. The microkeratome almost never cuts at the same point, and the reoperation can be approached like a primary procedure. One possible exception is the

Schwind microkeratome (Kleinostheim, Germany), which stabilizes the eye by applying direct suction to the cornea prior to performing the lamellar incision.

Some surgeons have advocated completing the lamellar keratectomy via freehand dissection when keratome arrest occurs. Although this may produce acceptable results in instances where the microkeratome has already cut across the optically important zone overlying the pupil, such practices are generally unwise because significant amounts of irregular astigmatism may result from such maneuvers.

Stromal Bed–Related Complications

Excessive Hydration or Desiccation of the Bed

Laser ablation should always be performed on a dry stromal bed. Hydration or desiccation of the bed alters the ablation rate of the tissue, leading to an unpredictable result. If for any reason (for example, temporary laser failure) there is a time lapse between creation of the flap and laser ablation, the flap can simply be reposited to its original position during this interval. With the flap in place, the cornea can be irrigated without affecting stromal hydration. Laser ablation can proceed as usual, even after a delay of 30 minutes. The same recommendations apply if laser failure occurs during stromal ablation.

Before laser ablation, it is important that the conjunctival cul-de-sac be dried with cellulose sponges. In one case, we encountered undercorrection postoperatively as a probable sequela of excessive lacrimation during laser ablation. In such instances, the ablation should be stopped, the bed and the cul-de-sac dried with sponges, and ablation then resumed on dry stroma. Similarly, if fluid is seen to arise from within the stromal bed during laser ablation, it is acceptable to interrupt the procedure briefly to dry the stromal surface with a cellulose sponge.

Rough, Irregular Surface

A rough or irregular stromal bed is another microkeratome-induced complication. In this situation, ablation is performed as usual. Irregularities in the interface usually fit in with each other when the flap is reposited. Irregular astigmatism may result but is usually transient, resolving after 3–5 months.

Laser-Related Complications

Laser Failure

If the laser fails and needs more than 30–60 minutes to be repaired, it is prudent to terminate the procedure. LASIK can easily be reattempted by lifting the flap after 48 hours with tying forceps. For a discussion of laser failure occurring during ablation, see Excessive Hydration or Desiccation of the Bed.

Decentration

Decentration recognized after laser ablation is a serious complication of PRK and LASIK. With decentration, the patient is forced to see through the periphery of the ablated area, which often manifests irregular astigmatism and undercorrection with regard to the target spherical equivalent. As with PRK, significant loss of best spectacle-corrected visual acuity is common with decentrations of greater than 1 mm. Decentration may also produce monocular diplopia and asthenopia. Active eye-tracking–assisted laser systems greatly reduce the incidence of this complication, which may be more likely to occur during LASIK given the need for prolonged (more myopic) ablation times in many cases and the increased difficulty of fixating a target light through the stromal bed produced by the microkeratome.

We have experienced three cases of decentration. One method of treating decentration is to transpose the ablation center with use of arcuate incisions. The arcuate incision is performed on the opposite side from the decentered ablation (i.e., if decentered medially, perform the cut temporally; if upward, then make the cut inferiorly). As shown in Figure 9-3, the effective ablation center is moved centrally following arcuate keratotomy. An alternative would be to apply eccentric PRK or LASIK in a graded fashion, with the assistance of masking agents as appropriate. For a more complete discussion of decentration and its management, see Chapters 5 and 6.

Ablation of Hinge

Hinge ablation can occur in the presence of a small flap diameter, a decentered flap, an incompletely reposited flap, a decentered ablation, or a large ablation zone diameter. Hinge ablation is common during hyperopic and toric ablations. To avoid this problem when treating hyperopia, a larger diameter flap (9–10 mm) can be created with the appropriate suction ring and microkeratome unit. When treating astigmatism, it is helpful to rotate the suction ring, and hence the orientation of the flap hinge, along or adjacent to the flat meridian of the elliptical toric ablation. Examples of the ablation profiles created during toric or hyperopic LASIK are shown in Chapter 7 (see Plates 28, 29).

Ablation of the hinge per se does not usually create any problems, especially if the flap thickness is adequate (130–160 microns). Theoretically, however, hinge ablation might lead to a somewhat prismatic effect at the edge of the flap that can induce halo phenomena, but this

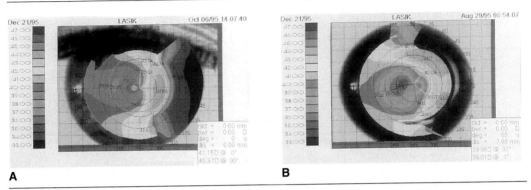

Fig. 9-3. A. Topography of a decentered ablation in a totally clear flap, causing irregular astigmatism. The best corrected visual acuity (BCVA) at this time was 20/40, with −1.0 sph, −3.0 cyl × 100. **B.** Arcuate cuts were performed and the ablation zone was shifted centrally. This resulted in regaining the preoperative BCVA of 20/20 with refraction of −1.0 sph, −1.0 cyl × 100.

has yet to be conclusively demonstrated clinically. Irregular thickness of the flap undersurface can also create irregular astigmatism. To avoid this complication, all steps of flap creation, reflection, and stromal bed ablation should be properly followed. It is wise to avoid extending the flap base manually, as it might lead to an irregular hinge with resultant irregular astigmatism. If the procedure is aborted after lamellar keratectomy is attempted, allow 3–6 months before repeating the procedure.

Postoperative Complications

Optical Complications

Overcorrection and Undercorrection

Unfortunately, there is still no definitive, universally accepted nomogram for LASIK, and therefore most LASIK surgeons use their own nomograms (which may vary for each brand of laser). PRK nomograms do not apply to LASIK in most instances. Using the PRK nomogram for LASIK (which is always corrected to the corneal plane) results in undercorrection for myopia of up to 6–8 D, whereas high myopia treatments yield overcorrections. This is probably due to a different ablation rate of the cornea stromal tissue at different depths (i.e., higher ablation rate as the blade goes deeper). Photoablation should always be performed on a dry stromal bed. No topical medications are added after the flap is reflected.

Management of undercorrection is usually not problematic. Eyes with undercorrection can be retreated within 3 months. We prefer to wait at least 1–2 months, especially for highly myopic eyes, as some regression can be anticipated. The advantage of early retreatment is that the flap can be easily reflected and manipulated manually. During our early experience, we retreated LASIK undercorrection in five cases (ranging from −1.50 to −7.50 D) with surface PRK. This was attempted between 5 and 11 months after LASIK. In all five cases, good results were achieved. We currently have follow-up data up to 31 months, with no regression or stromal haze greater than + 2 in any case. However, this series of patients who have undergone PRK following LASIK is too small to establish definitive conclusions, and these promising results await further confirmation in larger, prospective clinical trials.

A high myope turned hyperope is an unhappy individual. In a series of 325 eyes with myopia greater than −8.0 D, overcorrection was observed in 19 eyes (5.8%) with a range of +0.25 to +8.0 D. Overcorrection can be treated in the same manner as undercorrection. However, ablation centration of hyperopic treatments is difficult, especially if the original flap created for myopic treatment is small.

As a result of our initial experience with LASIK for high myopia, we have opted for a conservative approach, targeting −1.50 D as an initial refractive endpoint. Before any re-ablation is performed, the interface should be thoroughly cleansed of all epithelial debris. At the time of retreatment, 1 D is added to the attempted correction in residual myopia and 1.5–2.0 D for hyperopia, to account for the different ablation rate of the scar tissue in the stromal bed.

Regression

In our experience, refractive regression following LASIK is minimal. The refractive result stabilizes from the third month onward in most cases. In 14.8% of our cases, however, there was a regression of 0.5–1.5 D between the third and twelfth month and a further 0.25–0.5 D regression between the twelfth and twenty-fourth month. The maximum regression we have observed after LASIK is 2.0 D.

Unlike PRK, steroids are of no benefit in reversing regression after LASIK. Depending on the refraction, as well as the patient's needs, we prefer to intervene by treating regression with a second LASIK procedure, at least 6 months after the initial LASIK and after refractive stability has been documented.

Induced Regular Astigmatism

Regular astigmatism can sometimes be produced by spherical ablation profiles, minimal decentration of the ablation zone, and variations in flap healing. In our experience, the amount of preoperative versus postoperative regular astigmatism is not statistically different at 12 months after surgery. In 92% of our 325 cases, the induced regular astigmatism was 1.0 D or less, usually with the rule. In 8% of cases, the induced astigmatism was between 1.25 and 4 D. We recommend treating such regular astigmatism using arcuate keratotomy incisions after the third month.

Another cause of astigmatism is the presence of epithelial cells under the flap. The astigmatism thus induced generally has its flatter axis in the meridian of the epithelial cell deposits. By mobilizing the flap and irrigating away abnormal interface material, such astigmatism can usually be significantly reduced.

Induced Irregular Astigmatism

Induced irregular astigmatism is produced by eccentric ablation, suturing of the flap or cap, interface remnants, epithelial islands, or an irregularly reposited thin flap, which produces wrinkles. The underlying cause should be treated in each case. Epithelial remnants and islands causing irregular astigmatism should be removed within the first 3 months (Plate 36). The same prompt attention should be given to a thin flap that has been irregularly reposited (Fig. 9-4). During the first 3 months, the flap can be easily lifted by gently scratching through the epithelium at one point on the flap margin. A 30-gauge cannula is then pushed through the epithelial defect and under the flap while irrigating with BSS. The flap can then be lifted easily, and the bed is copiously irrigated. The flap then is reposited in its proper position.

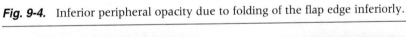

Fig. 9-4. Inferior peripheral opacity due to folding of the flap edge inferiorly.

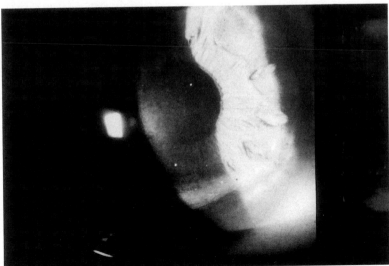

Glare, Halos, and Polyopia

Problems such as glare, halos, or uniocular polyopia are rare after a properly performed LASIK. In contrast to PRK, where a 5-mm-zone ablation might produce an effective central optical zone of uniform power measuring only 3–4 mm in diameter the effective central optical zone approaches that of the ablation zone diameter in LASIK. The fact that the ablated area is covered by a flap creates a cushioning effect at the edge of the ablation zone, allowing for a more regular and smooth transition of refractive power to the periphery. Glare, halos, or polyopia arise from eccentric ablations or very small ablation-zone diameters (< 4 mm), particularly in eyes with large pupils. Once diagnosed, the underlying cause can generally be treated. In eyes with large pupils, we recommend that ablation zones of at least 5 mm be performed. For retreatments, we use a 6-mm zone with transepithelial PRK or LASIK.

Decentration

The topic of decentration after LASIK is addressed under Intraoperative Complications.

Central Islands

Contrary to earlier opinions, central islands seem to be more common after LASIK than PRK. It may be difficult to recognize these islands, however, unless the color code of the topography is modified to the smaller steps (0.5 D is recommended) used with relative scales rather than the 1.0 D or 1.5 D steps recommended by Waring and Wilson/ Klyce, respectively.

Although little is known about the natural history of these topographic abnormalities when they arise after intrastromal ablation, observation is a prudent approach initially. If no sign of resolution is seen by 3 months after surgery, it may be reasonable to consider treating the island while the original lamellar flap can still be easily mobilized by manual blunt dissection. Prior to treating a topographic abnormality that appears by CVK mapping to be a central island, the surgeon should be absolutely certain that the changes observed arise from irregularities within the stromal bed rather than the flap itself. For a more detailed discussion of treating topographic central islands, see Chapter 5.

Medical Complications

Corneal Flap or Cap Loss

Loss of the flap or the cap, which results from incomplete adherence of the flap or cap to the bed, is a rare occurrence when proper air drying is performed after LASIK. Loosening of the pressure patch or eye rubbing may trigger flap or cap dislocation, and patients should be counseled accordingly.

There are two management alternatives for a lost flap or cap. The best is likely suturing a lamellar homograft to the stromal bed. The other alternative is to allow epithelialization of the bed, which can yield an acceptable result if excessive corneal haze does not ensue (capless technique). The cornea should be allowed to follow its natural course of healing. When the eye is quiet and stable, additional intervention can be considered. The capless technique, however, may be applicable only to myopic keratomileusis. In hyperopic keratomileusis, however, a lamellar graft is essential at the time of cap loss, and surgeons should be prepared for this possibility. Once corneal topography has stabilized, enhancement procedures (including RK, astigmatic keratotomy [AK], or homoplastic automated lamellar keratoplasty [ALK]) may be attempted.

We have experienced three lost caps. In one case where the cap was thick and the remaining cornea thin, keratophakia was performed using a donor cornea. This case developed an internal keratoconus and marked haze (scarring). The eye later underwent full-thickness penetrating keratoplasty. The other two cases were left capless, and later, severe haze developed, which was treated 10 and 12 months later using transepithelial PRK.

Irregular Flap (Wrinkled, Rotated)

Irregular flaps, whether rotated or wrinkled (Fig. 9-4), are almost always the result of a thin flap, usually with a thickness less than 90 microns. This defect can result from uneven or disrupted microkeratome advancement or from the blade engaging at shallow thickness and going progressively deeper as it advances across the cornea.

Reference marks made by an RK marker or specially designed LASIK marker at the edges of the flap at the beginning of the procedure act as intraoperative guides to proper flap reapposition. If wrinkling or rotation of the flap subsequently induces loss of best corrected visual acuity and/or irregular astigmatism, then action is taken as soon as the complication is recognized.

Irregular Bed

An irregular bed can be produced by interrupted automated keratome movement (Chiron, Irvine, CA), manual keratomes (due to unsteady speed and force applied during the cut), or a rotating system keratome (Draeger Storz, Heidelberg, Germany) that might go deeper as it advances (see Fig. 9-1 and Plate 35). If a complete flap has been created, it is usually wise to perform the photoablation because the flap, provided that it is of a proper thickness (130–170 microns), reduces the irregularities without producing significant irregular astigmatism. If astigmatism is encountered postoperatively, it is prudent to wait for at least 3 months before intervening unless it is obvious that the anatomic defect can be easily rectified. The irregular flap shown in Plate 36 initially produced an astigmatism of 7 D. At 3 months, the astigmatism was only 0.75 D.

Retained Particulate Debris

Debris may have its origin in the microkeratome head, glove dust, or filaments from cotton or cellulose sponges or other material (Plate 37). Early in our LASIK experience, we once used methylcellulose prior to ablation, and minute gel drops were still visible 12 months later, although vision was unaffected. Colored particles from the metal handles over which the laser mask rests in the Meditec laser have been observed in the epithelial-stromal interface, whereupon the handles were immediately changed to plastic by the manufacturer.

Interface debris rarely produces any tissue reaction, but it may induce an inflammatory reaction, local haze, and shrinkage of the flap (Plate 38). If inflammation does not subside with medical treatment, the material is washed out.

Any particles not inducing inflammation or affecting vision are left undisturbed. We usually prescribe combined antibiotic-steroid drops four times daily prophylactically during the first 14 days after surgery.

Haze and Scarring

Corneal haze following LASIK is rare. Scarring (Plate 39) is more often observed in cases in which thin, irregular flaps are associated with epithelial ingrowth or where sutures were used to fixate the flap. The best solution in these instances is to postpone further treatment with transepithelial PRK so that the abnormally thin and scarred flap is not manually manipulated during retreatment surgery.

Epithelial Ingrowth

At the outer edge of the hinged flap there is almost always some small ingrowth of epithelium (see Plate 36), although this may not be visible with slit-lamp biomicroscopy. Ingrowth that does not affect the center (pupillary region) or does not produce any optical effect is left untouched. When the process is more central and affects visual acuity (Plate 40), removal of the ingrowth is attempted. Be aware that epithelium in the periphery of the interface may cause thickening of one edge of the flap and may induce regular or, more commonly, irregular astigmatism. Removal of epithelial debris is best done by mobilizing the flap and simply irrigating the interface with BSS attached to a 30-gauge cannula. The most appropriate timing for removal of epithelial ingrowth needs further study.

Persistent Epithelial Defect or Erosion

We have never encountered a case of persistent epithelial defect or erosion following LASIK. LASIK leaves the epithelium, Bowman's layer, and anterior stroma intact. Preservation of anatomic relationships is probably the reason for the absence of such events following LASIK. If an epithelial defect within the flap is encountered, additional efforts should be made to ensure adequate flap adherence to the underlying stromal bed, such as application of a bandage contact lens or taping shut the eyelid during the first postoperative night.

Another complication resulting from a total cap is that the cap, if poorly adherent and not sutured, might be displaced into the fornix or over the lid margin. When this occurs, the corneal cap is usually de-epithelialized the next day. After suturing the cap or flap, the epithelium takes about 7–10 days to cover the denuded cornea. If the flap is sutured upside down, the defect will persist. This defect should be recognized as early as possible and the cap immediately replaced.

Infectious Keratitis

Infectious keratitis following LASIK is a genuine concern, despite the absence of any reported cases in the literature. There is certainly potential for contaminated debris to give rise to an intrastromal abscess. As such, perioperative antibiotics, meticulous surgical asepsis, and careful irrigation of debris from the stromal bed and flap undersurface are of paramount importance.

In our aggregate experience to date of 325 cases, only two inflammatory reactions have been observed after LASIK: one case of filamentary keratitis that developed on the first postoperative day and subsided spontaneously after 6 days and one case of inflammatory reaction due to retained surgical glove dust (see Plate 38), which subsided after a short course of topical steroids.

Subretinal Hemorrhage (Fuchs' Spot)

Two of 325 cases (0.6%) developed a macular Fuchs' spot at 1 and 3 months following LASIK. The incidence of this finding, as expected, seems to be double that of our PRK cases because LASIK is performed in higher myopias. A possible explanation is the sudden increase and decrease of the IOP during suction or release of the keratome suction ring. Another possible explanation is the effect that excimer laser shock waves may have on the choroid during ablation, although in vitro studies by Seiler et al. suggest that this would be unlikely given the distribution of mechanical forces within the eye during PRK.

Retinal Vascular Occlusion

We had one case of small branch vein occlusion 1 month following LASIK. The occlusion was near the macula and affected vision due to macular edema. The edema subsided 1 month later, and the eye regained the preoperative best corrected visual acuity with no treatment. A possible explanation of the mechanism for this complication is discussed under Subretinal Hemorrhage above.

Lacquer Cracks

Two eyes developed macular lacquer cracks that resulted in a permanent decline in visual acuity to 20/200. Both occurred 1 month following the operation. These cracks may perhaps be explained by the dramatic fluctuations in IOP observed during creation of the flap.

Endothelial Cell Count

There is no statistically proved loss of endothelial cell density following LASIK in our patient population, but we did observe one case of transient endothelial decompensation that persisted for 15 days following LASIK. This was probably a result of deep ablation due to a very thick flap. Treatment was steroid drops five times daily for 15 days. After 4.5 years of follow-up, the patient has a clear cornea without symptoms of endothelial dysfunction.

Conclusions

Knowledge of LASIK complications and their management is rapidly expanding. The evolution of LASIK procedures has many parallels to that of phacoemulsification in the early 1980s. As such, many complications believed to be serious or common at present may be unheard of in the future as technology and surgical skill advance in the years to come. We hope that the basic information and recommendations put forth in this chapter will help new LASIK surgeons acquire the knowledge and skill necessary to adeptly manage surgical complications of this procedure.

Bibliography

American Academy of Ophthalmology. Ophthalmic procedures assessment: Keratophakia and keratomileusis: Safety and effectiveness. *Ophthalmology* 99:1332–1341, 1992.

Bas AM, Onnis AM. Excimer laser in situ keratomileusis. *Refract Corneal Surg* 11(3):229–233, 1995.

Buratto L, Ferrari M, Rama P. Excimer laser intrastromal keratomileusis. *Am J Ophthalmol* 15(3):291–295, 1992.

Fiander DC, Tayfour F. Excimer laser in situ keratomileusis in 124 myopic eyes. *Refract Cornal Surg* 11(3):234–238, 1995.

Ibrahim O, et al. Automated in situ keratomileusis for myopia. *Refract Corneal Surg* 11(6):431–441, 1995.

Kremer FB, Dufek FB. Excimer laser in situ keratomileusis. *Refract Corneal Surg* 11(3):244–247, 1995.

Pallikaris I, et al. A comparative study of neural regeneration following corneal wounds induced by an argon fluoride excimer laser and mechanical methods. *Lasers Light Ophthalmol* 3(2):89–95, 1990.

Pallikaris I, et al. Laser in situ keratomileusis. *Lasers Surg Med* 10:463–468, 1990.

Pallikaris IG, et al. A corneal flap technique for laser in situ keratomileusis. *Arch Ophthalmol* 109(12):1699–1702, 1991.

Pallikaris IG, et al. Tecnica de colajo corneal para la queratomileusis in situ mediante laser. Estudios en humanos. *Arch Ophthalmol (ed Esp)* 3(3): 127–130, 1992.

Pallikaris IG, Siganos DS. Excimer laser in situ keratomileusis and photorefractive keratectomy for correction of high myopia. *Refract Corneal Surg* 10(5):498–510, 1994.

Pallikaris IG, Siganos DS. Corneal flap technique for excimer laser in situ keratomileusis to correct moderate and high myopia: Two year follow-up. Best paper of sessions. American Society of Cataract and Refractive Surgery Symposium on Cataract, Intraocular Lens, and Refractive Surgery, Boston, MA, 1994. Pp 9–17.

Rozakis GW. *Refractive Lamellar Keratoplasty.* Thorofare, NJ: Slack, 1994. Pp 111–122.

Seiler T, Schmidt-Petersen H, Wollensak J. Complications after Myopic Photorefractive Keratectomy, Primarily with the Summit Excimer Laser. In JJ Salz, PJ McDonnell, MB McDonald. *Corneal Laser Surgery.* St. Louis: Mosby–Year Book, 1995. Pp. 131–142.

Siganos DS, Pallikaris IG. Laser in situ keratomileusis in partially sighted eyes. *Invest Ophthalmol Vis Sci* 34(4):800, 1993.

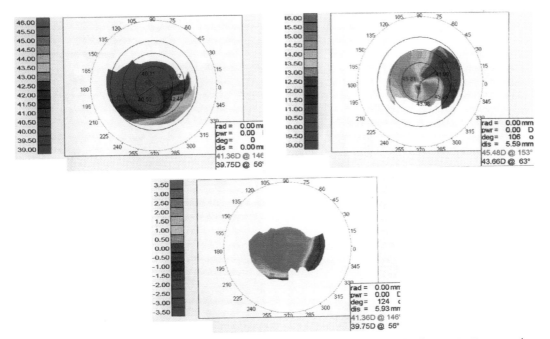

Plates 22 *(top left)*, **23** *(top right)*, **and 24** *(bottom)*. Induction of myopic shift after PTK. Preoperative topographic map showing flattening along the 56-degree meridian **(Plate 22)**. One month after PTK, the central cornea demonstrates steepening with minimal change in the axis and magnitude of astigmatism **(Plate 23)**. The difference map shows +3.5 D central steepening, presumably due to the edge modification treatment during PTK **(Plate 24)**. (See Chap. 6.)

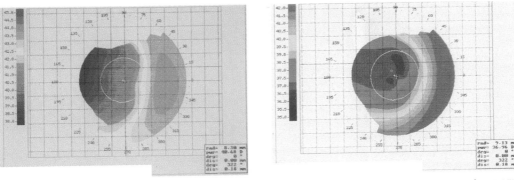

Plates 25 *(left)* **and 26** *(right)*. Treatment of ablation decentration and irregular astigmatism after PRK. One year following myopic excimer PRK, marked nasal decentration is present, with the temporal edge of the ablation zone near the pupil center **(Plate 25)**. BCVA was 20/30 with −1.5 D sphere. Retreatment was performed with a 6.0 mm, 200 pulse PTK ablation centered over the pupil to remove epithelium, followed by a 6.0 mm diameter, −1.0 D PRK ablation. Epithelial autofluorescence was monitored during the PTK portion of the ablation and confirmed that stromal ablation was greatest temporally. Methylcellulose 0.3% was then placed over the nasal two-thirds of the ablation zone and 100 more pulses were applied using a 4 mm PRK mode. Three months later, BCVA was 20/20 with +0.75 − 1.00 x 45, and CVK showed improved centration **(Plate 26)**. (From JH Talamo, MD Wagoner, SL Lee. Management of ablation decentration following excimer photorefractive keratectomy. *Arch Ophthalmol* 133:706–707. Copyright 1995, American Medical Association.) (See Chap. 6.)

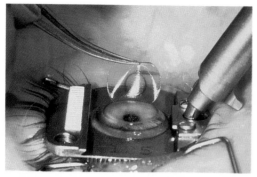

Plate 27. Demonstration of hinged corneal flap following lamellar corneal resection. (See Chap. 7.)

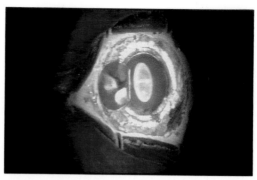

Plate 28. Visual augmentation of excimer photoablation with topical 2 percent fluorescein: Astigmatic ablation. (See Chap. 7.)

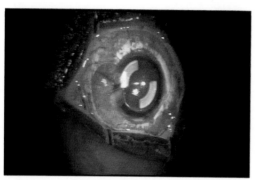

Plate 29. Visual augmentation of excimer photoablation with topical 2 percent fluorescein: Hyperopic ablation. (See Chap. 7.)

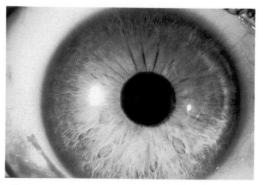

Plate 30. Typical day 1 postoperative appearance of an eye following LASIK. (See Chap. 7.)

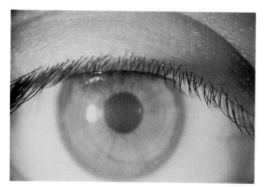

Plate 31. Slit-lamp photograph showing diffuse corneal edema secondary to increased intraocular pressure (IOP) 10 days following corticosteroid use after LASIK. The corneal edema and increased IOP resolved after the topical corticosteroid was discontinued. (See Chap. 8.)

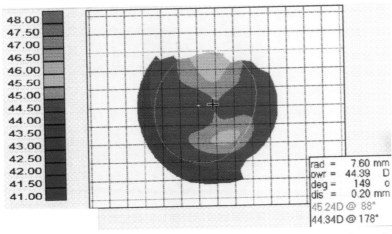

Plate 32. Computer videokeratography of an eye with −11.5 D of myopia prior to LASIK. (See Chap. 8.)

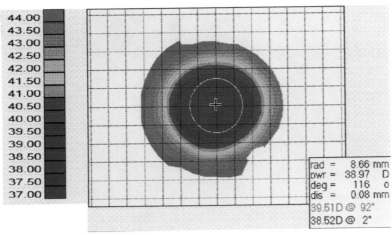

Plate 33. The same eye with a typical postoperative course at 1 week. (See Chap. 8.)

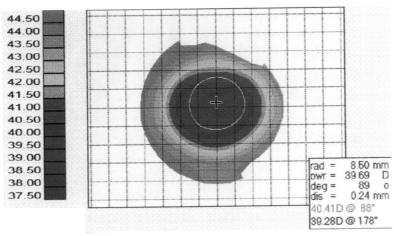

Plate 34. The same eye 3 months after the procedure. The eye regressed approximately 1 D between the first week and the third month after the procedure. (See Chap. 8.)

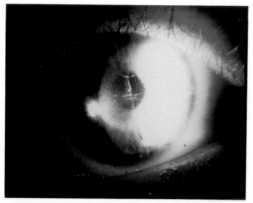

Plate 35. Prominent horizontally and vertically oriented central opacities due to arrrest of keratome. One line of best corrected visual acuity loss occurred. (See Chap. 9.)

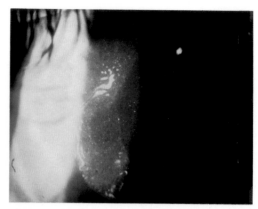

Plate 36. Epithelial islands under the hinge of a thin (60-micron) flap. The islands are oriented parallel and adjacent to the edge of the flap. (See Chap. 9.)

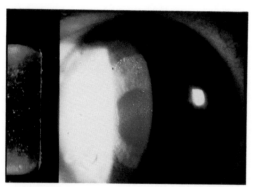

Plate 37. Intrastromal dust. (See Chap. 9.)

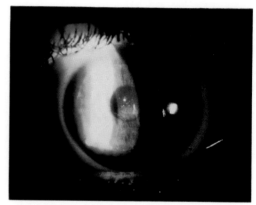

Plate 38. Cotton filament in the interface causing intrastromal reaction (steroids were given). (See Chap. 9.)

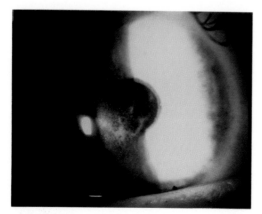

Plate 39. Intrastromal scarring. Despite the scarring, BCVA is 20/20 with plano −1.0 x 95. (See Chap. 9.)

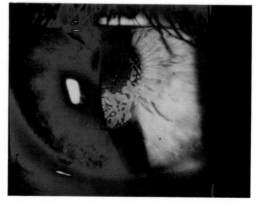

Plate 40. Prominent central foci of epithelial ingrowth beneath flap. (See Chap. 9.)

II Technical Considerations: Individual Laser Systems

In this part of the book, we examine the hardware and software features of the individual laser systems. While consideration of the various procedures and techniques of excimer laser surgery is important, careful consideration of the excimer laser systems commercially available for application in refractive surgery is equally important. Presently, there are at least nine systems available. The nine systems we will discuss comprise the principal list of lasers most readily available at this writing. Although other custom-made excimer lasers may be available for clinical use, their technical features and industrial support base are not readily accessible and so they are not addressed here.

The following chapters were written by experienced independent surgeons, who worked closely with representatives from the specific laser system manufactures to ensure the technical accuracy of each discussion. Much time and care was spent to achieve a balanced, uniform, consistent discussion of each system.

This part of the text is divided into three sections based on the major delivery system features and ablation approach of the excimer laser described: Wide Field Ablation, Scanning Slit Ablation, and Flying (Scanning) Spot Ablation. Each section is prefaced with a brief summary of the potential advantages and disadvantages of the ablation approach discussed. These comments are by no means exclusively characteristic of the laser systems described within each ablation approach; however, they should serve as good foundation for understanding basic strengths and weaknesses of the laser systems.

Wide Field Ablation

Lasers used for wide field ablation have the longest and strongest track record for technical dependability and clinical use in refractive surgery. This class of laser includes the Summit Apex Plus, Apex/OmniMed, and ExciMed (Chap. 10); the VISX STAR and 20/20 (Chap. 11); the Chiron-Technolas Keracor 116 (Chap. 12); and the Coherent-Schwind Keratom (Chap. 13). The principal feature that each of these systems share is their use of a broad circular beam of excimer laser light for the removal of corneal tissue, hence the term *wide field*. Although each system uses wide field ablation in a characteristically different way, general comments about this type of ablation can be useful in understanding the specific excimer laser described.

The primary advantage of wide field ablation is the shorter operating time, typically less than 30 seconds for a low myopic photorefractive keratectomy. Additionally, because the systems use a broad beam that does not need to be aligned relative to adjacent beams, eye-tracking features are not as important and can be considered optional for these systems. Most wide field lasers have been used for many years and have been both time tested and modified for improvement; they are thus further along in the U.S. FDA regulatory process than lasers used in scanning slit and flying spot ablation. Moreover, the simplicity of the expanding aperture in the wide field approach makes the correction of myopia and astigmatism rather easy.

A potential disadvantage of the wide field approach is the need for high output energy in order to achieve a therapeutic effect within the large area ablated. This need can result in higher costs and more frequent maintenance of the optical components subject to the higher energy. Good beam uniformity and homogeneity is also necessary to allow for a uniform pattern of ablation within the broad beam. Historically, the correction of hyperopia with the wide field approach has been more technically challenging and difficult than correction of myopia and astigmatism. In addition, the incidence of steep central islands is higher with wide field ablation than the scanning slit or flying spot approach.

10 Summit Apex Plus, Apex/OmniMed, and ExciMed Laser Systems

Uwe Genth, Ronald R. Krueger, Theo Seiler, and Alex Sacharoff

History

In 1985, Summit Technology opened its doors in Watertown, Massachusetts, with the goal of developing excimer lasers for a variety of medical applications. The Company was founded by David Muller, a former technical scientist at Lambda Physik, Acton, Massachusetts (a company that makes industrial excimer lasers). Summit's early research covered many medical specialties, including cardiology and dentistry. By 1991, however, the company had phased out these efforts and focused its attention on ophthalmology.

Summit was the first company to design and manufacture an excimer laser specifically for ophthalmic applications. Summit's first system, the ExciMed was first used clinically to perform routine excimer PRK in clinical trials in Europe, Asia, and the United States [1, 2]. Summit later introduced the OmniMed during the clinical trial process, and Apex (new name; identical to OmniMed). These were the first lasers approved for excimer photorefractive keratectomy (PRK) in the United States. The Apex Plus, which uses an erodible disk, is currently available for international sale only and is in clinical trials in the United States [3].

Among the major milestones of Summit is the U.S. Food and Drug Administration (FDA) approval of its SVS Apex laser for photo-therapeutic keratectomy (PTK) in March 1995, making it the first ophthalmic excimer approved for any use in the United States. In October of the same year, Summit received FDA approval to use its laser to perform PRK for myopia of −1.5 to −7.0 D, using a 6-mm optical zone. Summit was the first company to obtain PRK approval within the United States. Currently, Summit's Apex/OmniMed is one of only two lasers fully approved and sold for use in the United States.

At present, Summit has approximately 400 installations in 45 countries, and its lasers have been used to perform more than 500,000 PRK procedures around the world. The company manufactures its excimer laser workstations at its corporate headquarters in Waltham, Massachusetts, and at its European site in Cork, Ireland. Summit employs more than 200 people worldwide, including certified service technicians in more than 40 countries.

Unique Aspects of the Hardware

The Laser System

Each device in the Summit excimer laser series (Apex Plus, Apex/OmniMed, and ExciMed) is a compact laser that, although stationary, can be moved within a room if necessary (Fig. 10-1). Summit's objective was to design a commercial laser with all components integrated into one system. Rather than compiling laser components from

Fig. 10-1. Summit's Apex excimer laser, approved by the FDA for use in the United States in the treatment of low to moderate myopia without astigmatism.

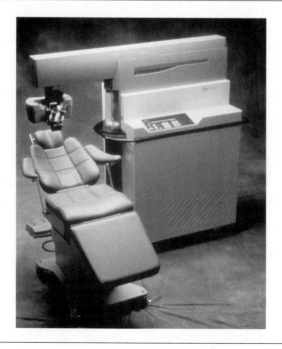

other laser companies, Summit designs and manufactures its own laser cavity and the laser's computer hardware system.

The software that operates the laser system is simple. Through a main menu one chooses submenus that define the treatment (e.g., PRK, phototherapeutic keratectomy [PTK], patient training, or laser disk for astigmatism or hyperopia). The main parameters required from the operator are the refractive data (sphere or, if necessary, cylinder) and the treatment zone.

The display system of the Summit series of lasers differs from that of other excimer lasers because of the absence of personal computer interfacing. The display consists of a window through which a single line of figures (42 letters or numbers) are digitally displayed. The letters are made up of a 5×7 matrix of light-emitting diodes (LEDs), which provides adequate resolution. Adjacent to the display is the keyboard, which has several function keys and a set of numerical keys.

An integrated thermal printer records the output information belonging to the last treatment as well as the actual laser parameters. The printout is from a typical narrow thermal printer roll.

All Summit systems, including the holmium:yttrium-aluminum-garnet (holmium:YAG) laser, have an internal water cooling system that emits waste heat to the environment by a cooler. There is no need for a water connection.

The active laser medium of an ophthalmic excimer laser is argon fluoride (ArF), which produces an ultraviolet beam of 193-nm wavelength. The Summit system works with a premix bottle that contains all components in the correct concentration for use in the cavity, namely fluorine (a toxic gas) and the rare gas components (e.g., helium and argon). The bulk of the premix is composed of inert gases, which are used as a buffer to stabilize the discharge process. The premix bottle is installed inside a secondary containment system. The capacity is approximately 40 fills of the cavity, but, if necessary, it will deliver five more fills. The customer is instructed to contact a Summit-trained technician to schedule a bottle change four or five fills before the cylinder becomes empty. Changing the gas bottle must be performed by an authorized technical representative from Summit. During the gas refill, the toxic component of the old fill is collected and bound in a filter. This filter is replaced with each gas bottle change.

The optical pathway in the Summit system is purged with pure nitrogen, which should be a minimum of 99.998% pure. To maintain purity, a steady connection to a nitrogen source is recommended instead of reconnecting the gas bottle.

The Summit systems are relatively small compared to other wide-field ablating lasers. The size of the Summit lasers is approximately

$165 \times 69 \times 186$ cm (L $\times$ W $\times$ H), and a typical system weighs 660 kg. The minimum room size is 10×12 feet. The electrical requirements meet both the American and European standard of 110 V, 15 amperes, and 60 Hz; or 220 V, 10 amperes, and 50 Hz, respectively. These are the two common standards, but each system could be adapted to other conditions if enough electrical power is provided.

Unlike other PC-based excimer laser systems, the Summit has a fixed microchip, so its software is permanently installed, and it is impossible to change or delete any part of it. To update the software, the microchip must be replaced. This provides a high level of security, protecting the system from breakdown caused by hard disk crash or software failure.

The surgical chair is reclinable, and the back rest and foot rest are moved into the horizontal position prior to the procedure. The patient's position beneath the laser can be adjusted and fine tuned by three pairs of foot switches for each direction of movement. The movements are made by electrically driven spindles. The chair has both high speed and fine (slow) speed movement. In addition, it is possible to adjust the distance of the head rest to the back rest and to position the head rest along two horizontal angles.

The Delivery System

The Summit lasers produce a full-size circular beam spot with a maximum diameter of 5.0 mm for the ExciMed and 6.5 mm for the Apex/OmniMed and the Apex Plus. An iris diaphragm provides a micron-step variable adjustment of the diameter, starting from less than 1.0 mm to the maximum spot size.

The optical portion of the beam delivery has no moving parts, except for the iris. Therefore, the center of the wide-field pulse is fixed, with all ablation circles being concentric to each other. There is no scanning or active movement of the beam, making active eye-tracking unnecessary.

The correction of myopia using a wide-field approach requires a homogeneous distribution of energy density within the circular ablation zone. The laser cavity itself produces a rectangular beam with a guassian energy profile that is determined by the shape and the arrangement of the laser electrodes. There are several optics in the laser rail, placed between the second turning mirror and the iris, which are used to shape the beam for proper illumination of the iris. In practice, it is often impossible to produce a completely uniform energy density, and consequently in early systems (e.g., ExciMed) the beam is shaped as the central part of a guassian curve. More recent systems (Apex/OmniMed and Apex Plus) utilize a larger optical zone size, which leads to a reduced tendency toward hyperopic overshoot. With the Summit ExciMed system, the small ablation zone diameter and gaussian energy distribution result in greater hyperopic overshoot in the early postoperative period [4, 5]. The Apex/OmniMed and Apex Plus produce less hyperopic overshoot. The optics, iris, and two turning mirrors are mounted on an optical bench, which provides a more stable beam profile over time in the 6.5-mm systems.

The whole optical pathway is enclosed and purged by nitrogen gas, beginning at the first turning mirror with the Apex Plus, and at the second turning mirror with the other Summit systems. During a 5-minute warm-up time after switching on the laser, a very high nitrogen flow removes all air from the rail. After the warm-up, nitrogen flow decreases, but flow continues during the period when the laser is turned on, except in the holmium:YAG laser. If the laser is not able to put out enough energy, it will not leave the "arming-laser" test procedure. If a refill is not possible, an adjustment of the pressure on the nitrogen valve to a higher value (4 bar, 60 psi) increases the purge and could activate the laser for a short period.

When the laser is running continually at a high voltage, the output energy can be improved by removing one attenuator. These small quartz plates are about 1 mm thick and do not have a refractive surface. They can be inserted automatically or removed with one keystroke.

The Summit lasers use a Zeiss microscope, providing a stereoscopic view with adjustable focus and four zoom factors, (0.6, 1.0, 1.6, and 2.5). In the ExciMed system, the last turning mirror for the microscope is placed behind the laser aperture, which prevents a confocal view for the surgeon because of parallactic error. To achieve a confocal view, the Apex/OmniMed system has two little mirrors, left and right, beside the laser aperture. The distance between these mirrors allows for passage of the excimer beam without ultraviolet (UV) exposure of any of the optics in the microscope head. Further improvements are seen in the Apex Plus, where there is only one mirror centrally mounted for both axes under the laser aperture. The mirror has a central hole to allow for passage of the laser beam.

Illumination of the patient's eye is achieved by an adjustable lamp on a flexible light fiber. The Apex/OmniMed and Apex Plus have an additional illumination source centrally, which is created by several tiny lamps arranged in a circular fashion under the laser aperture. Both illuminations are independently adjustable in their brightness.

The fixation target for the patient is a blinking green LED. This LED is mounted directly above the last turning mirror. Beneath the LED, there is also a lens that focuses the light onto the patient's eye. The advantage of focused fixation is that if the patient's eye deviates from the center, he or she experiences a drastic decrease in brightness. The green color and blinking feature also help to maintain fixation during the procedure. The ExciMed and Apex/OmniMed lasers have an additional red ring of light around the laser aperture.

The patient's eye is positioned and centered by using two helium-neon (HeNe) lasers. These HeNe beams converge at an angle of 45 degrees in the center of each ablation circle in the image plane. This means that the crossing of the HeNe beams defines the corneal height during treatment. After they merge, they diverge, placing two red spots on the iris adjacent to and on either side of the pupil. Decreasing the pupil size with a miotic agent facilitates better visualization of the two spots on the underlying iris. The small pupil also has the advantage of a higher depth of focus, which helps the myopic patient see the fixation target more easily. In cases where the center of the pupil does not correspond with the first Purkinje image during fixation, the centration of the HeNe beams should be made between the first Purkinje image and the geometric center of the pupil. The crossing point of the HeNe beams is not visible during ablation of the cornea, therefore, its position on the iris must be kept constant throughout the procedure.

The distance from the image plane to the laser aperture provides enough space to perform LASIK (17 cm), which is currently in clinical trials in the United States. The Apex/OmniMed system is also equipped to perform holmium:YAG treatments under the laser delivery system and microscope.

Maintenance Considerations

As with other wide-field excimer lasers, the high pulse energy of the Summit lasers results in high loading of the optics, with consequent susceptibility to damage and attrition. The optics near the output couplers of the cavity (including the output coupler itself, the first turning mirror, and the secondary-containment device [SCD] window) are especially vulnerable due to the high-UV energy exposure. The lifetime of these optics is variable, with the mean interval to change the optic being about 300,000–500,000 pulses for the output coupler, the turning mirror, and the SCD window. These three optics are not purged by nitrogen, except in the Apex Plus.

During the lasing process, the composition of the gas within the cavity changes slightly due to chemical reactions with the metal surface inside the cavity. Circulation and filtering of the gas is necessary to maintain the laser process.

As with most other excimer lasers, the Summit lasers require a change of the gas fill every day the laser is in use. If the system is not used for a long period, one gas exchange may not be sufficient to run the laser. The Summit lasers have an optional software feature to do a four-times gas exchange, whereby instead of fully filling the cavity (45 psi), the cavity is filled to 15 psi and evacuated to 3 psi pressure in each step. The premix gas bottle contains 40 fills but will deliver 5 more fills, if necessary. Evacuation of the cavity lasts approximately 4 minutes, and once the process is begun, it cannot be interrupted. Consequently, the gas-refill subroutine questions the user regarding the necessity of gas exchange to avoid a mistake.

When the laser is ready to begin treatment, a test of the fluence is automatically performed prior to each procedure. A shutter at the laser aperture closes, and the laser begins firing internally. All Summit systems have two power monitors, measuring the energy via a beam splitter. One monitor, installed before the optical rail, is placed between the first and second turning mirror. The beam splitter of the second monitor is mounted just in front of the laser aperture, to give the true output energy and to verify the condition of the delivery system optics by comparison with the other monitor. When both values are reduced, the voltage is adjusted on the cavity electrodes to achieve the level of fluence necessary to perform predictable PRK. The range within which the voltage is adjustable is 25–34 kv for the ExciMed, 20–29 kv for the Apex/OmniMed, and 22–29 kv for the Apex Plus. The actual voltage needed for a procedure can be checked afterward by requesting a printout of the laser parameters. With a fresh gas fill, the voltage should be within the lowest third of the specified range. As the gas quality decays during laser operations, the voltage can be increased until a fresh gas change is required.

Realignment of the cavity is necessary only when replacing or cleaning the laser resonator mirrors, the output coupler, or the high reflector.

The purchase of a Summit laser workstation includes a 1-year warranty. Summit offers a yearly maintenance contract for its machines. After 1 year or 600,000 shots, yearly maintenance contracts are available for approximately $36,000.

Safety Features

The premix bottle of laser gas, which includes fluorine, is installed inside the secondary containment device. This is a cabinet containing the main parts of the laser, excluding the optical rail; it is made of 5-mm-thick stainless steel. It is designed to protect the environment in case of a gas leak internal to the excimer laser system. During a gas change procedure, the used gas from the cavity has to pass through a filter, which is a type of charcoal scrubber. The toxic components are chemically bound in the filter, and the rare gas is emitted to the environment.

During a gas bottle change, the helium bottle must be connected to the nitrogen input valve. The helium must be of 99.999% purity. When switching the internal magnetic valves, the helium pressure is kept slightly above atmospheric pressure to prevent contamination of the pipeline and the cavity.

It is recommended that the nitrogen purge be permanently connected to a nitrogen source from a wall outlet. If this is not possible, a 50-liter gas bottle should be used. An additional small gas bottle should be kept nearby to prevent a possible break in procedure that could be caused by an empty bottle.

Calibration

On a daily basis, the fluence and the homogeneity of the laser beam should be checked by using a wratten gelatin filter. This gelatin filter is part of the calibration tool kit and is delivered with the laser. The filter is fixed on a white surface (paper) horizontally in the image plane. A standard PTK, using a beam diameter of 5.0 mm with the ExciMed or 6.5 mm with the Apex/OmniMed and Apex Plus, is then performed on the gelatin until the first perforation. Because the ablation rate (thickness of removed tissue per pulse) is determined by the fluence, the number of pulses necessary to perforate the gelatin should not vary significantly from day to day. Usually, 600–650 pulses are needed to ablate the gelatin to the point of perforation. Consistency regarding the required number of pulses over time is an important parameter for each individual system.

The homogeneity of the laser beam is judged by observing the uniformity of the ablated area during the calibration procedure. This area becomes more lightly colored (brighter) as the filter ablation progresses, signifying where inhomogeneities of energy distribution might exist. Continuing the ablation process beyond perforation allows for an objective assessment of homogeneity by counting the number of pulses required for near full perforation of the filter. The following points are important in this process, although they are covered in greater detail in the approved labeling of the system:

1. The first perforation must be in the center of the ablated area.
2. The progress of ablation must symmetrically extend outward.
3. The additional pulses required to ablate 90% of the area should not exceed 200 in number.

Once a week, it is necessary to check the position of the HeNe aiming beams and the fixation light while checking the fluence and beam profile. For checking the HeNe beams, a PTK with a small diameter (1 mm) is performed on exposed black photographic paper until the white layer appears. The position of the HeNe beams merging in the white circle can be checked separately to distinguish alignment by alternately covering the left and the right HeNe beams. If no photographic paper is available, it is possible to adjust the HeNe over the intersection of two lines drawn on a sheet of paper. The position of the small PTK in relation to the point of intersection can be checked during ablation. If the HeNe beams do not align or if there is a shift in their position, realignment of the HeNe by a service technician is absolutely necessary.

The fixation light for the patient also can be checked by using the intersection of lines on a piece of paper. The point of intersection can be aligned in the center of the merging point of the HeNe beams, and then, with the room darkened and the HeNe beams switched off, the projected blinking light is slightly visible on the paper.

Several additional safety considerations deserve mention. First, the electrical connection in the office should have a slow (sluggish) fuse or surge protector because a high-voltage surge occurs when the system is switched on. Next, excimer systems with a holmium:YAG laser should be installed in an air-conditioned surgery room with a temperature of less than 27°C (80°F). If there is no air conditioning, the holmium:YAG laser may not work on relatively warm days, in which case an error message, "Ambient Room Temperature Too High," is displayed.

Software-User Interface

There is no patient database or preexamination menu in the Summit systems. The lasers have a limited keyboard and display for inputting and reviewing numerical details of the treatment parameters (Fig. 10-2). The output information is scrolled along a single line of 42 numbers or letters on the digital LED display. There is no writing, deleting, or editing of the software components, and changes in the program plan can be made only by replacing the fixed microchip in the system. Operating Summit laser systems does not require a knowledge of computers, and the information is conveyed in English.

Ablation Parameters and Capabilities

The fluence of the Summit excimer lasers is 180 mJ/cm^2. To maintain this value, the voltage across the cavity electrodes is adjusted before each treatment. The stromal ablation rate (approximately 0.25 μm/pulse), is used in calculating the profile and pattern of ablation for

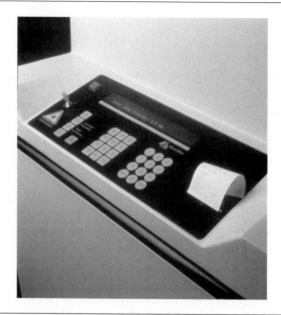

Fig. 10-2. Keyboard and display of the Summit Apex excimer laser.

correction of refractive error. A myopic ablation pattern is principally achieved by the stepwise opening of an iris aperture [6]. The diameter of these steps range from less than 1.0 mm to 5.0 mm with the ExciMed, and from less than 1.0 mm to 6.5 mm with the Apex/OmniMed and Apex Plus. A large number of steps helps to make the surface contour smooth, especially with the filling in of epithelium. An optional erodible laser disk feature for myopia is available with the Apex Plus laser, which helps to further enhance surface smoothness [3].

The ablation patterns for correction of astigmatism and hyperopia are only possible with the Apex Plus laser. The erodible (or ablatable) mask was first introduced with the ExciMed laser for the correction of astigmatism by placing the mask in an eye cup on the patient's eye [7]. This practice was discontinued because of difficulties in alignment, not only of the laser with the eye but also of the laser with the mask (disk) and the mask (disk) with the eye. Currently, only the Apex Plus offers this feature. The new laser disk is placed in an easy-to-use cassette, which is then inserted into a convenient port situated near the surgical microscope with the laser disk positioned to be coaxial with the laser beam [3]. This new laser disk feature, referred to as the *emphasis disposable laser disk,* is comprised of a thin-profile polymethyl-methacrylate (PMMA) disk encoded with the desired refractive correction. The disks have a diameter of 6.5 mm, which is the maximum

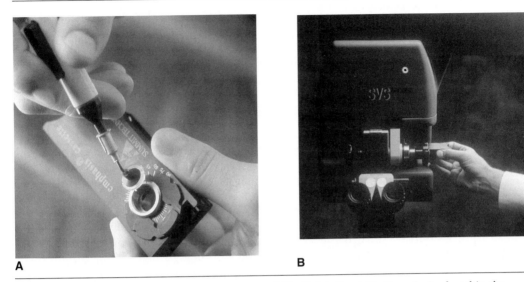

Fig. 10-3. A. Cassette in which the emphasis erodible disk is fixed. **B.** Cassette is placed in the optical rail just behind the laser aperture.

spot size of the Apex Plus and is applied on a quartz plate. The whole disk is fixed on a cassette (Fig. 10-3A), which is placed in the optical rail just behind the laser aperture (Fig. 10-3B) [3]. The PMMA absorbs the UV radiation and is ablated in a fashion similar to the cornea while the quartz substrate freely passes the laser light. As the PMMA ablation proceeds, an opening or hole in the disk allows the beam to pass and ablate the cornea. The shape of the hole is elliptic for the correction of myopic astigmatism and ring-shaped for hyperopic corrections. This method of laser delivery using a PMMA disk produces no step transitions on the corneal surface, making it much smoother than PRK with an iris and slit aperture [7].

For the correction of hyperopia, the maximum ablation depth is in the periphery, at a diameter of 6.0–6.5 mm. To allow the cornea to maintain a smooth profile, a transition zone is required that must be at least 1.0–1.5 mm in radius. To create this, an ablation zone of 8.0–9.0 mm is needed; Summit uses the reusable Axicon, a special optic to enlarge the beam size. Immediately following a 6.0- to 6.5-mm hyperopic treatment, the ablated disk is replaced by another cassette, containing this Axicon optic. The Axicon is a conical quartz optic that diverges the laser light and expands it to a ring-shaped beam on the corneal surface. The ring has an inner diameter of 6.0–6.5 mm, corresponding to the peripheral edge of the hyperopic correction, where its energy density is maximal. The energy density decreases outwardly to that of the ablation threshold at its outer diameter. Therefore, by applying a number of pulses corresponding to the maximum ablation depth of the hyperopic correction, a transition zone of up to 9.5 mm can be created. This method has been in clinical use since 1994 and achieves good alignment of the hyperopic ablation and the transition zone.

Advantages and Disadvantages

Preliminary Clinical Results

Demographics and Indications

In 300 patients, 398 eyes were treated for low to moderate myopia, ranging from −1.50 to −7.0 D, with a 6.0-mm ablation zone diameter as part of Summit's investigational device exemption (IDE) within the U.S. clinical trials. The minimum age was 21 years, and astigmatism was limited to 1.5 D of cylinder or less with a stable refraction. The mean age was 36.1 years (range 21–69), and 63.7% of patients were male and 36.3% female.

Efficacy

Uncorrected visual acuity (UCVA) was 20/40 or better in 95% (6 months) and 98.8% (1 year), 20/25 or better in 82.4% (6 months) and 89% (1 year), and 20/20 or better in 65.4% (6 months) and 80.5% (1 year).

Mean spherical equivalent manifest refraction was −4.37 ± 1.48 D (preoperative), +0.19 ± 0.82 D (1 month), −0.13 ± 0.66 D (3 months), −0.12 ± 0.70 D (6 months), and +0.08 ± 0.60 D (1 year). Predictability of outcome was within ± 2.00 D in 96.8% (6 months) and 100% (1 year), within ± 1.00 D in 89.4% (6 months) and 85.3% (1 year), and within ± 0.50 D in 64.8% (6 months) and 51.2% (1 year).

Safety

Re-epithelialization occurred within 3 days in 95.4% of eyes, with 100% closure within 1 week. Clinical success was defined as UCVA of 20/40 or better with a best spectacle-corrected visual acuity (BSCVA) of at least 20/25 or less than or equal to 1 line loss from the preoperative value. This was found in 91.8% of eyes (6 months) and 97.6% of eyes (1 year). BSCVA was 20/20 or better preoperatively in 97.4% of eyes, and postoperatively in 95.0% of eyes (6 months) and 100% of eyes (1 year). The remaining eyes were either 20/25 or 20/32. Loss of 2 lines of BSCVA was found in 4.7% (6 months) and 1.2% (1 year), and 3 lines loss in 1.8% (6 months) and 0% (1 year). Anterior stromal haze was recorded as trace (0.5) in 53.4% (6 months) and 43.9% (1 year), mild (1.0) in 7.3% (6 months) and 0% (1 year), and moderate (2.0) in 2.3% (6 months) and 0% (1 year). Glare and halos were reported in 10% of eyes (6 months) and 2.4% of eyes (1 year). IOP elevation of more than 5 mm Hg was seen in 1.8% (6 months) and 0% (1 year).

Adverse events occurred in less than 1% of eyes at any postoperative visit, including blurred vision, cataract, corneal epithelial defect, corneal scarring, corneal ulceration or infection, diffuse nebulae, dryness, edema, foreign body sensation, ghost images, guttae, iritis, irregular astigmatism, itching, lens opacity, microcysts, monocular diplopia, patient discomfort, photophobia, ptosis, reading difficulty, and superficial punctate keratitis.

Summary

PRK using the Apex/OmniMed excimer laser has been shown to be safe and effective for the treatment of low to moderate myopia. It is approved in the United States by the FDA for clinical use in treating myopia. The Apex Plus is in clinical trials in the United States.

Comparison to Other Systems

The Summit Apex excimer laser is currently one of only two commercially available systems that have been approved by the FDA for clinical use in treatment of low myopia in the United States. Summit was the first company to receive FDA approval of its laser, which can perform PRK for up to −7.0 D. Summit's track record demonstrates predictability and stability of outcome, as shown in the prospective clinical trials [8]. With regard to technical issues, the Summit Apex/OmniMed laser is effectively able to correct myopia and treat corneal opacities and irregularities. The treatment of astigmatism and hyperopia will be possible with a patented laser disk that has been in international distribution for nearly 2 years in the Apex Plus and has been modified in the Apex laser for clinical trials in the United States. In the future, it may be possible to upgrade this system to include the erodible disk feature.

The Summit Apex Plus is able to treat myopia, astigmatism, hyperopia, and therapeutic corneal opacities with its emphasis erodible laser disk. This technology, which is currently available internationally, has distinct advantages over other nonscanning wide-field systems in that it avoids the use of apertures or slits in achieving the ablation profile. This eliminates the step transitions on the corneal surface, making it the smoothest way to perform PRK [7].

Although scanning systems claim to produce a smooth corneal surface comparable to that achieved by the erodible disk, they require a sophisticated scanning motor and tracking system to do so. Should a scanning motor or tracking system fail to operate properly, it can concentrate the rapidly pulsing light at one location, resulting in corneal perforation within 2–3 seconds. Scanning laser systems also require a longer procedure time, which may contribute to unwanted corneal dehydration and unpredictable results [9].

The Summit series of excimer lasers is designed specifically for ophthalmic applications. Other commercially available excimer lasers for ophthalmic use incorporate industrial-based lasers, which require more optical components to achieve a homogeneous beam profile. The greater the number of optical components, the greater the energy losses from the laser head to the output, and the more frequent the need for maintenance and replacement of optical components.

The smaller size, vertical integration of the laser delivery system, and large number of service technicians in more than 40 countries make Summit's serviceability superior to that of its competitors.

Future Improvements

Technology continues to evolve. Continuing developments with the emphasis erodible laser disk, available in the Apex Plus, will improve this technology beyond its current state. In the future, it may be possible to treat not only myopic astigmatism and hyperopia but also hyperopic astigmatism and even irregular astigmatism.

References

1. Seiler T. Photorefractive Keratectomy: European Experience. In F Thompson, PJ McDonnell (eds.). *Color Atlas/Text of Excimer Laser Surgery: The Cornea.* New York: Igaku-Shoin, 1992. Pp 53–62.
2. Seiler T, Kable G, Kriegerowski M. Excimer laser (193 nm) myopic keratomileusis in sighted and blind human eyes. *Refract Corneal Surg* 6: 383–385, 1990.
3. Friedman MD, et al. OmniMed II: A new system for use with the emphasis erodible mask. *J Refract Corneal Surgery* 10(Suppl.):5267–5273, 1994.
4. O'Brart DPS, et al. The effect of ablation diameter on the outcome of excimer laser photorefractive keratectomy: A prospective, randomized, double-blind study. *Arch Ophthalmol* 113:438–443, 1995.
5. Seiler T, et al. Complications of myopic photorefractive keratectomy with the excimer laser. *Ophthalmology* 101:153–160, 1994.

6. Munnerlyn CR, Koons SJ, Marshall J. Photorefractive keratectomy: A technique for laser refractive surgery. *J Cataract Refract Surg* 14:46–52, 1996.
7. Maloney RK, et al. A prototype ablatable mask delivery system for the excimer laser. *Ophthalmology* 100:542–549, 1993.
8. Thompson KP, et al. Photorefractive Keratectomy with the Summit Excimer Laser: The Phase III U.S. Results. In JJ Salz (ed.). *Corneal Laser Surgery*. St. Louis: Mosby, 1995. Pp 57–63.
9. Dougherty PJ, Wellish KL, Maloney RK. Excimer laser ablation rate and corneal hydration. *Am J Ophthalmol* 118:169–176, 1994.

11 VISX STAR and 20/20 Laser Systems

Jonathan I. Macy, Shareef Mahdavi, and Andrew Garfinkle

History

Not long after the excimer laser was developed by IBM and successfully used in the semiconductor market, the founders of VISX (Santa Clara, CA) began investigating the possibilities of using this powerful new tool for vision correction. In 1986, just 3 years after Stephen Trokel and colleagues published the first article on the excimer laser for use in corneal surgery [1], VISX was founded and the first prototype excimer laser refractive surgical system was developed. Charles Munnerlyn and Terry Clapham, two of VISX's founders, worked to develop both the delivery system and the precise algorithms required to make the excimer suitable for use on corneal tissue. During the same year, the first U.S. Food and Drug Administration (FDA) clinical site was established at Louisiana State University and the first human eyes were treated with the VISX excimer laser.

Three years later, in 1989, the first VISX system was sold internationally while clinical investigations of the laser for phototherapeutic keratectomy (PTK) and photorefractive keratectomy (PRK) were well under way in the United States. By 1991, VISX was the first to apply for FDA approval to market the excimer laser system for PTK, and in 1993, it was the first to submit to the FDA its premarket approval application for PRK for myopia. During this time VISX was also active in clinical investigations of excimer PRK for both astigmatism and hyperopia. VISX received FDA approval to market its systems for PTK in September 1995 and for low myopic PRK in March 1996. Clinical studies for high myopia, astigmatism, and hyperopia are proceeding into more advanced phases in the United States.

While actively soliciting feedback from physicians who used the system, VISX continued to invest in research and development to refine both the system and the laser procedures. In March 1995, VISX introduced the STAR Excimer Laser System. STAR is less expensive to operate and easier to use and maintain than earlier systems. The STAR is clinically equivalent to the initial system but is just half the size of its predecessor, enabling it to fit easily into a variety of operating environments. Its improved gas management system and new optical configuration more than doubles the lifetime of the laser optics. STAR is equipped to treat myopia, hyperopia, and astigmatism without masks or ancillary products. Both the STAR and VISX 20/20 excimer lasers are discussed in this chapter.

Unique Aspects of the Hardware

The Laser System

Although there are 19 VISX 20/20B (Fig. 11-1) systems currently installed in the United States and several hundred more around the world, they are no longer being distributed. The STAR excimer laser system (Fig. 11-2) has replaced the VISX 20/20B. Although equivalent in performance and laser beam quality, the new system is more compact, more efficient, less expensive to maintain, and is computer integrated. The basic laser was made by Questec (Billerica, MA) in the past, but VISX currently manufactures and tests each STAR system on

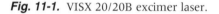

Fig. 11-1. VISX 20/20B excimer laser.

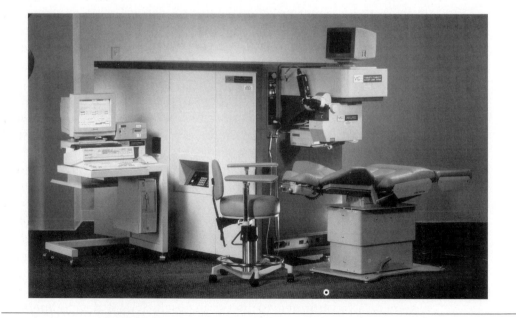

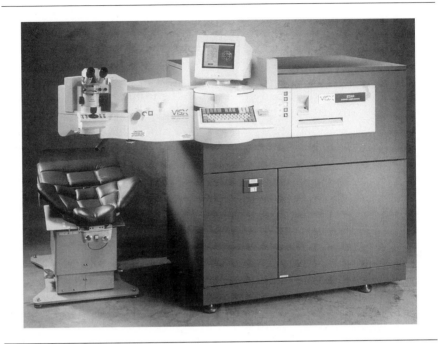

Fig. 11-2. VISX STAR excimer laser.

site in Santa Clara, California. Unlike the air-cooled 20/20B system, the STAR system is internally water cooled.

It is recommended that a separate room be set aside for the laser system. The STAR laser is 150-cm high, 110-cm wide, and 204-cm long, whereas the 20/20B laser is 141 × 84 × 271 cm. The main console weighs 726 kg, compared to the 955 kg 20/20B. The room housing the laser should be no smaller than 20 square meters, with the shortest room dimension being at least 3 meters. The ceiling materials should not shed particulate matter, and the floor should be tiled to keep dust to a minimum.

The conduit to the room must carry 220 VAC (volts alternating current) single phase, 50 or 60 Hz, and 30-ampere service. This system requires three gas cylinders: an argon-fluorine (ArF) laser gas mixture (premix), helium, and liquid nitrogen. The laser premix and the helium in the gas cabinet are used in the excimer laser. In the 20/20B system, liquid nitrogen is kept external to the system and chills the laser gases, trapping contaminants. The newer STAR system has eliminated the need for liquid nitrogen.

The external computer of the 20/20 system requires an assistant for treatments. No assistant is necessary in the STAR system because an IBM-compatible personal computer (PC) is integrated into the laser hardware. It is at the immediate right of the surgeon and swivels to comfortable positions. Windows 4.0 software is accessed with a mouselike trackball. Each screen provides appropriate prompting instructions to proceed through gas checking, fluence adjustment, lens calibration, VisionKey card, and treatment. A dot matrix printer has been upgraded to a laser printer. A continuous color display (CCD) camera and high-resolution monitor record and demonstrate each treatment.

The patient chair has a motorized joystick control with a foot release pedal that is unlocked prior to treatment. A back position switch raises and lowers the chair. An ergonomically improved chair has replaced the operating bed of the 20/20 system. Once the patient is properly positioned, the chair is rotated and locked into the treatment position because the laser does not fire otherwise.

The Delivery System

The VISX excimer laser system combines the submicron precision and nonthermal tissue removal qualities of an excimer laser with a sophisticated computer-controlled delivery system. Features include a coaxial operating microscope, a gas cleaning and detection system, a computer workstation with installed software, and a video camera with monitor.

It is believed that a smoother laser beam leads to faster and clearer healing [2]. In VISX systems, the light passes through a series of optical elements to create a uniform beam imaged onto the patient's eye. The laser beam is processed through an optical delivery system. The operating microscope is coaxial with the laser beam. The beam is homogenized by a rotating prism plus a spatial integrator, and the beam is shaped with an iris diaphragm and opposing slit blades. Ablation is begun with the smallest aperture, and the diaphragm is widened in many tiny steps to reach the desired optical zone. Up to 240 steps may be taken in a single ablation.

A Leica Wild operating microscope, coaxial with the laser beam, has been added to the STAR system to replace the Moller microscope from the 20/20 series. The Moller microscope has manual zoom and focus features in which the magnification is set at 14×/12× for final focus and final centering; the new microscope has three fixed magnification powers at 10×, 16×, and 25×. Therefore, the surgeon is able to select the desired magnification because each setting provides focus adequate for ablation.

The Moller operating microscope utilizes internal illumination for the treatment field. The Wild microscope and the associated controls have also been improved. New lighting provides the option of soft off-axis general illumination or direct illumination, as necessary during epithelium removal. The off-axis lighting allows the patient greater ease in fixating on the light-emitting diode (LED) fixation signal during the ablation. A new control pad contains a central joystick with x, y, and z (axis) controls. Speed of focus is determined by the amount the joystick is moved. The control pad also has locations for adjustments of microscope and reticle illumination. These controls are duplicated for right-handed and left-handed surgeons.

In both systems, there is a single coaxial LED patient fixation light between the two oculars. A reticle is used to adjust the surgeon's alignment of centration with a reflection of the patient fixation light on the cornea. The reticle, installed in the left eyepiece of the 20/20B device, is now a virtual image, seen in stereo. The reticle flashes when the system is not ready for ablation and becomes a solid red image when ready. There is also a digital readout on the virtual reticle. The top of the image shows percent of treatment remaining, and the bottom of the image shows depth of treatment.

The STAR system has an increased working distance from the microscope to the patient (13.3 cm) to allow laser in-situ keratomileusis (LASIK) to be done under the same operating microscope. Existing 20/20 systems have a working distance of 9 cm, which can be upgraded by the installation of an additional lens to allow a microkeratome to be maneuvered under the same operating microscope as the laser ablation.

Maintenance Considerations

The optical delivery system of the STAR excimer laser system has been redesigned to deliver laser energy more efficiently. The laser is mounted in the hardware so that the optical delivery of laser energy is at least three to four times more efficient. Moving the laser up in the cavity decreases the length of the optical pathway, allowing the use of fewer mirrors. Where six mirrors were required in the 20/20 system, three are used in the STAR system. Energy density is reduced, so the mirrors and the optical train last longer. By making the laser chamber smaller and using a ceramic insulator plate, the need for liquid nitrogen was eliminated. There is also a purge of the optical path, which was not available in the 20/20 series.

In the STAR system, the lifetime of the gases is increased, so the laser works more efficiently. The elimination of liquid nitrogen saves $100–700 per month in gas-related costs. The premix (ArF) now lasts 3–4 days per fill, as opposed to the 1–2 days in the 20/20 models. These machines use a gas boost to provide tiny amounts of premix to adjust fluence. The boost feature allows for approximately 18 fills per bottle of premix compared to 12 for the 20/20. This key feature should significantly reduce the cost of ArF premix.

Generally, maintenance costs are estimated to be approximately 10% of the purchase price of the laser system per year.

Safety Features

Fluorine gas is toxic and can be fatal if inhaled in large quantities. Two breathing masks should be present in the treatment room. The exhaust fan or room air purifier should be operative. The manufacturer recommends that safety glasses be worn by all personnel in the room. A "Laser On" light outside the treatment room is helpful. VISX has taken numerous steps to ensure operator and patient safety in the presence of ArF: The gas bottle is contained in a steel-walled gas cabinet that is part of the laser enclosure, and the air volume in the gas cabinet is continually circulated through an air purifier that neutralizes any potential fluorine leaks. Should there be a fluorine leak inside the enclosure, the gases are safely scrubbed internally. During servicing of the system and when the gas tanks are changed, fluorine could leak into the room. This health threat must be eliminated by installing an exhaust fan capable of removing the entire room's air volume within 2 minutes (VISX room purifier). Should outside venting be the solution of choice for elimination of room contamination, vertical venting through the roof is recommended. Either method should be activated by an easily accessible wall switch, which must be mounted next to the exit door.

Before treatment, a plastic calibration card is ablated and checked for centration, morphology, ablation zone size, and accuracy of correction. On the 20/20 system, the software is readjusted for cornea before treatment. This card should be read on a standard lensometer. The calibration table is built into the STAR system on an arm that swings into position beneath the microscope. The calibration for cutting plastic or cornea is programmed in the system software. When the arm is in position under the microscope, the machine "knows" plastic is being cut. Because it will only ablate the cornea with the armature safely out of the way, it likewise "knows" when the cornea is being treated.

Table 11-1 explains the proper procedure for turning on the VISX laser 20/20B system. To power up the STAR laser, a key is inserted in the front panel and the Systems Start button is pressed. A 10-minute warm-up cycle ensues. The Reset button remains lit at all times. As soon as the Systems Start button is pressed, the computer comes on line and is operational.

The first screen to appear is the Self-test screen (Fig. 11-3A). The status of the pressures in the premix gas cylinder and helium cylinder is displayed as is the status of the other devices that must be tested

Table 11-1. Turning on the VISX 20/20B laser system

A. Powering up
   1. Insert the System Power Key into the front of the control panel.
   2. Turn key to On.
   3. Press the green System Power On button.
      a. Green light should illuminate.
      b. Laser Emission light should illuminate.
      c. If light is not on, verify that doors are closed properly.
      d. The 10-minute warm-up cycle begins.
B. Gas exchange
   1. Press Code on laser panel.
   2. Press 14 on laser panel.
   3. Press Enter twice.
   4. Wait 15 minutes to ensure completion of exchange.
   5. Close cylinder valves.
C. Computer control station
   1. Press switch to right of monitor.
   2. Menu appears on computer screen.
   3. Verify that printer is on-line and has sufficient paper.
D. Patient management
   1. Patient fixation light should be on.
   2. Patient chair should function (the laser does not fire if chair is not locked in treatment position).
   3. Microscope illumination should be operative (spare bulb available).
   4. Microscope zoom and focus should be operative.
      a. Magnification setting is 14×/12× for final focus.
      b. Magnification setting is 14×/12× for final centering.

before attempting an ablation: VisionKey reader, videoboard, input/output (I/O) board, premix bottle, helium bottle, random access memory (RAM) battery, fluorine alarm, aspirator, illumination, dust covers, motors, laser, and swing arm. If the machine has not been used recently, a gas adjustment may be necessary.

The second screen displays the test of fluence (Fig. 11-3B). There is no laser emission because the testing is done internally. The laser is fired while the fluence is measured. If the fluence is not measured at the desired level of 160 mJ/cm^2, the computer adjusts the laser voltage or the gas mixture until the fluence is correct.

The third screen displays lens calibration (Fig. 11-3C). With the calibration arm in position beneath the microscope and the vacuum nozzle in its fixed position, the "new media" plastic is placed on the arm. No focusing is necesssary. A planned correction of −4.00 D is automatically set up and the foot switch depressed. The material is

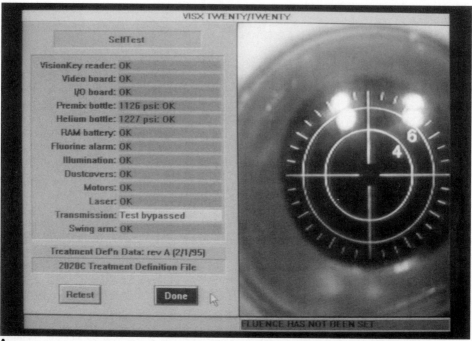

Fig. 11-3. **A.** Self-test screen indicates the status of all component devices before ablation. **B.** Fluence is then measured and adjusted internally.

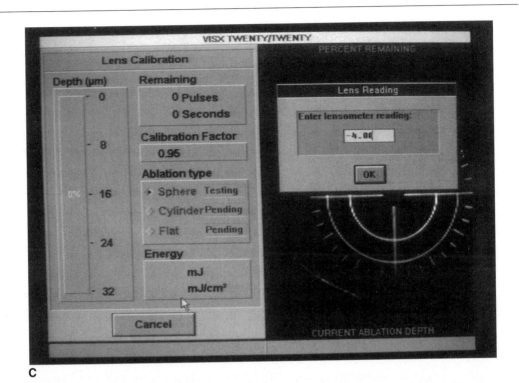

C

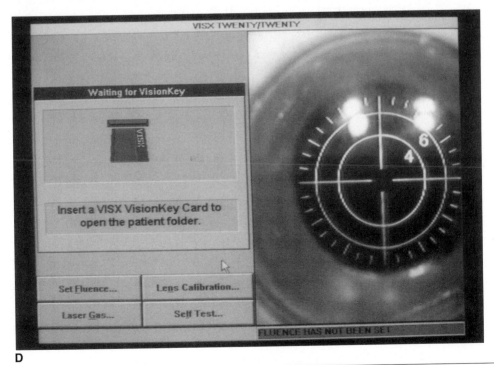

D

Fig. 11-3 (continued). **C.** A –4.00-D ablation completed on calibration arm, result measured on lensometer, and data entered on screen. **D.** VisionKey optical memory card imprinted for each patient with specific protocol.

evaluated at the lensometer and the reading entered on the screen. The computer then readjusts fluence for minor variations from intended corrections, and the desired spherical correction is then retested. A 50-micron PTK flat test is also done to check beam homogeneity. Cylindrical testing is a pass/fail test. A correction of −4.00 D at 0 degrees is entered and the result must fall within 0.50 D of the intended correction. If the machine fails the test, the interlock light signal comes on at the bottom of the screen, and service evaluation is required. The bottom right corner of the screen indicates the interlock conditions for potential problems, and if this information appears, the surgeon must return to the Self-test screen to attempt to correct the problem.

As before, the plastic material tested must be evaluated manually for centration, morphology, and shape. For centering, 30 laser ablation spots are automatically placed on the test card and the results evaluated within the virtual reticle. The reticle has 4-mm and 6-mm rings.

Once the reticle has been adjusted to ensure proper alignment of centration, the operating microscope is focused and positioned over the patient's pupil. In early protocols, physician fixation of the eye with a nitrogen-blowing handpiece was standard. Further experimentation determined that there was no benefit from physician fixation when compared to voluntary patient fixation on the LED light [3].

Once the patient is in position, a flexible aspiration nozzle is adjusted inferior to the operative field for effluent removal. Ablation is begun with depression of a foot switch. If there is movement or poor patient fixation, the surgeon removes his or her foot from the foot switch, and treatment immediately ceases. Treatment can be restarted at the point of discontinuation without adjustment of the software.

Software-User Interface

The integrated computer, keyboard, and monitor complex of the STAR system is conveniently located for the surgeon. It employs Windows software operated with a trackball and keyboard.

The VisionKey card has been added to allow quicker access to new techniques and algorithms. Multipass, which creates smoother surfaces and faster recovery of best corrected visual acuity by breaking down the procedure into steps, is now part of the VisionKey software. VisionKey also lets the surgeon preprogram patient information, preoperative information, and treatment data. Software systems have been updated to provide easier-to-use prompting and system calibration. Software access is restricted to regulatory approvals in each market (i.e., software includes only FDA-approved modalities).

The VisionKey card appears on the monitor screen after calibration is complete (Fig. 11-3D). An optical memory card (installed on most 20/20 systems) is generated for each patient, and the system will not operate without the appropriate card. Cards arrive from the factory programmed to each system and imprinted with the specific protocols allowed. Cards are not interchangeable between machines. Patient demographics and treatment outcomes may be entered onto the card at the computer terminal. System upgrades will be achieved with new cards rather than with new software for installation.

When the VisionKey is inserted, the patient information screen appears. Then the preoperative folder opens so that the treatment plan can be entered. The treatment plan includes the eye being treated, the vision without correction, vision with correction, corneal clarity, manifest refraction, cycloplegic refraction, autorefraction, and keratometry readings.

Treatment is the next choice. The new software displays not only the eye to be treated, but also the intended treatment and the depth of treatment. Video capture allows the camera video to be displayed simultaneously with the computer information. The left margin of the screen displays the available protocol options from the inserted VisionKey card.

At the conclusion of treatment, the VisionKey is ejected, and the machine is turned off.

Ablation Parameters and Capabilities

At the corneal surface, energy density (fluence) is set at 160 mJ/cm^2, and each pulse ablates approximately 0.25 μm of tissue. The ablation pulse rate is preset at 6 Hz in the 20/20B and at 10 Hz in the STAR system, but STAR is capable of 30 Hz if necessary. The pulse laser energy for a 6-mm ablation is 45 mJ/pulse. The spot size can be adjusted between 0.6 mm and 6.0 mm, and is expandable to 8.0 mm. Completion of an ablation for −5.00 D of simple myopia would take about 25 seconds with the STAR system and 40 seconds with the 20/20 series. Such ablations can be done with either laser or manual removal of the epithelium before stromal ablation.

The importance of a smooth transition zone was identified early in the development of the VISX excimer laser [4]. The tiny steps of ablation (240 steps are possible) are adjusted by the iris diaphragm to create a smooth ablation. PRK ablations begin centrally and widen to the 6.0-mm or 6.5-mm ablation zone. Addition of the multipass software to VisionKey has contributed to this progress.

VisionKey software is identified for each machine and specific for each protocol. Current potential options include PTK circle, PTK slit,

PRK, astigmatism, PRK enlargement, PRK variable, PRK hyperopia, and custom programs, subject to regulatory approval. *PTK circle* provides a central ablation in which the stromal depth, treatment zone diameter, and transition zone are separately selected. Self or patient fixation and epithelium removal manually or with laser are other options. *PTK slit* is designed for focal scars of rectangular shape. The number of pulses or ablation depth determines the amount of treatment.

Spherocylindrical (sequential) and elliptical ablations are the two methods used for treating compound myopic astigmatism. In a sequential ablation, the cylinder error is corrected first using rectangular apertures that change with each laser pulse. After a short pause, the spherical error is corrected by superimposing a 6-mm spherical cut over the existing cylindrical cut [5]. This two-step procedure may produce transition zones. Transition zones have the potential to induce flattening along the minor axis, where flattening may not be desired. The depth of the total correction is measured by adding the depths of the spherical and cylindrical ablations together.

Because of concerns about steep cuts causing potential transition zones, a unique VISX algorithm was designed to correct the cylinder without creating such zones [6, 7]. Using the new algorithm, cylinder is corrected simultaneously with sphere, creating a toric, or elliptical, ablation. The elliptical ablation occurs when rectangular apertures shorten in width and the iris diaphragm starts in and opens out as the laser pulses. The elliptical ablation has no transition zones and the major and minor axes have different lengths. Futher, the number of pulses and, therefore, depth of ablation needed to treat combined sphere and cylinder errors is equivalent to that required to treat spherical errors only. This method is more advantageous than spherocylindrical ablation because the ablation is not as deep. The VisionKey feature automatically defaults to the elliptical algorithm.

The relationship of sphere and cylinder in the correction of compound myopic astigmatism determines whether an elliptical program for treatment is the wisest choice. For the elliptical program to be effective, the minor axis (using minus cylinder notation) must be large enough to prevent glare and night vision problems. If the minor axis is less than 6 mm in length, then the width of the elliptical ablation may be too narrow to cover the optical zone adequately. Therefore, the minor axis length should always be set at 6 mm. The relationship of sphere to cylinder also determines the width of the ablation. When the error of sphere and cylinder is equal, assuming the minor axis is 6 mm, the ablation is 4.25 mm. Any width less than this might result in clinically significant glare. Therefore, the elliptical program for correction of compound myopic astigmatism should only be used for corrections where the cylinder is less than or equal to the sphere.

Advantages and Disadvantages

Preliminary Clinical Results

Indications

The FDA phase III PRK protocol for the treatment of low myopia (−1.0 to −6.0 D at the corneal plane) using the VISX 20/20B excimer laser began at 10 sites in April 1991. Astigmatism was limited to 1.00 D of cylinder or less. Best spectacle-corrected visual acuity (BSCVA) was 20/40 or better in both eyes, and all entrants were 18 years or older. Contact lens use was discontinued prior to final evaluation for at least 2 weeks with soft contact lenses, and for at least 3 weeks with hard contact lenses.

Effectiveness

The phase III trial included 2056 eyes; 909 of these eyes were treated using a 6-mm ablation zone and no nitrogen blowing across the cornea during the procedure. Eighty percent of the eyes were evaluated 1 year after PRK, and 61% were evaluated 2 years after treatment. Thirty-nine percent were female and 61% male. The mean age was 37.6 ± 9.2 years. The mean pretreatment myopia was −4.2 ± 1.5 D.

The summary of effectiveness is based on a single treatment using a 6-mm ablation zone (Table 11-2). After 1 year, 60% (278/464) of eyes had uncorrected visual acuity (UCVA) of 20/20 or better. After 2 years, 52% (115/223) had UCVA of 20/20 or better. After 1 year, 92% (429/464) of eyes had 20/40 or better UCVA, and 93% (207/223) had the same level of vision after 2 years.

At 1 year, 87% (374/431) of refractive errors and, at 2 years, 91% (194/214) of refractive errors were within 1 D of intended. Less than 1% (2/214) of eyes were overcorrected by more than 1 D after 24 months. No eyes had a spherical equivalent greater than 1 D after 24 months (Table 11-3). The results were extremely stable, demonstrating a mean spherical equivalent of −0.64 D at 12 months, −0.58 D at 18 months, and −0.58 D at 24 months. The mean deviation from intended correction of −0.4 D at 12 months, −0.43 at 18 months, and −0.46 at 24 months was equally stable (Fig. 11-4).

Safety

Based on the results of all 1160 eyes treated without nitrogen blowing across the cornea, acute and long-term outcome measures were evaluated. There was no intraocular infection, no hyphema, no hypopyon, no corneal perforation, no cystoid macular edema, and no

Table 11-2. Effectiveness of PRK for myopia based on a single treatment using a 6-mm ablation zone

Effectiveness parameters	12 months (n = 467)	24+ months (n = 226)
1. UCVA 20/20 or better (Pretreatment: 0%)	278/464 (60%)	115/223 (52%)
2. UCVA 20/25 or better (Pretreatment: <1%)	351/464 (76%)	169/223 (76%)
3. UCVA 20/40 or better (Pretreatment: <1%)	429/464 (92%)	207/223 (93%)
4. Deviation from intended within 1 D	374/431 (87%)	194/214 (91%)

UCVA = uncorrected visual acuity.

Table 11-3. Rare overcorrection more than 1 D after 24 months

Effective parameters	12 months	24+ months
Deviation from intended correction > +1 D	7/431 (1.6%)	2/214 (<1%)
Eyes with spherical equivalent > +1D	5/431 (1.2%)	0/216 (0%)

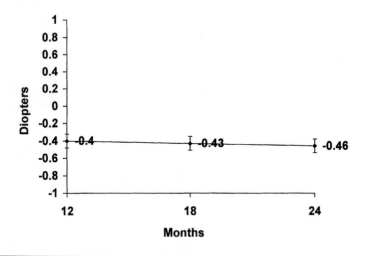

Fig. 11-4. Stable mean deviation from intended correction at 12 months, 18 months, and 24 months.

persistent corneal edema. About 1.5% (70/1160) of eyes experienced a two-line or greater loss of BSCVA at 12 months. Over time, 79% (11 of 14) of these eyes improved to less than a two-line loss. By 24 months, only 3 of 581 eyes (0.5%) experienced a two-line loss of BSCVA.

Eleven eyes had lens abnormalities reported that were not present before treatment. None of these had a 2-line BSCVA loss or loss to 20/25 at the last examination. Four eyes had lens abnormalities that were not seen on subsequent examinations. Three eyes experienced corneal infiltrates or infections. All had been given a contact lens after treatment. BSCVA in all three cases was 20/20 or better at last examination. Short-term and long-term endothelial cell studies demonstrated no significant change in cell counts ($p > 0.05$) at 6 months and 24 months.

Summary

PRK using the VISX excimer laser has been shown to be safe and effective for the treatment of low to moderate myopia. The elimination of nitrogen blowing across the cornea and the use of a large 6-mm ablation zone have produced excellent results. The VISX laser has also been shown to successfully modify astigmatism and hyperopia. Continued improvements in technology, such as the VISX STAR excimer laser, should provide greater reliability, greater user-friendliness, and greater accuracy for refractive physicians and their patients.

Comparison to Other Systems

Although other systems claim to have the potential to correct astigmatism and hyperopia, current VISX STAR excimer lasers already have this capability and are upgradable for astigmatism [8] and hyperopia [9], pending FDA approval. VISX plans a platform for eye tracking and an option for scanning treatments, which will also be available as an upgrade, thus reducing future obsolescence of the current systems.

With many years of use worldwide, the VISX excimer laser systems for photoablation have evolved into more compact, more efficient, more reliable, less expensive, and more user-friendly devices. Computer integration of treatments for PTK, PRK for myopia, PRK for astigmatism, and PRK for hyperopia provides an array of modalities found in no other system.

Future Improvements

Meeting demands in today's competitive medical environment requires not only state-of-the-art technology but also providing accessibility at a reasonable cost. The MobilExcimer is an attractive alternative for surgeons who practice in smaller communities with limited markets or for those who do not otherwise have the patient volume needed to support an excimer laser. With rapidly evolving technology and high support costs, the mobile system, once approved by the FDA, may provide a desirable alternative to a fixed site excimer laser.

The LaserVision system is delivered by a trailer truck, has a topography room, a waiting room, and an excimer surgical suite. The operating suite is larger than those at many fixed-base laser centers. The system is 48 feet in length and is totally self-contained, with optional hookups for water, telephone, and electricity. At the heart of the MobilExcimer unit is a patented laser mounting system that allows the laser to withstand repeated highway and patient traffic.

At the Canadian Ophthalmological Society meeting in June 1995, the first data ever presented on a mobile excimer laser for PRK surgery was reported [10]. Fifty patients aged 21–70 with preoperative spherical equivalents (SE) of −2.00 to −8.00 D and less than 3.00 D of astigmatism were recruited from July 1994 until January 1995. Patients randomly chose between a mobile (22/50) or a fixed-base excimer laser system (28/50), each with identical VISX 20/20 lasers with 402c central island software. The mean ages and SE were 42 and −6.19 (mobile), and 38 and −5.73 (fixed), respectively. All PRK surgery was done by Andrew Garfinkle at either the Montreal, Quebec LaserVision Center or in Cornwall, Ontario.

Stability of the laser after transport was repeatedly tested by VISX-approved technicians [11]. Beam alignment, diaphragm size calibrations, output energy, and beam profile required small adjustments, less than what would have been required at a new fixed-site laser installation. Although the mobile system was used both in winter and summer, environmental factors, such as temperature, humidity fluctuations, and air cleanliness, did not influence the stability of the laser. No significant service problems or part malfunctions were encountered. Normal traffic inside the unit during surgery did not necessitate recalibration or realignment of the laser.

After informed consent was obtained by the physician, excimer laser PRK was performed using 402c central island software, laser/scrape epithelial removal, and a postoperative bandage contact lens. Results were analyzed by analysis of variance (ANOVA) and showed no statistically significant difference between the mobile and fixed-site PRK surgery. In this series, the UCVA was 20/25 or better in 82% of eyes at 6 months and in 86% of eyes at 1 year in mobile and fixed-base groups.

PRK results in the mobile excimer subgroup revealed a mean SE of −0.59 D, whereas the SE was −0.52 in the fixed-base group at 1 year. At 6 months, 2 patients in each group had UCVA of 20/40 or less. The reduced visual acuity was caused by steep central islands of 3.0–6.0 D, all but one of which had resolved by 1 year. No overcorrections or clinically significant decentrations were noted. Haze measured grade 1 or less in all patients at any time point, and no patient lost 2 or more lines of BSCVA.

The MobilExcimer system is practical and versatile and it compares favorably with a fixed-base system. Physician and patient acceptance is excellent. The mobile technology offers a viable alternative to conventional fixed-site surgery centers.

References

1. Trokel SL, Srinivasan R, Braren B. Excimer laser surgery of the cornea. *Am J Ophthalmol* 96:710–715, 1983.
2. Campos M, Trokel SL, McDonnell PJ. Surface morphology following photorefractive keratectomy. *Ophthalmic Surg* 24:822–825, 1993.
3. Terrell J, et al. The effect of globe fixation on ablation zone centration in photorefractive keratectomy. *Am J Ophthalmol* 119:612–619, 1995.
4. Kerr-Muir MG, et al. Ultrastructural comparison of conventional surgical and argon fluoride excimer laser keratectomy. *Am J Ophthalmol* 103:448–453, 1987.
5. McDonnell PJ, et al. Photorefractive keratectomy to create toric ablations for correction of astigmatism. *Arch Ophthalmol* 109:710–713, 1991.
6. Shimmick J, Bechtel L. Elliptical ablations for the correction of compound myopic astigmatism by photoablation with apertures. *SPIE-PROC* 1644:32–39, 1992.
7. Spigelman A, et al. Treatment of myopic astigmatism with the 193 nm excimer laser utilizing aperture elements. *J Cataract Refract Surg* 20(Suppl.):258–261, 1994.
8. Campos M, McDonnell P. Photorefractive Keratectomy for Astigmatism. In JJ Salz (ed.). *Corneal Laser Surgery*. St. Louis: Mosby, 1995. Pp 65–76.
9. Macy JI, Nesburn AB, Salz JJ. Laser Correction of Hyperopia. VISX Blind Eye Study—United States Results. In JJ Salz (ed.). *Corneal Laser Surgery*. St. Louis: Mosby, 1995. Pp 256–260.
10. Garfinkle A. A comparison of VisX 20/20 PRK results using fixed-base and mobile excimer laser systems. *Can J Ophthalmol* 30(2):105, 1995.
11. Personal communication. Joel Zeger, Sigmacon Medical Products Ltd., Downsview, Ontario, Canada, 1995.

12 Chiron-Technolas Keracor 116

Jeffery J. Machat and Kristian Hohla

Overview and History

Although the Technolas Keracor 116 (Chiron-Technolas, Irvine, California) is basically a wide-field ablation laser, it also is able to scan both small and large beams, making it a hybrid system. This is the single most important feature of the Technolas Keracor 116. To understand the importance of this feature, one must first consider the inherent characteristics of scanning and wide-field excimer laser beams.

Because homogeneity of ablation depends on a uniform distribution of energy across the corneal surface, the wide-field deposition of laser energy in a single pulse is more subject to energy "noise" such as hot spots or cold spots than are scanning laser systems and may more frequently contribute to small irregularities in the ablation profile. Large irregularities, such as central islands, are also more frequent because of differential energy absorption across the wide field surface. These wide-field laser characteristics can be contrasted to the greater frequency and number of pulses required by scanning lasers and the need for sophisticated eye tracking or mechanical coupling to "lock on" to the corneal surface. These characteristics make the synchronized placement of laser pulses more challenging, and complex nomogram development is often necessary. As a hybrid laser, the Technolas Keracor 116 addresses the characteristics of both modes of delivery by limiting the number of pulses and crucial placement necessary while smoothing homogeneities in the beam with the scanning feature. The Technolas Keracor 116 bridges the transition in technology between wide-field and scanning delivery while using some advantages of both systems.

Unique Aspects of the Hardware

The Laser System

The laser cavity and system features of the Technolas Keracor 116 were designed and developed soley by Technolas and incorporate several unique features (Fig. 12-1). The laser cavity, gas cylinder, and internal controls for servicing are housed in a single compartment to the left of the patient bed. The unit is compartmentalized for serviceability, and the entire optical delivery system is accessible from the laser head to the arm that connects the left and right compartments. The system is fitted with a coaxial Zeiss operating microscope for surgical viewing. The right compartment is separate from the main housing and contains the external personal computer (PC) and the 220-volt power input, and it can hold a videocassette recorder. The surgeon can view the procedure while maintaining direct access to the PC on the right. The lighting and joystick controls, mounted on the optical arm next to the right hand of the surgeon, control fine patient-bed movements for alignment as well as three alignment lights. These include a single red light-emitting diode (LED) for patient fixation, a second red coaxial HeNe light in the center of the beam, and an angled green HeNe light for corneal vertex height control. Although the bulk of the left compartment is adjacent to the patient bed, a little more than 30 cm extends beyond the optical area toward the surgeon, serving as an instrument stand.

The Technolas Keracor 116 is cooled internally through a sophisticated dual mechanism that uses both water and air heat exchange systems. High-volume surgery requires external room cooling to 60° F for the most efficient laser functioning with good homogeneity and

Fig. 12-1. Chiron-Technolas Keracor 116 excimer laser system.

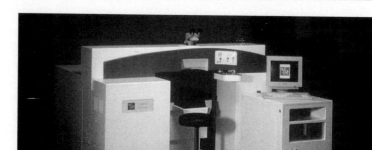

beam stability. An exhaust fan that empties the room every 10–20 minutes is advisable in case of a gas leak. All incoming air should be filtered through hospital grade (5-micron) HEPPA filters. The room size should be a minimum of 20 m², and ideally 30 m². The 220-volt electrical supply should ideally arise from the floor next to the surgeon's right foot, although this is not mandatory. It is, however, important to ensure that a true supply of 220 volts is obtained (it is not uncommon to have a true measurement of 208 volts). A step-up transformer can be used to achieve this voltage. Reduced voltage has a direct impact on laser functioning because the laser head draws considerable power. A very high voltage (approximately 30,000 volts) is used in the laser cavity. Rather than controlling the fluence by adjusting the voltage within the laser cavity, an optical attenuator is utilized, which helps to maintain better beam homogeneity by retaining this high voltage in the cavity. In this way, the fluence is controlled without being dependent on the homogeneity.

The system requires only a single argon-fluoride premix gas cylinder, which contains approximately 130 gas cavity refills. The premix cylinder is replaced by a technician. Considering that each gas refill is sufficient for 10–20 procedures on average, up to 2600 procedures are possible on a single cylinder if used efficiently. In reality, however, each cylinder is only capable of several hundred to a thousand cases. Filtered air is used to purge the optical pathway, which is maintained under positive pressure rather than creating a closed system filled with nitrogen gas. The argon-fluoride gas exchange process occurs by evacuating the gas cavity over several minutes using an internal vacuum to develop a negative pressure inside the cavity prior to refilling the cavity with fresh gas. The internal vacuum avoids the need for purging the cavity with helium, thus conserving gas. In this way, additional gas cylinders are not required (e.g., helium for gas cavity purging, nitrogen for the optical pathway and liquid nitrogen for prolonging gas longevity).

The operating bed is capable of fine adjustment and consists of a head rest and nonadjustable bed. Although alignment precision is excellent in all three (x, y, and z) planes, the movement is relatively slow. Patients appear to appreciate the stability of the flat bed relative to a reclining and rotatable chair.

The Delivery System

The Technolas Keracor 116 laser functions at a fluence of 130 mJ/cm² and a pulse repetition rate of 10 Hz. Its computer-controlled iris diaphragm in the delivery system is capable of up to 1024 steps. The iris aperture expands from 0.8 mm to 7.0 mm. The unique delivery system of the Keracor 116 incorporates a scanning mode, which is

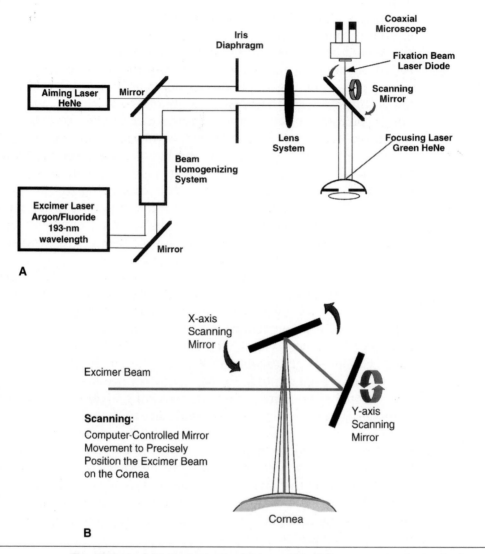

Fig. 12-2. **A.** Optical schematic of Keracor 116 delivery system. **B.** The dual-mirror (x, y) scanning feature.

based around the scanner block that houses the final polishing mirror optic (Fig. 12-2). The polishing mirror oscillates 50 microns about the point of fixation and therefore blends each pulse into previous pulses. Clinically, this oscillation effect (beam wobble) may have three benefits: (1) smoother ablation, (2) reduced regression, and (3) reduced haze formation. The classic circular ridges commonly observed from the expansion of the iris diaphragm following wide-field ablation are dramatically reduced. The scanner block also enables the system to perform a toric (astigmatic) ablation pattern, hyperopic ablation pattern, and a second myopic ablation pattern without the aid of the iris diaphragm. The astigmatic ablation pattern is produced by scanning across the minus cylinder axis with increasing diameter to create a 4-mm × 12-mm cylinder (Fig. 12-3A and B). A new pattern called *PlanoScan* achieves astigmatism correction while minimizing a hyperopic shift by using a small, fixed-diameter scanning beam (Fig. 12-3C). The hyperopic pattern is created by scanning a midperipheral trough, which is blended centrally and peripherally to reduce regression and haze (Fig. 12-3D and E).

The beam homogenization process depends on an optical system composed of seven optical components plus an optional condensing lens for use in phototherapeutic keratectomy (PTK). These components consist of three mirrors (two bending, one scanning block) and four lenses (two cylindrical, one spherical, one condensing). The laser head output consists typically of a rectangular 11-mm × 22-mm beam that encounters the first bending mirror and directs the beam toward the optical dielectric attenuator. The fluence or beam energy delivered to the eye is controlled at this attenuator during the recalibration procedure. The beam then enters the beam homogenizer, which consists of three optics (two cylindrical lenses and one condensing lens). The beam is essentially square at this point and quite homogeneous, with a flat beam profile. The coaxial red HeNe light is introduced and continues into the beam. The mechanical iris diaphragm then creates a circular beam of 14 mm or less in diameter. An additional condensing lens is interposed between the scanner block and final polishing mirror optic and the iris diaphragm. This lens makes a physical picture of the diaphragm on the cornea with a ratio of 2 : 1.

The Technolas Keracor 116 is equipped with a Zeiss coaxial microscope that has three levels of magnification. A reticule complete with 180-degree axis markings is fitted inside one ocular to aid alignment. When the patient fixates, aligning the visual axis, a brighter reflection of the target laser diode is observed. Height alignment is obtained by overlapping the corneal reflection of the red target laser diode and the angled green HeNe light, signifying that the correct corneal height is reached. The green HeNe light is emitted from the right side of the scanner block and appears to the left of the reflected target laser diode if the patient must be elevated and to the right if the patient must be lowered. In this way, precise alignment in all three planes can be achieved. The red coaxial HeNe light remains in the center of the beam and is seen to oscillate during all photorefractive corrections and to scan during toric or hyperopic ablation patterns, while the red target laser diode remains stationary. The beam alignment system allows the user to realign the red coaxial HeNe light with the red fixation target laser diode through a software interface with the scanner block. In the phototherapeutic mode, the surgeon controls move-

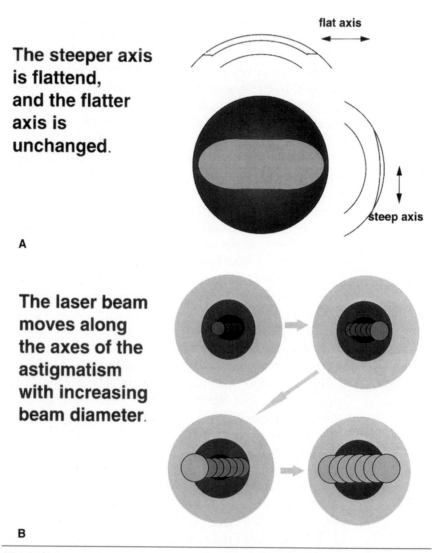

The steeper axis is flattend, and the flatter axis is unchanged.

flat axis

steep axis

A

The laser beam moves along the axes of the astigmatism with increasing beam diameter.

B

Fig. 12-3. Scanning pattern for wide-field correction of myopic astigmatism, with a progressively increasing beam diameter (**A, B**), PlanoScan correction of astigmatism with a small fixed-beam diameter (**C**), and hyperopia correction with an annular scanning pattern (**D, E**).

ment of the scanner block and beam with a joystick, which is highlighted by the movement of the red coaxial HeNe light while patient fixation is maintained on the stationary red target laser diode.

The eye-tracking system of the Keracor 116 is a prerequisite for complex scanning ablation patterns. It consists of an infrared camera that monitors the pupil-iris margin contrast difference and can be locked at any position (Fig. 12-4). The eye-tracking software actively

The laser beam moves over the cornea with a fixed diameter.

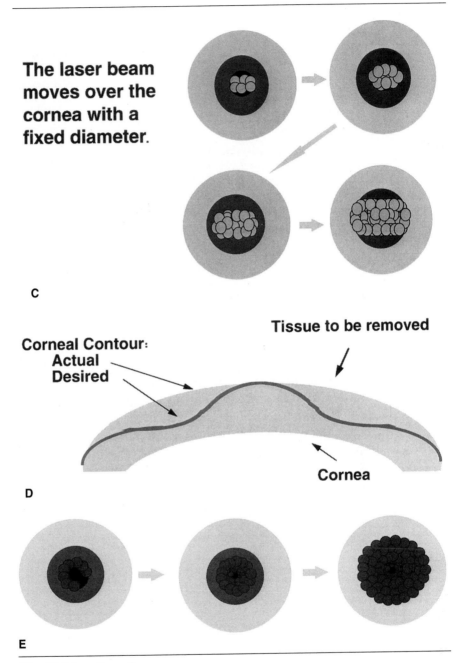

C

Corneal Contour:
Actual
Desired

Tissue to be removed

Cornea

D

E

Fig. 12-3 (continued).

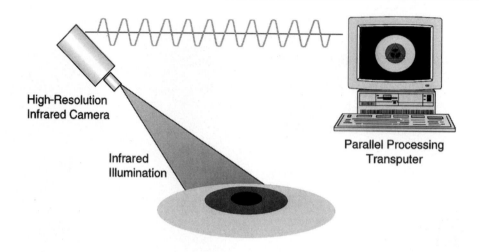

Fig. 12-4. Eye-tracking system of the Keracor 116 demonstrating hardware features and software capabilities.

follows the eye within a 3-mm triangulated area and deactivates the laser outside the 3-mm area if the scanning mirror can no longer track eye movement. The sophisticated system monitors the eye position every 20 milliseconds, and adjusts and reacts to position changes every 25 milliseconds.

There is no vacuum nozzle for effluent removal, but there is a suction ring, which can be placed on the eye to evacuate the plume. The alteration in stromal hydration from effluent removal may offset any benefit from plume removal. The optional attachment is available but rarely utilized. The working distance is more than adequate to perform more complex procedures, such as laser in-situ keratomileusis (LASIK).

Maintenance Considerations

The Technolas Keracor 116 has relatively low maintenance needs, but all excimer lasers require continual maintenance, which increases with an increasing volume of procedures. In general, wide-field delivery systems require more maintenance because they have greater energy requirements in laser head design and a more complex optical pathway for beam homogenization. Optic degradation is a natural event because the laser energy damages the lens and mirror coatings and decreases beam quality. The importance of the hybrid delivery system of the Technolas Keracor 116 is that future obsolescence is avoided through software modification toward a scanning laser system design, which also reduces maintenance requirements.

The optical components are replaced every 300–500 procedures and require replacement at variable intervals. Similarly, the monthly volume of procedures and the efficiency of laser usage determine the length of time a gas cylinder lasts. Performing several procedures per day is more efficient than doing the same number of procedures over several days. An average center performs 500 procedures per year and therefore requires a gas cylinder exchange and replacement of optical components almost yearly. In contrast, a high-volume center, performing more than 2000 procedures per year, would require replacement of optical components every 6–8 weeks and use two premix gas cylinders per year. Most maintenance visits by a service technician are required for realignment of the optical pathway and replacement of an individual lens or mirror. The ability to assess the laser beam both quantitatively and qualitatively during the recalibration procedure has a significant impact on the frequency of unscheduled visits because the surgeon is able to detect small beam misalignments and abnormalities. In a high-volume center with a single surgeon, minor maintenance, such as optic realignment, is required monthly. Systems that lack the capacity for qualitative examination of the beam have a higher threshold for unscheduled maintenance and more undetected beam abnormalities.

The Technolas maintenance contract is $40,000 annually and does not include the cost of optics, which varies from $15,000 to $150,000 annually, depending on the center volume and quality of beam desired. The annual cost of premix gas varies from $7000 to $14,000, which is equivalent to about $10 to $20 per case.

Safety Features

The most important safety feature of the Technolas Keracor 116 is the recalibration system, which allows the surgeon to examine the beam energy output quantitatively and qualitatively. The recalibration system consists of a phototherapeutic or fixed 5-mm diameter ablation of a fluence test plate, which consists of a thin 16-micron layer of foil glued onto a red test plastic. The fluence test plates are calibrated by fully ablating the foil and glue so that a homogeneous red end-point pattern is seen. A predetermined number of pulses indicate that the correct fluence is achieved. The normal number of pulses required to reach the end point for a fluence of 130 mJ/cm^2 is 65. If more pulses are required to reach the end point, then the fluence is too low; whereas, if fewer than 65 pulses is required, the fluence is too high. The fluence can be adjusted from the computer keyboard by altering the energy control bar, which adjusts the optical attenuator. The fluence test applies pulses at 10 Hz for the first 50 pulses, then at 2 Hz, thus the entire fluence test requires less than 15 seconds. Fluence adjustments can be made within seconds by depressing the right and left shift keys to increase and decrease energy output. The fluence test is then repeated to ensure that the precise fluence is maintained for each procedure. The fluence test also examines the energy output qualitatively, and the pattern of ablation of the foil and glue accurately represents the beam homogeneity, both with respect to macrohomogeneity (overall energy beam profile) and microhomogeneity (local energy beam hot and cold spots). The degree of inhomogeneity can also be quantified with respect to the number of pulses required to reach the ablation end point from one point to the next. A pulse difference greater than 6 (1.5 microns) from breakthrough to end point is considered unacceptable and requires maintenance, such as an alignment of the optical pathway or replacement of the optical components. There is no specific refractive check because polymethylmethacrylate (PMMA) plastic is a poor model to assess the ablative behavior of the beam on the stroma.

The other safety features of the Technolas Keracor 116 include a closed containment system for the laser cavity and gas exchange unit to control any potential halogen leakage. The two-step filtration system has containment filters that extract fluorine gas. There is no external ventilation mechanism other than that for servicing the unit, which further helps to prevent accidental gas leakage. Pressure gauges are computer controlled, further ensuring safety and serviceability.

Software-User Interface

The software of the Technolas Keracor 116 system has tremendous flexibility. Although many of the data screens are under continual development, the software is easily updated in minutes by entering a new floppy disc or, in future, via modem. The dual software control of the iris diaphragm and scanner block allows for a virtually unlimited number of ablation patterns of varying complexity, including toric, hyperopic, and potentially asymmetric patterns, with various blending and transition zones.

Currently, the Technolas Keracor 116 is equipped with the pretreatment multizone software program, which is the best modality for myopic corrections with a homogeneous wide-field delivery system (Machat 1993). The pretreatment software applies additional pulses to the central 2.5–3.0 mm of stroma beyond the full refractive correction to prevent central island formation and improve qualitative vision (Machat 1992). The myopic ablation pattern is then applied in a multizone pattern, in several steps, with increasing optical zone size from 3.0 to 7.0 mm. Toric ablation patterns are introduced at the second step to allow the successive spherical component to blend the cylinder into the new anterior corneal curvature. Each successive zone is larger than the preceding zone and begins at fixation with a closed iris diaphragm. Therefore, this application pattern provides for maximum smoothing, with each pulse blending the previous pulse and each zone blending the previous zone. The scanner block also oscillates each pulse about the point of fixation to further improve blending. The primary benefit from the multizone technique is that it allows for a 7.0-mm optical zone with a substantially reduced ablation depth. The large optical zone is essential to reduce night glare and reduce myopic regression. If the entire correction were applied in a single-zone fashion, the depth of ablation would not only be far greater but the contour would be much less stable. For example, a −10.00 D correction with a single 7.0-mm optical zone penetrates to a depth greater than 200 microns, whereas the Technolas multizone technique literally reduces the ablation depth by 50% while achieving the benefits of the large optical zone. Future software developments center on scanning programs designed to avoid the limitations of wide-field delivery systems, specifically central island formation, sensitivity to beam homogeneity, and difficulty with asymmetric ablation patterns.

The flexibility of the pretreatment multizone program is exceptional, allowing the user to manipulate the optical zone parameters, such as the number, size, and dioptric power distribution. The user can alter the parameters for a specific case, such as increasing the dioptric correction at 7.0 mm for a patient with excessively large pupils and sensitivity to night glare. Similarly, the pretreatment amount may be increased to account for alterations in the energy beam profile or the surgical technique that will counteract any increase in the incidence of central island formation. For example, an experienced surgeon using rapid mechanical debridement of the epithelium requires a greater pretreatment zone to account for increased stromal hydration compared to either a slower, less experienced surgeon or one whose patient is experiencing the dehydrating effects of alcohol on the stroma. The tremendous flexibility also enables new multizone or continuous curvature aspheric patterns to be quickly formulated for new procedures, such as LASIK. The software program offers proven standard parameters for various degrees of myopia, cylinder, and hyperopia corrections, but it also enables an experienced user to modify the nomogram to fit his or her particular technique. In addition to the flexible software, the screen walks the user through various steps of patient identification and ablation pattern development. These include the attempted correction, multizone parameters,

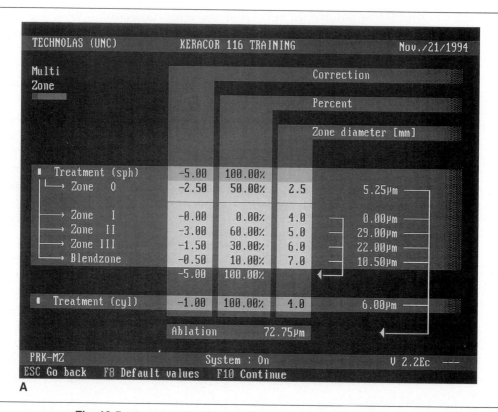

Fig. 12-5. Keracor 116 software screens reviewing preoperative multizone parameters (**A**) and cross-sectional graphic depiction of the ablation pattern (**B**).

and a review of the preoperative data with both surface and cross-sectional graphic depiction of the ablation pattern (Fig. 12-5). The fluence test mode screen is designed to simplify the beam testing process. Single keyboard keys control the entire testing process, from S for start, to G for gas exchange. Once fluence recalibration is completed, the achieved fluence is entered and retained by the computer program. Beam realignment can then be adjusted if the red coaxial HeNe light controlled by the scanner block and the red target laser diode are not aligned. A test mode for patient training or treatment mode can then be selected.

The optional eye-tracking system involves a series of screens that engage the system and allow the surgeon to lock the system into the desired position. The system can be realigned if the incorrect position is selected, in a process similar to that for beam realignment. The continuous color display (CCD) camera pupil image is displayed on the computer screen to simplify these maneuvers. The system may also be disengaged for certain procedures, such as LASIK, where reduced pupil image clarity and lowered ablation height affect eye-

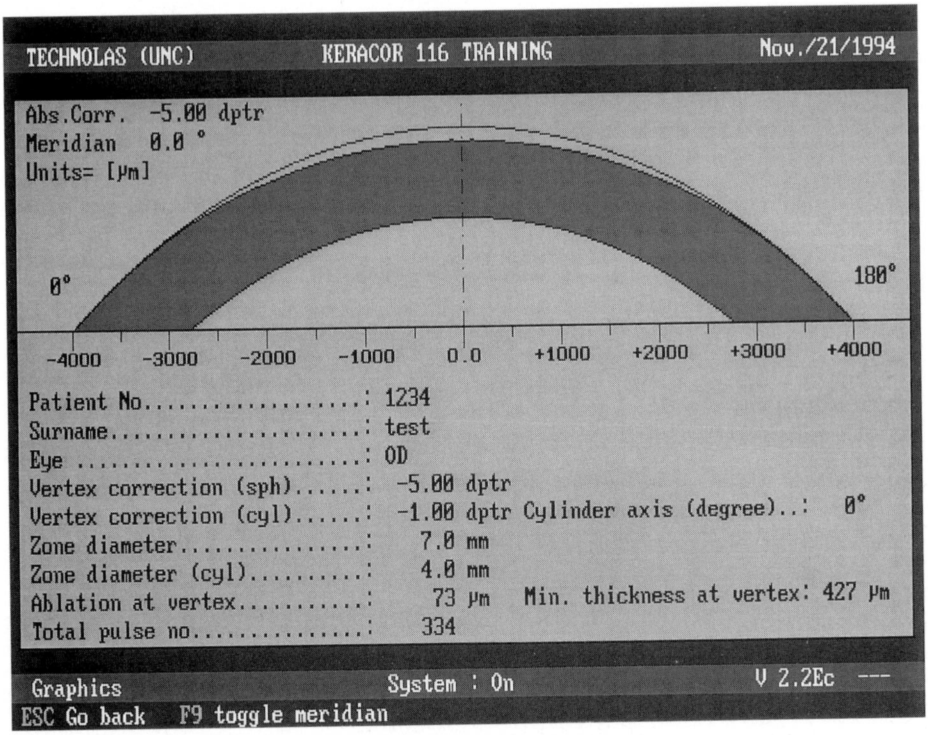
TECHNOLAS (UNC)
KERACOR 116 TRAINING
Nov./21/1994
Abs.Corr. -5.00 dptr
Meridian 0.0 °
Units= [μm]
0°
180°
-4000 -3000 -2000 -1000 0.0 +1000 +2000 +3000 +4000
Patient No..................: 1234
Surname.....................: test
Eye ....: OD
Vertex correction (sph)......: -5.00 dptr
Vertex correction (cyl)......: -1.00 dptr Cylinder axis (degree)..: 0°
Zone diameter...............: 7.0 mm
Zone diameter (cyl).........: 4.0 mm
Ablation at vertex..........: 73 μm Min. thickness at vertex: 427 μm
Total pulse no..............: 334
Graphics
System : On
V 2.2Ec ---
ESC Go back F9 toggle meridian

B

Fig. 12-5 (continued).

tracking sensitivity. When activated, the eye-tracking screen displays a green light when the point of fixation is within the active 3-mm triangulated area and the laser is active, a red light when outside the laser active triangle, and a blue light when disengaged. The red coaxial HeNe light can be observed to remain stationary within the locked visual axis or pupil center position during real or simulated eye movement. The scanner block literally tracks the eye during movement within the 3-mm triangulated laser active region, applying well-centered pulses even in cases of nystagmus.

The patient training and treatment screens display the patient name, designated eye, refractive error attempted, and multizone steps used. The multizone steps are displayed, including the dioptric breakdown with the corresponding number of pulses and time required for each step. As each step (zone) of the treatment progresses, a blue bar sweeps across the red screen indicating the proportion of each zone completed. At the completion of each zone, the user is instructed to redepress the foot pedal to begin the next step of the procedure. By breaking down the procedure into multiple steps (zones), patient fixation and comfort is enhanced by reducing the maximum time the patient must continuously fixate. Overall centration is also improved in that each zone begins centrally, thus affording the surgeon an opportunity to more accurately reevaluate centration.

Several other features have been incorporated into the software interface to improve user friendliness, such as Help screens, vertex distance calculators, and the statistical analysis of preoperative, intraoperative and postoperative data. The PTK software interface has been similarly designed for entering patient data into the program and adjusting the fluence. The PTK program is just as flexible as that of PRK, with features not widely available on other excimer laser systems. The spot diameter is variable from 0.8 mm to 7.0 mm, with an adjustable pulse frequency varying from 2–10 pulses per second. Most important, the joystick control of the scanner block allows for superb surgeon control of the treatment area. The patient continues to fixate on the target laser diode while the surgeon is about to ablate any area of the cornea denoted by the red coaxial HeNe light. The joystick control also allows the surgeon tremendous blending capabilities compared to moving the patient's head, as has been recommended with other systems. An adjustable number of pulses are preset to avoid overtreatment, which requires that the surgeon reconfirm the parameters once the initial treatment is completed. The number of variables that can be preset in combination with the scanning capabilities of the laser and joystick control affords an unparalleled degree of refinement for therapeutic cases.

Ablation Parameters and Capabilities

The Technolas Keracor 116 utilizes a fluence or energy density of 130 mJ/cm^2 and an ablation pulse rate of 10 Hz, with an ablation rate of 0.25 microns per pulse. The spot size varies from 0.8 mm to a maximum of 7.0 mm. Depending on the program and optical zone distribution utilized, the total time for a 5-D myopic correction varies from 19 to 26 seconds. The laser delivery system is unique in that it possesses both wide-field and scanning spot capabilities. The current software packages consist of either the pretreatment multizone technique or an aspheric continuous curve for myopia correction with a programmable transition zone of up to 7.0 mm. Software control of the scanner block also enables a fine oscillation to be introduced into all PRK modalities, blending each pulse into the next by a random displacement of 100 microns about the point of fixation. The pulse oscillation effect serves to smooth the ablative surface, reducing the incidence of clinically significant haze and regression. Cylindrical corrections are currently performed utilizing the scanning mode, which ablates across the minus cylinder axis. Hyperopic ablation patterns also engage the scanning mode, creating a midperipheral trough with central blending and a peripheral transition zone to reduce regression. All PRK toric and nontoric programs create a blended contour, which helps to improve refractive stability and to reduce any sharp or steep edges that may promote aggressive wound healing. The Keracor 116 has been documented to correct up to 9.0 D of cylinder with toric PRK and more than −20.00 D of sphere with myopic PRK. Hyperopic PRK has been less successful because regression remains a problem above 3.0 D. The Keracor 116 has a sufficient working distance (13 cm) for performing LASIK. LASIK and other in situ techniques have further improved clinical results, with corrections of close to −30.0 D having been obtained. Early results of hyperopic LASIK have been encouraging as the future direction for correcting moderate and severe degrees of hyperopia.

Advantages and Disadvantages

Preliminary Clinical Results

Preliminary clinical results have demonstrated exceptional safety and efficacy. The preliminary 6-month data representing the overall Canadian Keracor 116 experience treated at five investigational sites are reviewed.

Spherical and Toric Corrections: Myopia Less Than 6.00 D

In the Canadian experience, for myopic eyes less than −6.00 D, with less than 1.00 D of cylinder, 93% (97/104) achieved 20/40 or better and 75% (78/104) achieved 20/25 or better uncorrected visual acuity (UCVA). Mean preoperative myopia in this group was −3.79 D. Only 1 eye (1%) lost 2 lines of best spectacle-corrected visual acuity (BSCVA). Eighty-eight percent (92/104) of eyes were within 1 D of the intended correction.

Toric ablations were performed on an additional 112 eyes with a mean sphere of −3.41 D with up to 5.00 D of preexisting cylinder. The results reveal 86% (96/112) achieving 20/40 UCVA or better and 69% (77/112) achieving 20/25 UCVA or better. Preoperative mean cylinder was reduced from 1.58 D to 0.65 D at 6 months. Eighty percent (90/112) of eyes were within 1.00 D of the planned refraction at 6 months.

Spherical and Toric Corrections: Myopia −6.00 to −10.00 D

Forty-two myopic eyes in the range of −6.00 to −10.00 D (mean −7.70 D) received nontoric ablations with 83% (35/42) achieving 20/40 or better UCVA and 49% (20/42) achieving 20/25 UCVA or better. No eyes lost 2 lines or more of BSCVA. Seventy-nine percent (33/42) of eyes were within 1 D of the target correction.

Toric ablations were performed on an additional 36 eyes with 6-month data and a mean sphere of −8.03 D. Preoperative cylinder ranged from 1.00 to 12.00 D and was reduced from a mean of 1.74 D to 0.53 D at 6 months. UCVA was 81% (29/36) for 20/40 or better and 55% (20/36) for 20/25 UCVA or better. Three percent (1/36) of eyes with a toric ablation and 6.00–10.00 D of myopia lost 2 or more lines of BSCVA at 6 months. Seventy-nine percent (28/36) were within 1 D of the attempted correction.

Spherical and Toric Corrections: Myopia Greater Than −10.00 D

Only 8 eyes with more than −10.00 D of myopia and less than 1.00 D of cylinder had 6-month data available within this series (mean −11.49 D). UCVA of 20/40 or better was achieved in 83% (5/6), and none of the eyes lost more than 2 lines of BSCVA. Only 50% (4/8) of eyes were within 1 D of the attempted correction.

There were an additional 11 eyes with 6-month data that were treated for myopia greater than 10.00 D and cylinder ranging from 1.00–5.00 D. The preoperative mean cylinder was reduced from 2.43 D to 0.61 D. Less than half of all eyes (5/11) reached 20/40 UCVA or better and only 18% (2/11) had 20/25 UCVA or better at 6 months. Twenty-seven percent (3/11) of eyes with this severity of myopia and astigmatism lost 2 or more lines of BSCVA after 6 months.

Comparison to Other Systems

In comparison to other systems, the Keracor 116 is one of the most advanced laser systems available. It is one of the few lasers with an optional active eye-tracking system, 7.0-mm optical zone capability, joystick control for PTK, and sophisticated qualitative and quantitative recalibration system. The innovative hybrid laser delivery system allows this laser unparalleled ablation pattern flexibility and the beam oscillation and multizone program provide for an exceptionally smooth ablative surface. The software adaptability and scanning potential dramatically reduces the fundamental risk of technology obsolescence.

Future Improvements

The most recent improvements by Chiron-Technolas were primarily centered around the development of a fully automated scanning laser delivery system, which resulted in a new excimer laser workstation, the Technolas Keracor 217 C-Lasik. This system uses the new Plano-Scan, an all-scanning mode with a fixed diameter for myopia, hyperopia and toric ablations, which eliminates the need for an iris diaphragm. Complex ablation patterns are now possible with this flying spot ablation pattern without the increased maintenance and homogeneity dependence of the wide-field ablation beam. High pulse repetition rates are required; therefore, a new ceramic laser head was developed that is capable of a repetition rate of up to 50 Hz.

The PlanoScan has the ability to correct myopia, hyperopia, and myopic and hyperopic astigmatism in any combination. The major advantage of the PlanoScan algorithm compared to wide-field ablation is the much smoother ablated surface. This is demonstrated by the comparison of both treatment types on PMMA. The PlanoScan profile shows a much better correspondence with the theoretical calculated profile than with wide-field ablation. The algorithm is optimized in such a way that two consecutive pulses do not strike the same spot. This pattern minimizes the thermal and mechanical load to the cornea, thereby reducing the potential for corneal trauma, edema, or steep central islands.

Early results with PlanoScan in several hundred eyes have confirmed the improved quality of refractive surgery with this technology. Follow-up at 6 months for low myopia with an astigmatism up to 1 D demonstrates 100% of the eyes with UCVA of 20/40 or better, 85% with 20/25 or better, and 69% with 20/20. The mean preoperative refraction at −2.85 D was reduced to a mean postoperative refraction of −0.09 D. No eyes lost more than 2 lines. These results highlight the strength and accuracy of the PlanoScan scanning algorithm.

An additional feature of the Keracor 217 C-Lasik is its emphasis on the LASIK procedure. It has both an integrated Chiron Automated Corneal Shaper and special LASIK software. The built-in checklist for the Automated Corneal Shaper guides the surgeon in the steps for proper assembly of the microkeratome and correct performance of the LASIK procedure. The laser ablation itself is modified for LASIK, taking into account that LASIK ablation properties are slightly different from those of PRK. Consequently, the software distinguishes between both procedure types. Because the patient's bed can be rotated 90 degrees, the refractive workstation is also suitable for performing other refractive and ophthalmic surgical procedures.

Lastly, Chiron Technolas has integrated the corneal topography of the individual patient to the excimer laser treatment. This topographic link is possible due to the special flexibility of the scanning technology that enables a customized treatment. The surgeon can decide whether to add or subtract pulses at the cornea to adapt the procedure to the patient's unique surface structure for better results.

Future improvement in software and nomogram development, laser head stability, and systems to reduce maintenance requirements are expected. In general, smaller, more reliable and efficient lasers will be introduced, as will solid-state technology, once methods to truly stabilize these frequency-multiplied energy sources are developed.

13 Coherent-Schwind Keratom

Werner N. Förster, Gerhard Stenger,
and Ahmad Abu-Shumays

History

Herbert Schwind GmbH & Co. KG was founded as an ophthalmic instruments company in Kleinostheim, Germany, in 1958. Distribution of the Keeler ophthalmoscope and vision aids soon grew to include the sole distribution of Haag Streit products in 1963 and the introduction of proprietary Schwind examination units for the ophthalmologist in 1964. In this same year, Herbert Schwind started manufacturing contact lenses in collaboration with Titmus Eurocon of Aschaffenburg, Germany. In 1971, Titmus became wholly owned by Schwind, with production facilities in Switzerland, Italy, and Brazil, and with manufacturing licenses in France, Taiwan, and Argentina. Schwind/Titmus soft contact lenses entered the U.S. market in 1978, following U.S. Food and Drug Administration (FDA) clearance. This business grew to become the largest contact lens manufacturer in Europe, with 700 employees by 1980. The operation was diversified and began manufacturing intraocular lenses (IOLs) in 1982. Ciba Vision, a division of Ciba Geigy of Basel, Switzerland, acquired this business from Herbert Schwind in 1983.

Herbert Schwind was cognizant of the development of the new excimer-based refractive correction technology in the late 1980s. He initiated the development of the Schwind Keratom in 1989 by enlisting the participation of scientists, engineers, and ophthalmologists from universities and technology firms in Germany, including Lambda Physik, a division of Coherent Inc., Göttingen, Germany, specializing in excimer lasers. Following extensive clinical studies of the system at the University Eye Hospital in Münster, the Keratom was introduced in Europe and Asia Pacific in the summer of 1992.

Technical and business collaborations between Herbert Schwind and the Coherent Medical Group began shortly after the introduction of the Keratom. Because Coherent is the world's largest medical laser company, having pioneered the use of argon lasers in retinal photocoagulation more than 25 years ago, their expertise and worldwide network in laser distribution offered much to the Keratom's development. A comprehensive distribution relationship was formulated between the two companies in early 1994, granting Coherent the responsibility for selling the Keratom in most countries of the world.

Scientific publications regarding the Keratom were introduced as early as 1993, with a description of the system and its features for the correction of simple myopia [1]. In 1994, the correction of myopic astigmatism [2] and hyperopia [3] were introduced as well. As of June 1996, there are 95 Keratom installations around the world, with more than 80,000 eyes having been treated with the laser.

The Keratom combines Coherent's proven excimer laser with Schwind's advanced optical delivery system in a modern modular design with high performance, safety, and reliability. The modular design will allow new features and enhancements to be added to the system as technical and clinical capabilities in reshaping the cornea expand.

Unique Aspects of the Hardware

The Laser System

Figure 13-1 shows the Keratom excimer laser system, including the excimer laser (Novatube, Lambda-Physik), delivery system, microscope, monitor, and the operating bed. The unit measures 202 cm × 145 cm × 153 cm and weighs about 700 kg. Electric power requirements are single-phase 230 V, 3.5 kW (maximum) power, 16 ampere current. The 193-nm excimer laser is air-cooled and needs no water supply. A halogen-(fluorine) generator and external argon-neon gas bottle are required. The excimer pulse repetition rate can be selected from 1–30 Hz. The output energy from the excimer cavity may be adjusted up to 500 mJ/pulse (normally 300 mJ/pulse is used). The energy output is self-stabilized and is monitored by an internal power meter. Pulse-to-pulse fluctuation of the energy is less than 5%, and the pulse length is 23 nsec. Gas lifetime for each filling of the laser is approximately 20 days. An internal communication interface is connected by an optical glass fiber to the controlling computer. The specially designed operation bed has x, y, and z (height) control and can be moved using a joystick or a foot pedal. The resolution of bed adjustment is 20 μm.

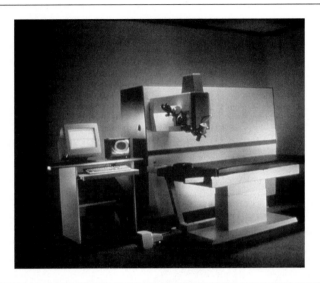

Fig. 13-1. The Keratom excimer laser system consists of a main cabinet containing the Novatube excimer laser, and auxiliary modules, the beam delivery system, the stereomicroscope, the eye monitor and tracking system, the computer station, and the patient's bed.

The Delivery System

Figure 13-2 shows the beam delivery system. Three mirrors, four lenses, and a special beam integrator are included in the delivery optical system, which is purged with pure nitrogen. The original rectangular excimer laser beam from the Novatube has a cross section of approximately 8 mm × 28 mm, with a top-hat profile in the long direction and a near gaussian energy distribution in the short direction. A mechanical shutter allows the laser beam to pass through the system. The shutter system consists of two independently actuated shutter blades. The excimer laser beam is expanded by two cylindrical lenses and directed by a 90-degree mirror onto a prismatic integrator element (Fig. 13-3). The integrator is used to homogenize the laser beam [1]. It consists of an array of 19 wedge plates or prisms, each 10 mm in diameter. The wedge plates are optically contacted on a base plate in such a way that the beam parts that pass through each individual wedge are superimposed in the focal plane of the integrator. The superimposed beams uniformly illuminate the apertures on a moving steel band (Fig. 13-4A). The apertures on the steel band are imaged on the cornea by the zoom lens, and thus determine the ablation profile on the eye. The apertures are etched into a 50-μm-thick stainless steel foil, which is moved by a special mask transport system. Index holes on the steel foil are used with light emitters and

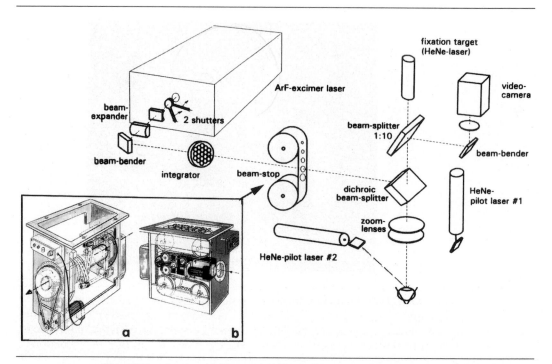

Fig. 13-2. Diagram of the beam delivery system and the fixation alignment system. A specially designed steel band module (a) provides rotation of the treatment axis in astigmatic correction. Alternately, a fractal mask module (b) can be installed in place of the steel band. (Modified from W Förster, R Beck, H Busse. Design and development of a new 193-nm excimer laser surgical system. *Refract Corneal Surg* 9:293–299, 1993.)

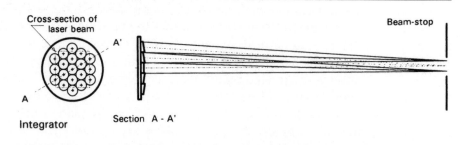

Fig. 13-3. Diagram of the integrator system. The nearly square cross section of the laser beam is transformed into an array of circular beams that are superimposed in the plane of the beam stop to produce a homogeneous intensity profile. (From W Förster, R Beck, H Busse. Design and development of a new 193-nm excimer laser surgical system. *Refract Corneal Surg* 9:293–299, 1993.)

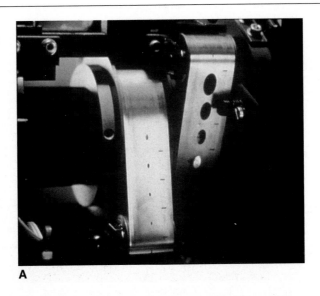

A

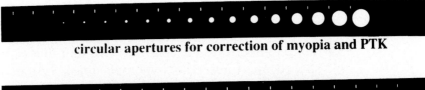

circular apertures for correction of myopia and PTK

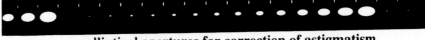

elliptical apertures for correction of astigmatism

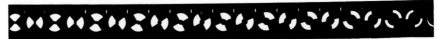

opposite sector apertures for correction of hyperopia

B

Fig. 13-4. **A.** Module showing orientation of steel bands. **B.** Steel bands illustrating aperture patterns for correction of myopia, myopic astigmatism, and hyperopia.

sensors to precisely position each aperture in the path of the excimer beam.

Three types of steel band apertures are included in the Keratom system (Fig. 13-4B), resulting in the following patterns on the cornea. Round apertures from 0.6–8 mm diameter correct simple myopia. Oval apertures from 0.6–8 mm correct myopic astigmatism. For the correction of hyperopia, it is necessary to block the center of the beam.

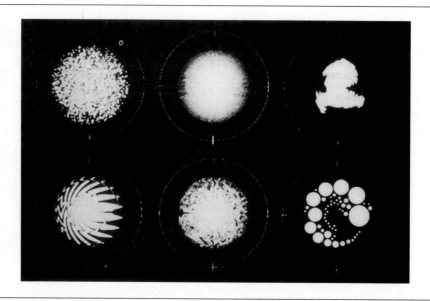

Fig. 13-5. Examples of possible fractal masks for use in correction of various refractive disorders.

The annular apertures are split into two half-masks, which resemble pie-shaped apertures. The hyperopic mask system produces ring-shaped ablations with rings of varying inner diameter. The ablation size is 8.0 mm in the outer ring and 0.6 mm in the inner ring. A specially designed module using fractal masks (Fig. 13-5) can be installed in place of the steel band module (see Fig. 13-2b). Fractal masks offer unique advantages to refractive correction (discussed in Future Improvements below). For phototherapeutic keratectomy (PTK) procedures, round apertures from 0.6 to 8.0 mm can be used.

After passing through the beam stops in the mask band, the laser is reflected downward by a dichroic beam-splitter and through two planoconvex lenses that focus the beam onto the cornea of the patient. The lenses function as a zoom-projection system (telescopic zoom) to provide a continual transition in the ablation diameter. The patient's eye is monitored by a continuous color display (CCD) camera through the dichroic beam-splitter. The imaging factor of the zoom-optic (i.e., demagnification from the aperture size to the image on the cornea) can be varied from 0.8× to 0.67×. The fluence variance caused by the zoom lens is taken into account by the controlling software. All components transparent to the ultraviolet (UV) radiation are made from synthetic quartz (Suprasil II) and are specially coated to minimize reflection losses at the 193-nm excimer wavelength.

To align the patient's eye for treatment, the patient fixates on a blinking red diode laser target (670 nm). The excimer treatment plane is located at the intersection of two helium-neon (HeNe) laser alignment beams. A passive eye-tracking system interrupts the treatment when the patient's eye moves. The tracking sensitivity has an adjustable range from 100 to 1000 μm. The working distance from the laser output aperture to the patient's eye is 28 cm below the delivery system, providing ample space for performing laser in-situ keratomileusis (LASIK) procedures under the laser.

The system is equipped with a special coaxial stereomicroscope with a cross-hair reticle. It uses a normal binocular eyepiece (Moller-Wedel) with two separate optical arms for the right and left objectives, designed so that the observation plane is coincident with the plane of the excimer and HeNe alignment beams (Fig. 13-6). The stereo angle

Fig. 13-6. The coaxial stereomicroscope. (From W Förster, R Beck, H Busse. Design and development of a new 193-nm excimer laser surgical system. *Refract Corneal Surg* 9:293–299, 1993.)

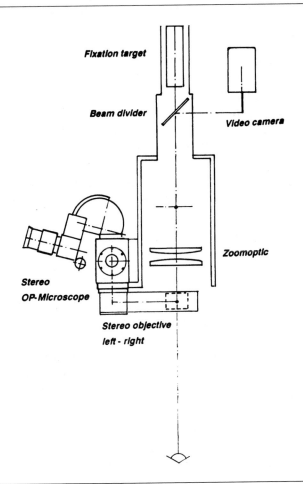

between the viewing directions is 22 degrees. The microscope provides magnifications of 3.5×, 6×, 11×, 20×, and 32×.

A special slit-lamp illumination module is built into the delivery system. It provides adjustable slit height and width (0–20 mm). Filters are provided for blue, yellow, and white illumination.

To allow a change of the axis in astigmatic procedures, a new mask transport system, called the *astigmatic module* [2], has been developed. Rotation of the module is possible in 2-degree steps between 0 and 180 degrees. In the delivery system, the apertures on the steel band are translated on this module (see Fig. 13-2a).

Maintenance Considerations

After 2 million pulses (approximately 5000 procedures), the optics require cleaning. This is normally done during routine service. The cleaning procedure can be repeated 10 times before the optics require replacement. The lifetime of the halogen generator and the argon-neon gas bottle is approximately 2 years, which is significantly greater than the 4- to 6-month lifetime of a typical argon-neon-fluorine premix cylinder used by other excimer lasers. The lifetime of the gas in the laser cavity, after a new filling, is approximately 20 days. The lifetime of the laser tube is 200–300 million pulses. The significance of these statistics is illustrated by considering the number of pulses during typical use: assume 100 eyes per week are treated, with an average of 400 pulses per procedure: These 40,000 pulses per week are equivalent to 2 million pulses, or 5000 patients per year. This is only 1% of the useful life of the excimer laser! To maintain optimum operation of the system, routine service and safety checks are performed twice yearly.

Safety Features

All major functions of the excimer laser system are controlled by computer. The patient fixates on a blinking laser target. To improve the centration of the ablation zone, an automatic passive eye-tracking device is provided. It has been in clinical use since 1992. When the surgeon starts the treatment by pressing the foot pedal, the position of the ablation zone is captured as a reference. The passive eye-tracking device stops the laser from firing if the deviation from the desired center of the ablation is beyond a preselected threshold. This threshold can be set by the user in the range of 100–1000 μm.

The argon/neon gas bottle is nontoxic, the halogen-(fluorine) generator produces only a small amount of fluorine at low pressure during the gas exchange. So long as no gas exchange is requested, the fluorine source remains in a solid phase, which is nontoxic. Outside ventilation is not necessary because the exchanged gas is neutralized by an active filter system.

In addition to the energy monitor, which measures the excimer output and stabilizes it through a feedback control system, Keratom has a second energy monitor after the beam integrator. This redundant energy monitoring further increases system safety. Another safety feature disables motion of the patient bed when the foot switch is depressed.

All critical operating parameters in the system are monitored to ensure safe and reliable operation. These include the laser energy, the positions of the steel band and zoom lens, and the nitrogen flow. All voltage levels from system power supplies are also monitored to ensure proper operation. Finally, a hardware emergency button is provided that shuts down the system in an emergency.

The actual fluence of the excimer laser just before surgery is very important for the calculation of the ablation profile. A fluence sensor was developed [1] to measure the ablation rate per pulse. The excimer laser fires at a material with a known thickness, such as a Wratten filter. To obtain consistent results, it is important to store the test material under dry conditions and to avoid the exposure of the test material to light. The fluence sensor consists of a cylindrical cavity with an aperture at the top, across which the test material may be fixed. The inner bottom surface of the cavity is covered with a fluorescing material. When the Wratten filter is perforated by the laser, the inner surface fluoresces. This fluorescence is measured by an optical detector. The number of pulses required to ablate the film of known thickness is automatically counted by the system computer. Results of the fluence test (ablation depth in μm/pulse) are used for calculation of refractive profiles. Additionally, it is recommended that a polymethylmethacrylate (PMMA) platelet be ablated periodically and sent to the company for measurement and verification of surface profile and corresponding refractive power.

An optional air or nitrogen blower or circumferential laminar flow evacuator may be used to remove ablation by-products. Care must be taken to place the blower or evacuator far from the patient's eye to minimize its effect on the water content of the corneal surface.

Software-User Interface

To start a treatment, specific data, such as name of the patient, sex, date of birth, and refraction, must be entered into the system. The complete database can be used for preoperative and postoperative

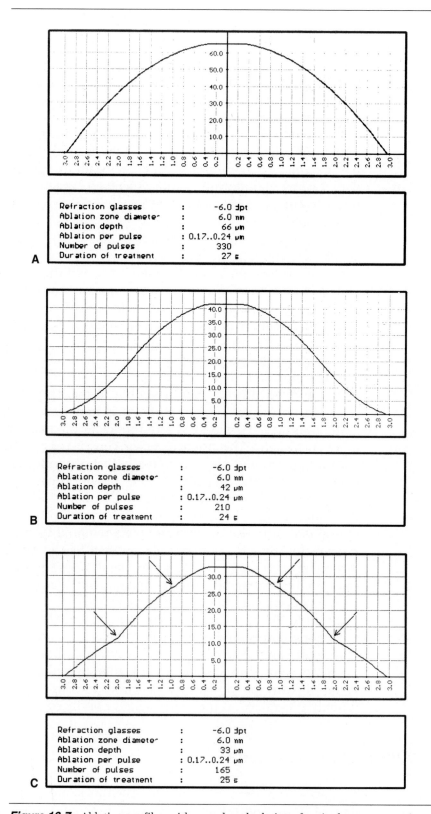

Figure 13-7. Ablation profiles with sample calculations for single-zone myopic PRK (**A**), aspheric myopic PRK (**B**), multizone myopic PRK (**C**), astigmatic PRK (**D**), and hyperopic PRK (**E**).

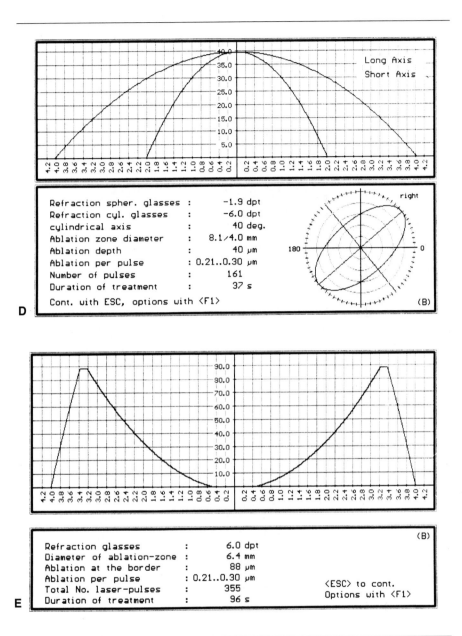

Refraction spher. glasses :   -1.9 dpt
Refraction cyl. glasses   :   -6.0 dpt
cylindrical axis   :   40 deg.
Ablation zone diameter   :   8.1/4.0 mm
Ablation depth   :   40 μm
Ablation per pulse   : 0.21..0.30 μm
Number of pulses   :   161
Duration of treatment   :   37 s
Cont. with ESC, options with ⟨F1⟩

D

(B)

Refraction glasses   :   6.0 dpt
Diameter of ablation-zone   :   6.4 mm
Ablation at the border   :   88 μm
Ablation per pulse   : 0.21..0.30 μm
Total No. laser-pulses   :   355   ⟨ESC⟩ to cont.
Duration of treatment   :   96 s   Options with ⟨F1⟩

E

Fig. 13-7. *(continued).*

data storage and analysis, with the maximum limit of data entry being 2 million procedures. The programming language is Pascal and Assembler, and the user language may be English, Spanish, French, or German. The software uses customized windows with a main menu, a mouse interface, and modem support capability for data communications and for remote servicing from the factory.

Ablation Parameters and Capabilities

The imaging factor (demagnification) between the steel band aperture and the cornea is varied from 0.8× to 0.67× using the zoom-optic lens. Thus, the system does not operate with constant fluence. The impact of fluence changes on the ablation depth by each pulse is taken into consideration by the software in determining the overall ablation profile. The range of fluence is 150–220 mJ/cm^2. If the fluence falls below 150 mJ/cm^2, system operation is interrupted, and a laser refilling cycle is required before continuing. The maximum zone size for PRK treatments is 8 mm. An optional 11-mm diameter is available for PTK.

Myopic Photorefractive Keratectomy

Different types of ablation profiles can be chosen by the surgeon to correct myopia: (1) a single-zone ablation profile (Fig. 13-7A), (2) an aspherical ablation profile (Fig. 13-7B), and (3) a multizone ablation profile (Fig. 13-7C). There is no limitation to the amount of myopia that can be corrected, although a warning message appears if the intended correction is more than 9 D. The time for a −5 D single-zone myopic correction depends on the chosen diameter of the ablation zone. For a 6-mm zone, the time is about 25 sec.

Myopic Astigmatism

For the correction of myopic astigmatism, dimensions of the elliptical ablation zone can be varied from 0.6 mm to 8.0 mm. Normally an elliptical zone with axial dimensions of 5.1 mm × 8.0 mm is used. As with myopia, the elliptical ablation pattern is generated by using band apertures. However, a new mask transport system is included to change the axis of astigmatic treatment by 2-degree steps between 0 and 180 degrees. Figure 13-7D shows a calculation example and profile for an astigmatic elliptical ablation.

Hyperopic PRK

For hyperopia treatment, the ablation depth varies from zero in the center of the zone to a maximum depth at a diameter of 6.4 mm, followed by a transition zone back to zero depth at 8.0-mm diameter. A calculation example and profile for hyperopic (annular) ablation is shown in Figure 13-7E.

Phototherapeutic Keratectomy

For PTK, the diameter of the ablation zone is 0.6 mm up to 8.0 mm (optional 11 mm). Each laser pulse ablates a uniform 0.25-μm thickness without inducing a refractive correction. The PTK mode is particularly useful for treating corneal diseases, including anterior pathologies and superficial opacities, and for smoothing of the corneal surface.

Advantages and Disadvantages

Preliminary Clinical Results

There are 95 Keratom installations around the world as of June 1996. The first systems were installed in the spring of 1992. The number of eyes treated with the Keratom is estimated to exceed 80,000.

PTK Treatments

In a 3-year PTK study of 252 eyes, Förster [1, 2] examined the use of the Keratom for treating recurrent erosions, corneal irregularities postpterygium surgery, band keratopathy (deposits), and other miscellaneous indications, such as scarring, amyloid deposits, alkali burns, keratitis, dystrophy, and protuberance. No recurrence was observed during the 12- to 36-month follow-up period in 90% of patients diagnosed with recurrent erosions. No change in refractive outcome or best spectacle-corrected visual acuity was observed at the 6-month follow-up period. Fifty-six percent of the pterygia patients had no recurrence within 12 months after PTK treatment; 72% of patients treated for deposits had no recurrence during the 9-month follow-up period, and haze in all cases was less than grade +1. Finally, 96% of patients in the miscellaneous group achieved their treatment goal, but one alkali burn and one dystrophy case were not successful.

PRK Treatments

In a retrospective review by Krueger et al. of 175 eyes treated with the Keratom excimer laser in former Czechoslovakia, where preoperative myopia ranged from −1.0 to −7.5 D, and astigmatism was limited to less than 1.0 D, 98% (138/141) of eyes were 20/40 or better, 88% (124/141) were 20/25 or better, and 66% (93/141) were 20/20 or better at the last evaluation (between 3 months and 1 year) [4]. Although some overcorrection existed, spherical refraction was within 1.0 D of emmetropia in 88% (131/149) of eyes and within 0.5 D in 68% (101/149) of eyes at the last evaluation. Division of these eyes into lower myopia (−1.0 to −3.0 D) and medium myopia (−3.25 to −7.5 D) reveals better results in the former (98% [± 1.0 D] and 84% [± 0.5 D]), than in the latter (83% [± 1.0 D] and 60% [± 0.5 D]). Only 0.7% (1/139) of eyes had loss of 2 lines of best spectacle-corrected visual acuity (BSCVA). Corneal haze was grade +1.5 or greater in approximately 3%, whereas less than 1% had grade +2.0 or greater throughout the postoperative period.

In a retrospective study of Vidaurri-Leal and co-workers, the results of both myopia and astigmatism were reported [5]. At the sixth postoperative month, uncorrected visual acuity (UCVA) was 20/40 or better in 94% (34/36) of the low myopic eyes (−1 to −6 D) and 82% (14/17) of the astigmatic eyes (−2.75 to −6.75 D spherical equivalent, with −1 to −4.5 D cylinder). About 81% (29/36) of the myopic eyes and 88% (15/17) of the astigmatic eyes were within 1 D of target spherical equivalent refraction. None of the myopic eyes lost 2 lines of BSCVA, but loss of 2 lines was noted in 12% (2/17) of the astigmatic eyes.

These findings are comparable to results of similar studies reported by investigators of other excimer systems.

Comparison to Other Systems

The Keratom has several distinct advantages over other wide-field excimer lasers. First, the beam-shaping iris apertures seen with the Summit, VISX, and Chiron Technolas lasers are similar in principle to the band apertures of the Keratom in that a steplike pattern is projected onto the corneal surface. In corneas treated with the Summit and VISX systems, these steps are imprinted onto the surface, thus affecting the overall smoothness because there is no scanning or wobbling feature. Although the Technolas has this feature, it includes movement of the beam with scanning components and active eye tracking. The Keratom laser system does not have these features but instead has a telescopic zoom system, which varies the fluence to provide continual and smooth change in the ablation profile with no ablation steps. It does this with a passive tracking system to ensure centration with eye movement. The Keratom system also has a prismatic optical integrator to ensure beam homogeneity prior to the beam's passing through the telescopic zoom.

The additional hardware required for both scanning and active tracking, as seen with the wide-field Technolas, as well as the scanning slit and flying spot lasers, give the Keratom an advantage in that it can achieve a very smooth ablation profile without use of complex mechanisms. As a wide-field laser, it does require more energy than the scanning slit and flying spot lasers, but it also operates much more quickly, completing the procedure in only a fraction of the time.

In relation to the other wide-field lasers, the high pulse energy required for ablation does not shorten the lifetime of the laser optics because the beam is expanded in the optical delivery system to an area 30 times larger than the ablation aperture in order to maintain an energy density well below the damage threshold of the optics.

Finally, the built-in solid-state fluorine generator and Novatube together make the safety and maintenance of the Keratom far superior to that of other excimer laser systems. The halogen generator liberates fluorine molecules under a vacuum to fill the ceramic Novatube laser cavity under highly pure gas conditions. Once filled, the laser may be used for approximately 3 weeks without further filling, which is several times longer than that required for other excimer systems. The fluorine generator eliminates the need for high-pressure toxic argon-fluoride gas tanks, which need to be replaced every 4–6 months. In contrast, the halogen generator lasts about 2 years before requiring replacement. These and other unique features of the Keratom are summarized in Table 13-1.

Table 13-1. Unique features of the Keratom

Features	Benefits
Solid-state halogen generator is used in place of argon-fluoride tank	No toxic gas tanks, sealed chambers, or ventilation systems
Laser gas fill lasts approximately 20 days; **halogen source and argon-neon tank** last approximately 2 years	Reliable uninterrupted operation over long periods; significant savings ($8000/year)
Calibration is required only once per day; two energy detectors stabilize and verify laser output	Energy detection and control ensure stable output; stable calibration gives consistent results and saves time (3 min/procedure)
Long optics life due to large beam, nitrogen purge, and hard coatings	Minimum downtime and expense related to replacing optics; savings are $7000/year
19-prism integrator produces homogeneous beam profile	Provides smooth profile without irregularities that impair visual acuity
Zoom lens provides continual and smooth change in ablation diameter	Smooth surface ensures minimal glare and light scatter and facilitates uniform healing
Large-zone ablation: each pulse is capable of ablating 8.0 mm diameter	Moves transition zone further away from visual axis; minimizes halos and distortions
Blinking fixation laser	Ensures accurate alignment of patient's visual axis with the excimer treatment beam
Passive eye-tracking interrupts treatment if eye moves	Ensures that ablation zone is centered on patient eye
Built-in slit-lamp capabilities	Allows diagnostic examination of the cornea
Large working distance (28 cm) between microscope aperture and eye	Ensures patient comfort; provides space for LASIK procedure

Future Improvements

The modular design of the Keratom makes it possible to upgrade the system with new features and improvements. A software program that integrates aspheric ablation zones and multizone approaches is currently under investigation. The large working distance between the beam exit aperture and the patient's eye makes the system particularly suitable for LASIK treatments. The development of fractal masks for use in the Keratom offers several advantages, including (1) an even smoother and more uniform ablation profile, (2) significantly faster treatments, and (3) new modes of treatment, such as for hyperopic astigmatism and irregular astigmatism. Keratom systems with fractal mask modules entered clinical investigations in June 1996.

References

1. Förster W, Beck R, Busse H. Design and development of a new 193-nm excimer laser surgical system. *Refract Corneal Surg* 9:293–299, 1993.
2. Förster W, et al. Correcting myopic astigmatism with an areal 193-nm excimer laser ablation. *J Cataract Refract Surg* 21:278–281, 1995.
3. Beck R, Förster W. Excimer Laser Delivery System for Astigmatic and Hyperopic Photorefractive Surgery. In JM Parel O*phthalmic Technologies IV Proceedings SPIE* 2126:212–216, 1994.
4. Krueger R. Photorefractive keratectomy for low and medium myopia with the Coherent/Schwind excimer laser. Presented at International Society of Refractive Surgery Mid-summer Symposium, Minneapolis, July 28, 1995.
5. Vidaurri-Leal J, Cantu-Charles C, Talamo JH. Excimer PRK for myopia and astigmatism with the Coherent-Schwind Keratom. *Invest Ophthalmol Vis Sci* 36:S190, 1995.

Scanning Slit Ablation

Rather than using a stationary system that delivers a broad beam of energy through apertures of varying size, scanning slit ablation uses a rectangular slit-shaped beam of light that scans across an aperture within the path of the beam, thereby allowing for uniform removal of tissue over the course of several pulses instead of just one pulse. The amount of tissue removed with each scan, however, may differ depending on the amount of overlap experienced between pulses. The systems utilizing this scanning slit approach, the Nidek EC-5000 (Chap. 14) and the Meditec MEL-60 (Chap. 15), are described in detail.

The advantages of scanning slit ablation include a lower required pulse energy output than that of wide field ablation and excellent beam uniformity and homogeneity because a smaller area is ablated with each pulse. The smaller area within the slit also appears to reduce the incidence of steep central islands, virtually eliminating this side effect during a scanning slit procedure.

A disadvantage of scanning slit ablation is that it requires a complex scanning system and takes longer for completion than wide field ablation. Consequently, eye tracking or mechanical fixation plays a more important role in scanning slit ablation. The eye-based mask used in the Meditec MEL 60 system may be cumbersome because it needs to be placed on the eye, unlike masks used in other systems.

14 Nidek EC-5000

Daniel S. Durrie, Paul M. Karpecki, Robert J.S. Mack, and R. Ray Sayano

History

The research into the development of an ophthalmic excimer laser system at Nidek Co., Ltd. (Gamagori, Japan) started in 1985. In 1986, a research and development project was formally initiated under the guidance of Carmen A. Puliafito and Roger F. Steinert, both then at the Massachusetts Eye and Ear Infirmary and Harvard Medical School, Boston. The result of that project in 1987 was a prototype linear incision system with slit-lamp delivery for radial keratotomy (RK) and arcuate keratotomy (AK) for myopic and astigmatic correction, respectively.

In 1990, the research and development evolved into the inclusion of large-area ablation and a photographic panel of the prototype was displayed at the 1991 American Academy of Ophthalmology (AAO) meeting in Anaheim, California. The development of the system continued with the incorporation of a transition zone proposed by Paolo Vinciguerra of Monza, Italy. The first commercial model was the EC-5000.

Even though the EC-5000 has been commercially available and used clinically since late 1992, development and refinement of the design have continued. At the 1994 AAO meeting in San Francisco, the prototype of the hyperopic correction feature was demonstrated, and at the 1995 AAO meeting in Atlanta, the auto-alignment and eye-tracking module was exhibited.

Unique Aspects of the Hardware

The Laser System

The Nidek EC-5000 excimer laser system is shown in Figure 14-1. The laser head used in this system is made to Nidek specifications by Lambda Physik (Göttingen, Germany). The dimensions of the internal laser are 75 cm in height, 120 cm in depth, and 37.5 cm in width. The system is controlled by an IBM personal computer (PC) with input of all patient data and control functions. The cooling system for the Nidek laser is ambient air cooling. The laser gases are a premix of fluorine (F_2), neon (Ne), and argon (Ar), and helium gas makes up the balance. This premix allows the gas to be highly reactive but it can also combine chemically and become ineffective. Therefore, the gas in the chamber has a finite lifetime whether the laser is fired or not.

The dimensions of the main body of the laser are 152 cm in height, 137 cm in depth, and 75 cm in width, and the whole system, which includes the computer workstation, is 152 cm in height, 137 cm in depth, and 141 cm in width. The device weighs 650 kg and occupies a minimum floor space of 280 cm × 205 cm. The Nidek laser uses a single-phase 208-volt AC, 50/60 Hz 15-ampere line source. The minimum door width to accommodate the Nidek EC-5000 is 80 cm.

The computer interface is an external IBM PC or model PS2 compatible PC with a VGA display and controller and a standard keyboard arrangement. The operating bed can either be supplied by the manu-

Fig. 14-1. Nidek EC-5000 excimer laser corneal surgery system.

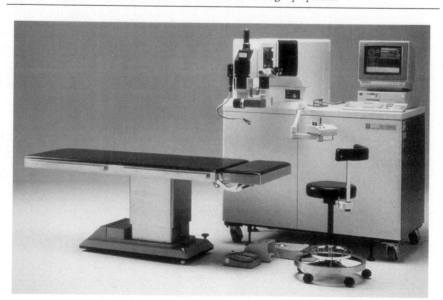

facturer or purchased separately. Fine movement control of the bed is not essential because the EC-5000 provides laser movement control in all directions.

The Delivery System

A schematic of the Nidek EC-5000 delivery system is shown in Fig. 14-2. The shaping system of the beam involves a rectangular cross-sectional beam of up to 2 mm × 9 mm and an opening diaphragm. Beam homogenization is achieved by linear scan of 10 overlayed rectangular cross-sectional beams, combined with rotation of the linear axis on completion of each scan (Fig. 14-3). The astigmatism correction combines the opening diaphragm with an opening slit in the direction of the cylinder. The hyperopic correction is achieved by an offset rectangular beam rotation about a central axis and mechanical diaphragm.

The Nidek EC-5000 has 11 pieces in its optic system and requires a nitrogen purge system. The constant flow of nitrogen across the optics allows higher transmission of ultraviolet (UV) light than in an air system. The Nidek EC-5000 features a Zeiss microscope with a variable illumination intensity, variable magnification, and focusing in x, y, and z axes.

The patient fixation target is a single coaxial, green light-emitting diode (LED) that is 3 mm in diameter. An optional eye-tracking and auto-alignment system is available internationally but is not part of the investigational studies in the United States. The system auto-

Fig. 14-2. Schematic diagram of the Nidek EC-5000 laser delivery system.

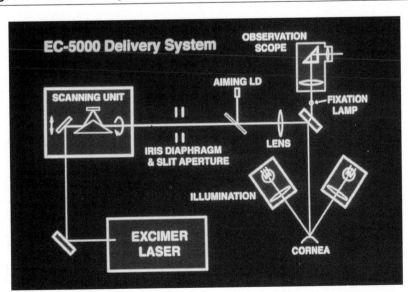

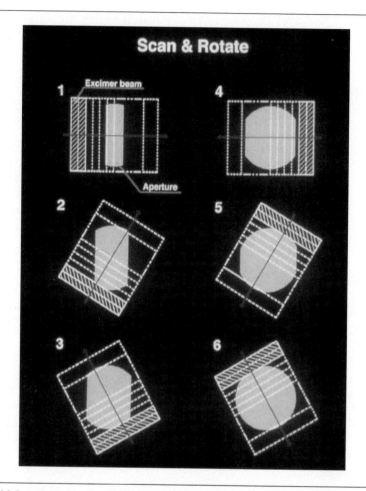

Fig. 14-3. Schematic diagram of beam scan/homogenization with cylindrical ablation.

matically aligns to the center of the patient's pupil and actively tracks the eye with automatic shutdown on significant eye movement.

A vacuum ring is also available for eye stabilization, which is not presently being used in the U.S. clinical trials.

The EC-5000 has an adjustable scanning rate of 0.5–5.0 scans per second. Scanning involves both linear and rotational movements to maximize ablation smoothness. A single scan pattern utilizes the full width of the rectangular beam to sweep across the optical zone in 10, slightly overlapping pulses of energy. As one pass is completed, the beam rotates clockwise by 60 degrees, and the scan is repeated. This sequence continues until ablation is completed, effectively avoiding localized overtreatment, which could otherwise occur as a result of laser beam profile irregularities or hot spots.

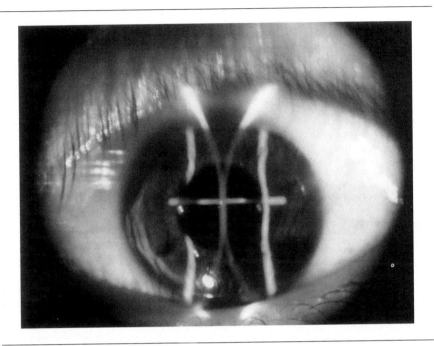

Fig. 14-4. Surgeon's view of alignment for centration of the Nidek EC-5000 excimer laser beam.

Another feature is the surgeon alignment system for centration. The system has two projected oblique slit images, which are aligned in the x, y, and z axes. The patient's pupil is centered in the surgical field, and the vertical center of the pupil is aligned with a horizontal line that is moved by the joystick. Next, the horizontal center of the pupil is aligned with the horizontal lines of the two cross-shaped illuminations, as shown in Fig. 14-4. Finally, the two vertical lines, which appear on the rounded surface of the cornea as arcs, must overlap at the center. This is adjusted by the focus control. The standard working distance for the system is 10 cm, but a 17.5 cm working distance can be special-ordered with the system to allow for adequate space for microkeratome use during a laser in-situ keratomileusis (LASIK) procedure.

Maintenance Considerations

The optics of the EC-5000 encompass 11 elements. Their effective lifetime is approximately 1 year, at which point the system needs to be replaced. The gas cylinders also have a lifetime of 1 year, and there are approximately 18 refills per cylinder of the premix gas. The lifetime of the gas in the cavity itself is about 1 week, or 1 full week of treatments.

If realignment of the laser cavity is necessary, it is performed at the regular preventive maintenance checks, as part of both the limited and comprehensive maintenance contracts.

The maintenance contract fees range from $17,000 per year for the limited service agreement (which includes five service calls and no parts) to $40,000 per year for the comprehensive service agreement. This agreement is a 1-year or 5 million laser pulse full coverage service and includes full preventive maintenance, all labor, travel expenses, and parts for the laser, excluding gases and consumables.

Safety Features

One of the safety features of the EC-5000 is the active tracking system. This adds to the safety by minimizing the chance of off-center ablation, should the patient move his or her eyes during the procedure. If the movement is significant, the tracking system interrupts laser beam transmission. For example, if the patient should lose sight of the fixation target and look away, the auto-tracking system follows the eye's movement to maintain central ablation. If the patient's eye moves significantly, the procedure stops immediately.

Some of the gas containment safety features include a halogen filter, which removes toxic fluorine from spent gas in the laser head, an emergency valve, and noncorrosive tubes and regulators that do not break down with excessive exposure. There is also a fluorine leak detector, which sounds an alarm if there is any gas leak from the laser head or the premix bottle.

Another safety feature is the preoperative calibration check, which involves ablation of a 3.00-D lens into a polymethylmethacrylate (PMMA) plate. The power as measured on a lensometer is compared to the desired settings internally, and the calibration is self-correcting. An optional effluent removal accessory (used for fumes during calibration of PMMA plates) is available.

Software-User Interface

The software interface has a patient identification and preoperative data menu (Fig. 14-5). The patient identification field has a maximum of 40 characters. Its range of programming capabilities includes the potential to change the frequency, scan rate, treatment zone size, and transition zone size, and to choose between programs for myopic, astigmatic, and hyperopic photorefractive keratectomy (PRK) and phototherapeutic keratectomy (PTK). Many of these program capabilities are fixed and unavailable in clinical trials.

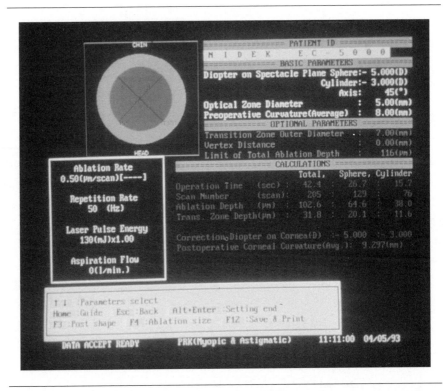

Fig. 14-5. Computer screen for inputting surgical parameters.

The software language is C language, and the standard set up is IBM compatible with keystroke entry.

Ablation Parameters and Capabilities

The average energy density of the EC-5000 is 140 mJ/cm². The laser pulse rate is 5–50 Hz, which is 0.5–5.0 scans per second that can be controlled by the user. The maximum ablation spot size is 9 mm, including the transition zone that is incorporated into the standard procedure. The transition zone is ablated as part of the actual treatment, not as a separate procedure. The range of astigmatism correction with the Nidek EC-5000 is from 0.5–20.0 D, myopia from −0.5 to −20.0 D, and hyperopia from +0.5 to +10.0 D. With regard to hyperopic PRK, the Nidek EC-5000 laser uses an expanding iris with a scanning and eccentrically rotating beam (Fig. 14-6).

Using 40 Hz, or four scans per second, the time for completion of ablation for a −5.0-D myope would be 27.2 seconds. Using a standard 5.5-mm optic zone with a 7.0-mm transition zone, an average keratometry of 44.0 D, and a 12.5-mm vertex, this would involve 109 scans during 27.2 seconds. However, the laser's scan rate can be varied

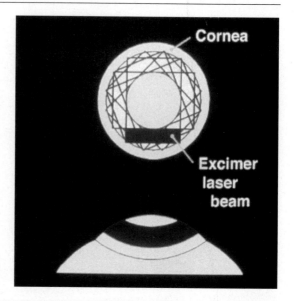

Fig. 14-6. Diagram of hyperopic photorefractive keratectomy with the Nidek EC-5000 system.

from 0.5–5.0 scans per second and still function with an oscillating-rotation combined pattern.

Advantages and Disadvantages

Preliminary Clinical Results

Nidek's clinical study of their EC-5000 excimer laser is being conducted at ten centers, located in the United States, Ireland, Italy, Brazil, and Canada. As of November 1995, almost 2500 procedures have been performed in these centers and results have been impressive. Most notable is the absence of corneal haze postoperatively and the virtual absence of central islands. According to Nidek engineers, this may be attributable to the laser's scanning beam technology, which is said to effectively reduce ablation beam–induced irregularities by sweeping the ablation area in six directions per cycle.

Of the 238 patients treated with the Nidek excimer laser for mild myopia (−1.5 to −6.0 D) and examined 1 year postoperatively, 97% have achieved 20/40 or better visual acuity, 89% have achieved 20/25 or better visual acuity, and 79% have achieved 20/20 or better visual acuity (Fig. 14-7). The loss of 2 or more lines of best corrected visual acuity is only 2% at 6 months and zero at 1 year (Fig. 14-8).

In the United States, the investigational study of the EC-5000 continues as protocols for hyperopic correction and the LASIK procedure are altered for commencement in 1997. These procedures are already being performed with Nidek's excimer laser in clinical study sites outside the United States.

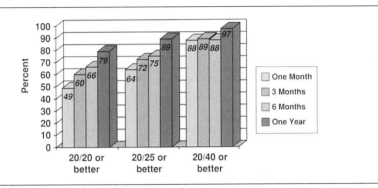

Fig. 14-7. Uncorrected visual acuity at 1 month, 3 months, 6 months, and 1 year following low myopic photorefractive keratectomy with the Nidek EC-5000 in 238 eyes.

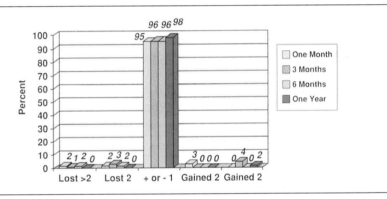

Fig. 14-8. Change in best corrected visual acuity at 1 month, 3 months, 6 months, and 1 year following low myopic PRK with the Nidek EC-5000 in 238 eyes.

Comparison to Other Systems

In comparison to other excimer laser systems, the Nidek EC-5000 laser has a smaller footprint, longer gas life, and larger potential range of surface ablation. The scanning slit beam technology may provide smoother ablations compared to the wide-field ablation of first-generation excimer lasers. The rapid pulse frequency allows for a short treatment time similar to wide-field ablation and faster than that of flying-spot ablation. Other superior features include the large working distance, large transition zone, Zeiss operating microscope, and surgeon-alignment feature.

Future Improvements

Although not yet fully implemented in their EC-5000 laser system, Nidek has two new system features that will be readily available in the near future: hyperopia correction and an eye-tracking system.

Hyperopia Correction

The EC-5000 hyperopia correction is accomplished by ablating a convex surface on the cornea. The method by which this is accomplished is as follows (see Fig. 14-6):

1. The shape of the laser beam is rectangular in cross section, which is perpendicular to the axis of the beam.
2. The rectangular beam is rotated at a fixed angle each time the laser is pulsed.
3. On completion of one revolution, the beam is offset from its axis, and the process is repeated.
4. The size of the optical zone is determined by a stationary aperture.
5. The smooth transition zone is achieved by increasing the diameter in a programmed manner from the size of the optical zone to the transition zone.

The specifications of hyperopia correction include a correction range of +0.5 to +10.0 D, optical zone sizes from 4.3–5.5 mm, and transition zone sizes from 7–9 mm.

A typical ablation time for a +0.5 D hyperopic correction with a 5.5 mm optical zone and 9.0 mm transition zone is 12 seconds. The laser repetition rate is 46 Hz, and the maximum ablation depth is 60 µm.

Eye-Tracking System

The EC-5000 eye-tracking system comprises two functions: (1) auto-alignment, which is active before ablation, and (2) eye-tracking, which operates during the ablation process.

Auto-Alignment

The auto-alignment function automatically aligns the axis of the laser-delivery system to the center of the patient's pupil. The range of the auto-alignment is ±30 mm from the central position of the laser delivery arm. This function is active prior to the start of ablation of the cornea.

Eye-Tracking

When the laser ablation is initiated, any eye movement within ±5 mm from the start position is tracked. If the eye movement is greater than ±5 mm, the laser irradiation is automatically interrupted. The ablation can be resumed after realignment of the laser and on depressing the footswitch.

Specifications

Detecting position	Center of pupil
Detecting area	14.1 × 10.6 mm
Auto-alignment range	±30 mm from central position of delivery arm
Eye-tracking range	±5 mm from start position of laser irradiation

15 Meditec MEL 60

Neal A. Sher and Eckhard Schroder

History

Although not well known in North America, the development of the Aesculap Meditec excimer laser system (Heroldsberg, Germany) began in 1985. In 1983, Stephen Trokel persuaded the Meditec company to develop an excimer laser for radial keratotomy (RK). Early work in Germany by Theo Seiler and Meditec was initiated, and a preliminary delivery system to perform slitlike keratectomies of variable depth and width was developed to perform radial and arcuate keratotomies and T cuts. In 1986 in Germany, Dardenne, Neuhann, Tenner, and Schroder began clinical studies on excimer laser RK in human eyes [1, 2]. It soon became apparent that this approach to incisional keratotomy was not predictable and that the procedure would be better performed with a blade. The research continued, and in 1986 Seiler performed the first phototherapeutic keratectomy (PTK) procedure on a Salzmann's nodular degeneration using an earlier model of the Meditec excimer laser [3]. In 1987, Dausch began to use the excimer laser to treat pterygia, corneal erosions, and herpes simplex keratitis [4]. In 1989, he performed the world's first laser keratoplasty, both penetrating and lamellar [5].

The concept of large-area ablation took hold in 1986–1987 and work on large-area ablation by scanning slit technique was continued. Over the next several years, the equipment was refined and the latest model of the Aesculap Meditec excimer laser—the MEL 60 laser—was introduced in 1990. A series of clinical studies have been completed (mostly in Europe) on the use of the MEL 60 excimer laser in myopia, hyperopia, astigmatism, presbyopia and PTK [6–9]. In 1996, there are over 150 Meditec excimer lasers in service in Europe, Asia, and South

America. In late 1994, this laser was introduced in Canada and Mexico. Clinical trials in the United States began in August 1995.

Unique Aspects of the Hardware

The Laser System

The system operates using a Meditec-produced laser cavity, which generates 193-nm laser output. It uses 230-V, single-phase, 25-amp electrical service. It has an internal closed-loop water cooling system with water-to-air heat exchanger. The system uses a 50-liter gas cylinder of premixed argon-fluorine and does not require nitrogen. It is relatively compact, with a space requirement of $270 \times 142 \times 150$ cm, and weighs 607 kg (including the surgical bed and the integrated surgical chair). The operating bed has x, y, z axis control, and the back rest can be lifted up to a chairlike position (Fig. 15-1). The integrated computer has a graphic display of parameters (Fig. 15-2).

The Delivery System

The MEL 60 excimer laser creates a large-area photoablation by using a scanning technique of an adjustable 9×1 mm^2 slit. The laser works at a fluence of 250 mJ/cm^2 and a repetition rate of 20 Hz. The laser

Fig. 15-1. The MEL 60 laser system.

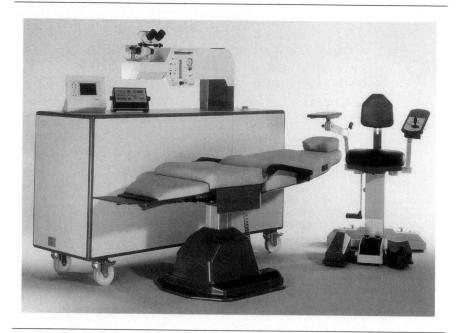

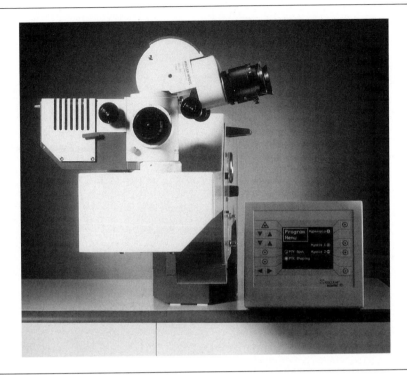

Fig. 15-2. The microscope and control panel graphic display of the MEL 60 laser system.

energy is coupled to the eye by a series of unique handpieces. Each handpiece (Fig. 15-3) is attached to the laser with conduits for the electronic control of the apertures as well as vacuum and plume aspiration lines. Some of the rings have been adapted to accommodate microkeratomes for ease of performance of laser in-situ keratomileusis (LASIK).

The handpiece serves two distinct purposes. First, with a suction ring on the bottom of the handpiece affixed to the sclera, active fixation of the eye is achieved, obviating the need for an active tracking system. There is a variable-control vacuum port on the laser that connects to the handpiece to adjust the level of suction on the eye. The surgeon is in full control of eye movement and eye position. The computer-controlled handpiece allows for debris plume evacuation during the surgical procedure, eliminating debris that could cause an irregular ablation pattern. The handpiece also allows the user to change surgical masks, which come in different patterns, for the appropriate correction desired. The mask for myopia without astigmatism is spherical. Figure 15-4 shows the mask for myopia with astigmatism.

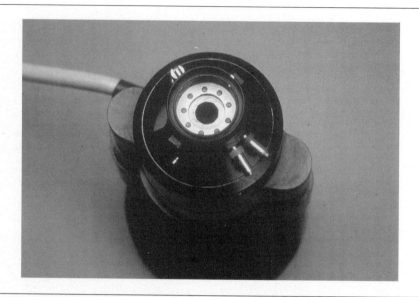

Fig. 15-3. Meditec MEL 60 handpiece (suction ring not attached).

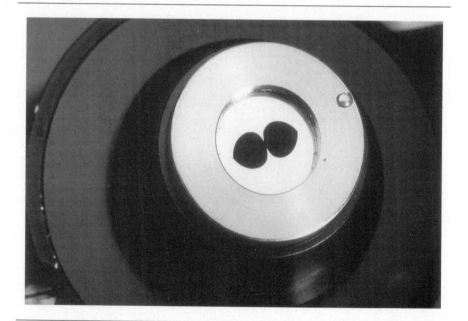

Fig. 15-4. The mask for myopia with astigmatism (see Fig. 4-13 for the mask for hyperopia and astigmatism).

The theoretic advantages to the scanning slit are a smoother ablation and less energy per pulse delivered to the surface of the cornea or within the stroma in LASIK techniques. The average energy is approximately 15 mJ/pulse, compared to as much as 50 mJ/pulse with other systems using a 6-mm treatment zone. Each sweep of the slit beam usually takes 2 seconds and ablates 1 μm of tissue. The scanning process is adjusted to achieve considerable overlap of adjacent laser shots to ensure a smooth surface.

There are seven optical elements in the optical beam path, and no purging is required. The operating microscope is a Moller-Wedel with magnification steps of 3.5, 6, 11, 20, and 32× and a cobalt blue filter. Illumination is adjustable in three steps. The working distance is more than 100 mm, which is adequate for LASIK procedures.

Maintenance Considerations

The gas cylinder is adequate for 120 cavity fills. Each fill is adequate for 6–8 patients. The optics have an expected lifetime of approximately 2 years. Preventive maintenance is suggested four times a year. The cost of a maintenance contract is approximately $40,000 per year.

Safety Features

All gas-containing parts are made from stainless steel and are built into a leak-tight gas containment area with an attached charcoal scrubber.

Calibration of the laser is achieved by test ablations on a special test foil. A special aluminum test paper with a red base is used. The laser handpiece is placed on the foil and the laser placed in calibration mode. The aluminum covering should be ablated by the ninth pass of the slit beam, revealing the red base. The ablated circle should be 1.0–1.2 mm in diameter. If necessary, the energy fluence can be adjusted. This test gives information on beam homogeneity as well as fluence.

Software-User Interface

The laser is not controlled by a personal computer (PC) with a high-level language but, rather, by a microcomputer (Z80 180) with a customized plasma display for user-friendly data input (see Fig. 15-2 for display). The laser has a wide range of programming capabilities, including myopia, myopia with astigmatism, hyperopia, hyperopia with astigmatism, and presbyopia, as well as a spot mode for therapeutic applications.

Ablation Parameters and Capabilities

The laser delivers 250 mJ/cm^2 at 20 Hz through a slit with a maximum opening of 9 × 1.5 mm. The linear slit scans at a rate of 2 seconds per scan across the surface to be treated. On average, it takes 90 seconds to complete a −5 D ablation. The treatment diameter can be chosen from 4 to 7 mm. For correction of higher myopia (> 6 D), a treatment diameter of 5 mm plus an additional 2 mm for a transition zone is used.

Depending on the type of astigmatism, the apertures are 5 to 9 mm in diameter. After each angular increment, the laser traverses the aperture. If the mask rotates regularly through 360 degrees, a symmetric tissue ablation will occur with maximum flattening in the corneal center. If the angular increments are not uniform and the angular distances are changed, the depth of the ablation can be increased along any axis. This leads to a correction of myopia with simultaneous correction of an astigmatism. The rotating masks are useful for correcting cylinders when a small spherical component has to be corrected, but if only the cylinder has to be flattened or steepened, a more oblong aperture is needed. The mask is rotated only through a small range (20 degrees).

By altering the shape of the masks as well as the angular rotation speed, corrections for myopia, myopic astigmatism, hyperopia, and hyperopic astigmatism can be achieved. When the mask is rotated with equidistant angular steps over 360 degrees, the profile of the ablated tissue is symmetric with the flattest part in the center, thus correcting myopia. These angular steps do not have to be equidistant. By varying the angular distances, the ablation depth can be increased in any desired axis during the rotation, resulting in a profile with a myopic and an astigmatic component.

The decreased energy per pulse delivered to the cornea reduces shock-wave rehydration of the central cornea. The fluid waves produced by the large-diameter excimer laser beam result in fluid pushed centrally as well as peripherally. This excessive central hydration, thought to be the result of larger-diameter excimer beams striking the cornea, ablates at a slightly lower rate than more dehydrated corneal tissue. This leaves the central cornea slightly under-ablated and is the best explanation of central islands. A scanning approach moves fluid across the cornea is a manner similar to a windshield wiper rather than a ripple effect. This may result in more even hydration. Central islands are not typically seen with the Meditec laser system. In a recent series of 75 cases, there were no steep central islands seen at 3 months.

Preliminary Clinical Results

Myopia

Studies for both low and high myopia have been completed. Recently, Ditzen, Anschutz, and Schroder presented a multicenter study on 325 eyes with varying degrees of myopia ranging from −1.0 to over −15.0 D myopia [6]. These eyes were placed in group I (n = 93), with myopia of up to 6 D; group II (n = 97), from −6.25 to −10.0 D; group III (n = 87), −10.25 to −15.0 D, and group IV (n = 48), more than 15.25 D. Table 15-1 summarizes the preoperative and postoperative refractions of the 325 eyes in the study. There was considerable regression in the higher-myopia group. In the lower two groups, there was almost no loss of best corrected visual acuity.

Laser In-Situ Keratomileusis

Ioannis Pallikaris at the University of Crete has been credited with first suggesting this modification of PRK in 1990. He applied the Meditec laser to the stromal bed after using a lamellar microkeratome to make a flap or cap in the anterior cornea. More recently, a hinge flap technique has been used. In 1994, using the MEL 60 excimer laser, Pallikaris reported a series of highly myopic patients treated with LASIK with a better outcome than with PRK alone [10]. Eighty-eight percent of the patients had correction within 2 D of attempted. The Moller-Wedel microscope and adequate working distance gives added flexibility for the surgeon to perform LASIK under the integrated

Table 15-1. Pre- and postoperative refraction of 325 eyes after PRK for myopia

Group	Mean pre-operative (D)	Mean postoperative (SD)					
		2 weeks	1 month	3 months	6 months	9 months	12 months
1	−4.1	+0.6 (1.4)	+0.4 (1.2)	0 (1.1)	−0.5 (1.0)	−1.0 (1.2)	−0.8 (0.8)
2	−8.3	+0.6 (2.1)	+0.5 (2.3)	−0.3 (1.8)	−0.7 (2.0)	−0.8 (2.2)	−1.7 (2.3)
3	−12.5	+0.5 (2.6)	0 (2.8)	−1.4 (2.6)	−1.9 (2.9)	−1.9 (2.8)	−2.0 (2.8)
4	−19.9	−4.5 (3.7)	−4.2 (3.7)	−5.2 (4.0)	−6.5 (3.6)	−8.1 (4.7)	−9.9 (6.5)

SD = standard deviation.
Source: K Ditzen, T Anschutz, E Schroder. Photorefractive keratectomy to treat low, medium, and high myopia—A multicenter study. *J Cataract Refract Surg* 20(Suppl.):234–238, 1994.

operating microscope rather than having to switch to a separate microscope for the lamellar keratectomy portion of the procedure. There was a higher rate of complications in this series, mostly related to problems from the microkeratome.

Astigmatic Corrections

Dausch and colleagues have reported on their extensive experience in correcting myopic astigmatism, simple and compound, and simple and hyperopic astigmatism [8]. In a series of 36 eyes with myopic astigmatism treated by Dausch, the mean preoperative cylindrical refraction was −2.10 D ± 0.93 (range −1.00 to −5.00 D). The mean cylinder at the last visit was −0.08 D ± 0.23 (range 0 to −2.25 D), which was significantly different from the preoperative cylinder. The mean preoperative spherical refractive error was −6.10 D, which was reduced to −0.12 D at 12 months.

Hyperopia

The surgical treatment of hyperopia represents a significant challenge to the refractive surgeon. Anschutz, in his comprehensive 1994 review of this subject, summarizes the early attempts at correction of hyperopia with the excimer laser [11]. The concept of peripheral steepening of the cornea has been credited to L'Esperance in 1989. The early prototype of the Taunton Technologies excimer laser (Monroe, CT; now VISX, Santa Clara, CA) had a set of apertures designed to steepen the peripheral cornea. Sher demonstrated some usefulness of peripheral steepening in excimer phototherapeutic keratectomy using the Taunton laser in attempts to reduce the hyperopic shift [12]. Using the Meditec laser, Dausch reported that in attempted corrections of +2.0 to +7.5 D, 80% of eyes achieved corrections within 1 D of attempted [7]. Attempts at higher corrections were not successful. Anschutz reported comparable results using similar techniques at the 1993 European Society for Cataract and Refractive Surgery meeting in Paris.

More recently, Meditec has adapted larger ablation and optical zones, which has led to more predictable and stable results. Dausch et al. began using a new rotating hyperopic template in 1993 with the MEL 60 laser for treatment of hyperopic astigmatism. This template had a 9-mm ablation zone and a 6-mm optical zone. Corrections up to +7.5 D were routinely achieved. Fig. 15-5 shows the results of 34 hyperopic eyes treated with this new mask. Compound hyperopic astigmatism has also been treated with good success.

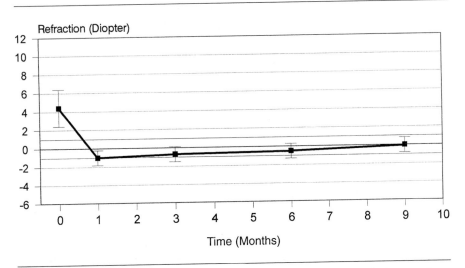

Fig. 15-5. Refraction versus time after photorefractive keratectomy in hyperopia in 34 eyes, range +2.0–7.5 D. (From D Dausch et al. Photo-refractive keratectomy for correction of astigmatism combined with myopia and hyperopia. *J Cataract Refract Surg* 20:252–257, 1993.)

Presbyopia

Anschutz first proposed the feasibility of intentionally producing a multifocal cornea in 1990. Techniques were developed to combine myopic and hyperopic PRK with a sectoral aspheric inferior ablation called a semilunar keratectomy. Starting in 1992, good stability was seen at least until 18 months after surgery in a preliminary series of patients with a baseline refraction of +1.0 to +4.0 D. Anschutz points out the need for an improved transition zone and aspheric profile [11]. In a new computer program developed by Meditec, it is possible to sculpt a defined partial aspherical steepening of the cornea by combining rotation speed of the mask with small-angle steps in the 60-degree sectoral zone combined with larger-angle steps in the transition zone. More recent clinical results show that this technique is more effective in hyperopia and presbyopia than it is in presbyopia alone. This technique is still considered experimental, and considerable additional work is needed before it is widely used.

Phototherapeutic Keratectomy

In his 1991 textbook, Dausch describes a number of conditions that can be treated with PTK using this laser [13]. Dausch was the first to suggest and demonstrate the effectiveness of excimer PTK in treating recurrent corneal erosion syndrome. Sixty of 63 cases of this disease improved after excimer treatment [5, 9, 13]. He also suggested the use of excimer PTK for the treatment of persistent corneal epithelial defects after burns and in grafts. The laser has been used to treat a variety of corneal conditions involving the anterior third of the cornea.

References

1. Tenner A, et al. Excimer laser radial keratotomy in the living human eye: A preliminary report. *J Refract Surg* 4:5–7, 1988.
2. Schroder E, et al. An ophthalmic excimer laser for corneal surgery. *Am J Ophthalmol* 103(3):472–473, 1987.
3. Seiler T, et al. Excimer laser keratectomy for correction of astigmatism. *Am J Ophthalmol* 105:117–124, 1988.
4. Dausch D, Schroder E. Erste Keratoplastiken am menschl. Auge mit einem Excimer-Laser. *Der Augenspiegel* 6:12–18, 1989.
5. Dausch D, Schroder E. Die Behandlung von Hornhaut-und Skleraerkrankungen mit dem Excimer Laser. *Fortschritte der Ophthalmologie* 87:115–120, 1990.
6. Ditzen K, Anschutz T, Schroder E. Photorefractive keratectomy to treat low, medium, and high myopia—A multicenter study. *J Cataract Refract Surg* 20(Suppl.):234–238, 1994.
7. Dausch D, Klein R, Schroder E. Excimer laser photorefractive keratectomy for hyperopia. *Refract Corneal Surg* 9:20–28, 1993.
8. Dausch D, et al. Photorefractive keratectomy for correction of astigmatism combined with myopia and hyperopia. *J Cataract Refract Surg* 20:252–257, 1993.
9. Dausch D, et al. Phototherapeutic keratectomy in recurrent corneal epithelial erosion. *Refract Corneal Surg* 9:419–424, 1993.
10. Pallikaris IG, Siganos DS. Excimer laser in situ keratomileusis and photorefractive keratectomy for correction of high myopia. *J Cataract Refract Surg* 10:498–510, 1994.
11. Anschutz T. Laser correction of hyperopia and presbyopia. *Int Ophthalmol Clin* 34(4):107–136, 1994.
12. Sher NA, Bowers RA, Zabel RW. Clinical use of the 193 nm excimer laser in the treatment of corneal scars. *Arch Ophthalmol* 109:491–498, 1991.
13. Dausch D, Klein RJ, Schroder E. *Ophthalmic Excimer Laser Surgery*. Strasbourg, France: Editions du Signe, 1991.

Flying (Scanning) Spot Ablation

This ablation approach differs from the wide field and scanning slit methods. The small amount of energy required, the limited area of energy deposition, and the multiple directions in which the beam must be scanned have yielded the term *flying spot*. While scanning slit approach requires scanning in a single direction across the cornea, the flying spot approach requires scanning in multiple directions before a uniform layer of tissue is removed. The Laser-Sight Compak-200 Mini-Excimer Laser (Chap. 16), Autonomous T-PRK (Chap. 17), Novatec LightBlade (Chap. 18) are discussed. In addition to the sophisticated scanning features unique to each system, there are numerous differences among these lasers.

A principal advantage of flying spot ablation is that only a small output energy is required, allowing for a smaller laser cavity size and a reduced need for optics maintenance. With the sophisticated scanning system, the spot placement in select cases can be custom-designed beyond that of a typical ablation pattern. Also, a hyperopic correction is easier to achieve with the flying spot approach because of the ease in creating a peripheral annular pattern. Moreover, the solid-state features of the Novatec system obviate the need for toxic gases that are required in all excimer lasers; this is because the Novatec laser is not an excimer laser even though it delivers ultraviolet laser light.

A disadvantage of flying spot ablation is that it requires the longest operating time. As a result, active eye tracking is important and necessary in most systems. Unlike the wide field and scanning slit approaches, both sophisticated scanning and sophisticated eye tracking are required in flying spot ablation. Although toxic gases are not used with the Novatec system, the maintenance requirements of the solid-state laser optics have yet to be determined. Because flying spot lasers are among the newest excimer laser systems introduced, the clinical data are somewhat limited and, therefore, flying spot lasers may be considered more investigational than wide field or scanning slit lasers.

16 LaserSight Compak-200 Mini-Excimer Laser

Penny Asbell, Craig F. Beyer, and Martin P. Nevitt

History

The LaserSight Compak-200 Mini-Excimer laser uses the same wavelength of ultraviolet (UV) light (193 nm) to photoablate corneal tissue for photorefractive keratectomy (PRK) as do other excimer lasers. The original concept for this laser was developed by J.T. Lin. In 1990, Dr. Lin and others evaluated the idea of using a frequency-quintupled neodymium:yttrium-aluminum-garnet (Nd:YAG) solid-state laser that operated at 213 nm to perform PRK [1]. A flashlamp-pumped Q-switched Nd:YAG (1064-nm) laser operating at 10 Hz, 10 ns per pulse with an output energy of 50 mJ per pulse was used. The fundamental beam was focused into a nonlinear optical crystal to obtain the second harmonic frequency of 532 nm. The fourth harmonic was obtained by frequency doubling the green (532-nm) radiation in a beryllium boroxylate (BBO) crystal. Frequency mixing the fundamental (1064-nm) wavelength and the fourth harmonic (266 nm) in another BBO crystal resulted in the fifth UV harmonic (213 nm).

Before 1991, there were several problems that slowed the further development of the LaserSight solid-state 213-nm laser. After frequency quintupling, an output level of only 0.4 mJ per pulse was obtained. To perform wide-area ablation PRK like the VISX (Santa Clara, CA) or Summit (Waltham, MA) lasers, much more energy would be required (at least 32 mJ per pulse). In 1991, LaserSight was able to obtain up to 5 mJ per pulse from the solid-state 213-nm LaserHarmonic laser, but the energy remained too low for wide-area ablation. To solve this problem, a paradigm shift was necessary regarding the delivery of laser energy to the cornea. By developing a computer-controlled galvanometric scanning delivery system that was capable of precisely and rapidly scanning a 0.5- to 1.0-mm-diameter ultraviolet (UV) laser beam on the corneal surface, the LaserHarmonic achieved the same corneal fluence as its predecessors (160–180 mJ/cm^2), and the laser achieved the same wide-area effect.

Ren and colleagues used the prototype solid-state LaserHarmonic LaserSight laser (213 nm) with the computer-controlled scanning delivery system to perform in vitro [2] and in vivo animal studies [3]. The authors concluded that the laser was capable of reshaping the corneal surface with a smooth transition on human cadaver eyes [2]. In rabbits [3], the LaserHarmonic resulted in a clinical course and histopathologic findings similar to the 193-nm excimer laser ablations. For a 3.00-D ablation over a 5-mm ablation zone, 1618 pulses at a repetition rate of 10 Hz required 162 seconds.

The advantages of a scanning spot delivery system became readily apparent.

1. As mentioned above, significantly less energy (nearly 10 times less) is required from the laser head to attain ablative threshold at the corneal surface. The resulting acoustic shock wave is also more localized, minimizing the acoustic sound heard during ablation and the focusing of acoustic waves in the eye.
2. Virtually any pattern can be scanned onto the corneal surface by merely making a change in the software; no hardware changes are necessary. Current software designs strive for spatially resolved, aspheric, customized ablations that optimize the quality of vision and decrease the chance of regression.
3. The scanning approach produces an extremely smooth corneal surface compared to wide-area beams that tend to accentuate surface irregularities after each pulse. With a scanning delivery system, each scan layer can be oriented in such a way that the peaks and valleys of the previous layer are smoothed out by the succeeding scan layer.
4. With a scanning spot, laser beam homogeneity and corneal fluid dynamics are less important in determining the final surface ablation quality. For instance, wide-field ablation beams must be extremely homogeneous to prevent the production of iatrogenic surface irregularities. In addition, wide-field beams force corneal fluid centrally, which decreases the ratio of the central ablation rate to the peripheral ablation rate, leading to central island formation.
5. Once corneal imaging techniques become sophisticated enough to provide "real-time" corneal topography and surface elevation, this information can be fed directly into the computer-controlled delivery system so that even the most highly irregular corneal surface can be made spherical with a customized ablation pattern.

Other problems continued to delay the commercialization of the LaserHarmonic system. The solid-state laser technology remained prohibitively expensive, and the frequency ranging from 10–50 Hz was too slow: procedures would last minutes instead of seconds. Therefore, using the same scanning delivery system as the LaserHarmonic laser, the 193-nm Compak-200 Mini-Excimer laser was developed in 1992. The Mini-Excimer laser was significantly cheaper and operated at ten times the frequency of the LaserHarmonic (100 Hz). Due to its decreased energy requirements, the Mini-Excimer possessed the same advantages as the solid-state laser (decreased maintenance and decreased operating expenses). The Mini-Excimer operated at the same wavelength (193 nm) as previous lasers and therefore, mutagenicity concerns were not as much of an issue as they were with the longer wavelength (213 nm) of a solid-state laser.

The Mini-Excimer was first used in the United States under the auspices of Penny A. Asbell at Mount Sinai Medical Center in New York. Her phase I study of blind eyes in 1994 showed that the Mini-Excimer could ablate the cornea and create a smooth, clear refractive surface [4].

More than 50 Mini-Excimer laser systems have been installed worldwide, and more than 5000 procedures have been performed. In the past 4 years, solid-state laser technology has advanced while the price continues to decline. LaserSight anticipates the commercial availability of its new version of the LaserHarmonic solid-state laser approximately 1 to 2 years from the time of this writing. The new LaserHarmonic operates at 200 Hz, twice as fast as the Mini-Excimer, and should sell for nearly the same price.

Unique Aspects of the Hardware

The Laser System

One of the most unique features of the Mini-Excimer laser is the small size of the laser cavity. Because the laser cavity uses only 1.7 liters of gas at 8 bars of pressure, the gas lifetime is significantly improved. One tank of argon-fluoride premix (0.19% fluoride, 4.2% argon, 95.61% neon) lasts for approximately 600 procedures or between 6 months and 1 year at a cost of $1000–2000. Like other excimer lasers, a gas refill procedure is performed on the Mini-Excimer each day prior to its use. The refill is performed manually by control knobs on the laser panel, although, an autofill option will soon be available.

The laser is compact and weighs only 136 kg (300 lb) (Fig. 16-1). It is 113 cm (3.7 ft) high, 67 cm (2.2 ft) long, and 46 cm (1.5 ft) wide

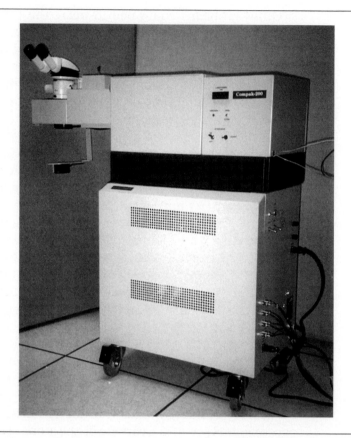

Fig. 16-1. Photograph of the LaserSight Compak-200 Mini-Excimer laser.

and so can roll through a standard door. The electrical requirements are 110 or 220 V AC with a frequency of 60 or 50 Hz and a current of 10 or 5 amperes. Thus, a standard electrical outlet is all that is required. There are no special cooling or ventilation requirements, but regular air conditioning is recommended to decrease room humidity in locations with humid climates. A standard external 486 IBM-compatible personal computer (PC) controls the scanning delivery system as well as the routine startup and calibration procedures.

The patient is positioned under the laser in a swing-out reclining electrical chair. The chair foot switch provides the vertical movements for focus, and the joystick, mounted on the laser and controlling the laser table, provides for x-y directional positioning movements.

The Delivery System

Because of the increased number of components in their delivery systems, typical wide-area–ablation UV lasers must rely on high-energy excimer lasers to achieve ablation threshold (120–180 mJ/cm^2) at the corneal surface. Utilizing a large-diameter beam (≥ 5 mm), more than 350 mJ of energy may be required from the laser head to achieve 30–35 mJ at the corneal surface. This represents an energy efficiency of approximately 10%; the remaining 90% of the energy is absorbed by the laser's optics and other mechanical components of the delivery system, which can decrease the overall lifetime of these systems.

As previously mentioned, decreased energy requirements, increased treatment flexibility, and increased surface smoothness are the prime advantages of the unique LaserSight scanning delivery system. The Mini-Excimer laser head produces a 193-nm beam with a maximum laser output energy of 5 mJ per pulse. The pulse duration is 2.5 ns, and the maximum frequency is 100 Hz. The delivery system utilizes an approximately 1-mm-diameter raw beam emitted from the laser head without incorporating numerous optics or other mechanical beam-shaping or beam-homogenizing devices, such as iris apertures, slits, rotating dove prisms, optical integrators, or telescopic zooms. Instead, the Mini-Excimer delivery system relies on four basic components to create a broad, smooth, ablative surface: (1) an energy attenuator, (2) a condensing lens, (3) a pair of computer-controlled galvanometric (x and y) scanning mirrors, and (4) a 45-degree mirror.

The Mini-Excimer delivery system has an energy efficiency of 50%. For example, when 2 mJ of laser energy passes through the delivery system, 1 mJ emerges. Because the beam diameter is less than 1 mm, 1 mJ of energy at the corneal surface exceeds the corneal ablation threshold and is equivalent to the energy density (160–180 mJ/cm^2) produced by other excimer lasers utilizing a 5-mm, 30- to 35-mJ wide-field beam.

The first component of the Mini-Excimer delivery system is the attenuator. Immediately after a gas refill, the laser head operates near its maximum output of 5 mJ. Therefore, the attenuator decreases the beam energy from 5 to 2 mJ to maintain 1 mJ of energy at the corneal surface. As the laser output diminishes after several procedures, less attenuation is required. One important point to remember is that the optics of the Mini-Excimer delivery system, which follow the attenuator, are never exposed to more than 2 mJ of energy, which extends their lifetime.

The condensing lens is the second component of the Mini-Excimer delivery system. It improves the gaussian beam profile and focuses the beam to a 0.85-mm diameter. The third component in the delivery pathway are the x and y mirrors driven by the computer-controlled galvanometric scanning motors. These mirrors overlap the gaussian laser beam profile on the corneal surface by 30–50% in both x and y directions. A larger overlap increases the smoothness of the ablated surface but also increases the duration of the procedure. The computer software not only determines the degree of beam overlap, but also can be programmed to ascribe nearly any pattern or sequence of ablative patterns on the corneal surface. The fourth component, the 45-degree mirror, changes the horizontal direction of the laser beam into a downward vertical direction perpendicular to the patient's cornea.

Currently, the unit is fitted with a Topcon operating microscope (Paramus, NJ) with a manual magnification changer. Two diode lasers converge on the patient's inferior limbus once the ideal patient chair height is obtained. The surgeon ensures that the eye is parallel to the floor while the patient fixates on a single coaxial light-emitting diode (LED). For PRK, centration is maintained by an active, integrated, ocular tracking system. The eye is illuminated by low-level infrared (IR) light and then scanned by an IR-sensitive videocamera. Under these conditions, the pupil appears as a dark hole, or sink, to the illumination. The dark pupil image is input to a real-time eye-tracking system consisting of a digital image processor that outputs pupil size and position. The eye-tracking system is currently being developed, and a prototype has been released for investigational use only. The information is fed into the computer, controlling the preprogrammed scanning x and y mirrors. By adding plus or minus gain to the laser scanning mirrors, the tracking system coordinates preprogrammed laser ablation patterns with real-time ocular movements. Because many surgeons are performing laser in-situ keratomileusis (LASIK), they may prefer not to purchase the tracking option. Instead, these surgeons rely on centration and fixation with a vacuum suction ring that is used with the microkeratome. For LASIK, the laser microscope is fitted with a different objective lens, which adds an extra 5 cm (15 cm total) of working distance to the focal point.

Maintenance Considerations

Due to the low energy requirements as well as the low level of complexity of the Mini-Excimer laser, maintenance costs and requirements are low. Optics last for 600–800 cases and are relatively inexpensive to replace (approximately $1000). If the laser head gas cavity is refilled each day before use, as recommended by the manufacturer, the gas cylinders typically last from 6 months to 1 year, and gas replacement costs range from $1000 to $2000 per year. For the first year, there is no charge for the service contract, which includes all parts and optics, laser head adjustments, gas, and labor. After the first year, the service contract costs from $25,000 to $45,000 per year depending on the type of contract purchased.

Daily operation consists of the following: Once the laser has been refilled, and routine software calibration tests have been performed, energy output is checked with a joulemeter at the end of the delivery system. Typically, at the beginning of the day, the energy level is greater than 1 mJ, and therefore, the attenuator must be increased. The *ideal energy range* for treatment is 0.8–1.1 mJ. Periodically throughout the day, the energy must be rechecked and the attenuator decreased so that the energy level remains within this range.

Before treating a patient, the desired dioptric power, the output energy, and an energy coefficient (0.4–0.8) is entered into the computer so that a test block of polymethylmethacrylate (PMMA) can be ablated. The resulting test block power is determined from the lensometer. If, for example, a −10.00 D correction was desired, a −3.00 D correction should be observed on the PMMA because the conversion factor between cornea and plastic is 30%. If an over-correction is observed on plastic, the energy coefficient must be decreased according to this formula:

$$\text{new energy coefficient} = \frac{D\ (\text{desired})}{D\ (\text{actual})} \times \text{previous energy coefficient}$$

The new energy coefficient must be verified by repeating the PMMA calibration procedure prior to treating the patient.

Safety Features

The Mini-Excimer laser system complies with the United States federal regulation 21CFR1040.10 and 21CFR1040.11 for the safety of class IV medical lasers. Government standards for the manufacture of lasers require warning labels and protective interlocks for all class IV laser products. The protective housings and safety interlocks guard against inadvertent radiation exposure and electrical contact. Most of the danger regarding excimer laser systems is related to the gas fluorine (F_2). However, the fluorine concentration used for the Mini-Excimer laser system is less than 0.2%; fluorine concentrations less than 3.7% are considered nontoxic. The other components of the excimer laser gas mixture are inert and would only be hazardous if inhaled without the presence of oxygen. Therefore, outside ventilation is recommended, but a charcoal scrubber is not necessary.

Software-User Interface

The computer workstation includes the computer, a monitor, and a keyboard (Fig. 16-2). Besides the computer terminal, the Mini-Excimer has three control areas: (1) the system (front) control panel

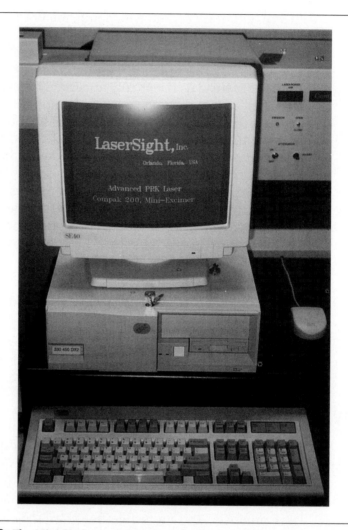

Fig. 16-2. The Mini-Excimer computer workstation, including the computer, monitor, and keyboard.

(on which there is an emission indicator light, attenuation switch, speed [fast/slow] switch, and shutter open/close switch), located on the front top right of the system, (2) the excimer laser head control panel (on which there are gas valve control knobs), located behind the access panel, and (3) the power control panel (on which there is the main power switch, the laser key switch, the x-y translation stage switch, and the pump switch), located on the right side of the system.

The computer hardware includes a 486/33, 4-MB RAM, 60-MB hard disk, with one 3.5-inch floppy disk driver, a 12-bit PC input/output board, a VGA monitor, and a keyboard. The software is designed to operate on the DOS platform. All software is preinstalled, configured, and tested at the factory. Installation by the user is not required unless updated Compak-200 software is issued by LaserSight.

The files that execute and support the Mini-Excimer system are located in the directory C:\laser. The following files reside in this directory:

FILE NAME	PURPOSE
ls.exe	The primary executable file
ls.cfg	Contains configuration data related to hardware settings
lscfg.bak	Backup file for ls.cfg
log.txt	Temporary file containing patient and surgery data; data for each surgery is appended to the end of this file

Ablation Parameters and Capabilities

The energy density (fluence) on the corneal surface is adjusted between 160 and 180 mJ/cm^2. The ablation pulse rate is 100 Hz, and the maximum spot size is 1 mm. For PRK, the laser automatically performs a surface ablation using the optical zones shown in Table 16-1. Only 30–40 seconds are required to achieve a −5- to −6-D myopic correction. Software is also available to treat compound myopic astigmatism. With this program, like other excimer lasers, the Mini-Excimer ablates along the flattest astigmatic meridian. Therefore, so as not to induce hyperopia, the patient must have a minus spherical equivalent preoperatively. LaserSight is currently developing software that would allow treatment of compound hyperopic astigmatism. For hyperopia, software has been designed that scans the cornea from a 5-mm diameter out to a 9-mm diameter, thereby steepening the cornea.

In the field of excimer laser PRK surgery, the ideal ablation profile, providing the best optics and the least chance of regression for any conceivable correction, remains unknown. A beta version of the LaserSight software allows investigators to create virtually any

Table 16-1. Optical zones for PRK surface ablation.

Desired correction (D)	Number of zones	Zone diameters (mm)
−1.00 to −2.00	1	7.0
−2.25 to −4.75	2	7.0, 5.6
−5.00 to −6.25	2	6.5, 5.2
−6.50 to −10.00	3	4.7, 5.8, 7.0

ablation profile on the corneal surface so that improved ablation profiles may be elucidated.

Advantages and Disadvantages

Preliminary Results

As of February 1, 1995, more than 6000 PRK procedures were performed in 18 PRK centers in China using the Mini-Excimer laser. One report from China [5], of myopic eyes (−2.50 to −7.50 D), revealed that the uncorrected visual acuity improved to 20/20 or better in 73% (105/143), 20/25 or better in 87% (125/143), and 20/40 or better in 97.9% (140/143). In the United States, the phase I U.S. Food and Drug Administration (FDA) clinical trials have been completed and LaserSight has begun phase IIa trials.

Prior to performing the phase I clinical trials in the United States, electron microscopy was performed on experimental eyes and showed both smoother ablation surfaces and smoother transition zones for the Mini-Excimer compared to the VISX laser. The 10 non-sighted eyes in the phase I trial also showed smooth ablation surfaces, as evaluated by corneal topography and slit-lamp examination. The average haze was 0.56 at 1 month, 0.33 at 3 months, and 0.28 at 6 months (measured on a scale of 0–5). Endothelial cell count was also stable by specular microscopy at the 2- and 6-month postoperative examinations, demonstrating the laser's safety [6].

As of January 1996, 50 eyes have been treated under a phase IIa protocol with the eligibility criteria based on a spherical equivalence of −1.50 to −10.00 D. Six-month data has been compiled on 26 eyes and at least 3-month data on the remainder, with over 80% having an uncorrected visual acuity of 20/40 or better. Based on the phase IIa data, the FDA has permitted expansion into phase IIb myopia clinical studies.

Comparison to Other Systems

Excimer laser systems for PRK have distinct differences, which can result in different clinical outcomes. These differences in excimer laser hardware and software result in various laser beam configurations that create characteristic ablation profiles on the corneal surface. The ablation profiles of three excimer laser systems were compared using the Tomey corneal topography system (New York, NY) [7]. Two of the lasers, the VISX 20/20 and the Technolas Keracor 116, were wide-field beam lasers, and the third was the LaserSight Compak-200 Mini-Excimer laser, which has a 1-mm scanning beam. Each laser treated 50 eyes, ranging from −1.00 to −8.00 D of myopia, with 100% follow-up at 1 month. Multizone algorithms were used for all lasers and central island pretreatment algorithms were used for the wide-field lasers. No central pretreatment was done with the LaserSight laser.

One month postoperatively, the ablation profiles could be classified into four major patterns by subtraction topography: (1) uniform, (2) semicircular, (3) keyhole, and (4) central island formation. The *uniform* pattern demonstrated concentric uniform flattening of the ablation zone, with the center flatter than the periphery. The *semicircular* pattern was a crescentlike nonuniform pattern of ablation with a power difference of 1.50 D or more between equidistant points along a meridian relative to the center of the ablation zone and extending for 90 degrees or more. The *keyhole* pattern was nonuniform, with a power difference of 1.50 D or more between equidistant points along a meridian relative to the center of the ablation zone and extending less than 90 degrees. The *central island* pattern was defined as a nonuniform pattern of ablation with a 1.50-D or greater increase in the central corneal power occupying at least a 2.50-mm diameter of the central cornea.

As shown in Table 16-2, the LaserSight laser produced the most consistently uniform ablation patterns on the corneal surface. Central islands, even with no pretreatments, were least frequent with the LaserSight laser (5%) compared to the VISX (15%) and the Technolas (20%), which had central island pretreatment ablations. In addition, the LaserSight central islands that did occur appeared transient and most likely were related to early epithelial closure and thickening at the wound margins. The LaserSight and VISX central islands were smaller and round, whereas the Technolas produced larger, vertically oval central islands. Although the LaserSight laser produced the most uniform patterns, the ablation profile was more aspheric (deeper and flatter toward the center) when compared to the VISX and Technolas. The advantage of an aspheric profile is that it reduces the overall depth of the ablation; however, if the ablation is too aspheric, loss in contrast sensitivity and halos around lights at night become more apparent for the patient.

Table 16-2. Tomey corneal topographic ablation profiles 1 month following excimer PRK with 3 laser systems.

Pattern	LaserSight	VISX	Technolas
Uniform	60%	38%	30%
Semicircular	15%	33%	40%
Keyhole	20%	14%	10%
Central island	5%	15%	20%

The authors conclude that the ablation characteristics of wide field lasers are primarily dependent on laser hardware, beam uniformity, and the fluid dynamics of hydrated corneal stroma. These factors are difficult to adjust and control. Because the LaserSight laser uses a significantly smaller (1-mm) scanning (flying) spot, beam uniformity and corneal fluid dynamics play a much smaller role in predicting the final ablation outcome. By reducing these uncontrollable variables, the LaserSight ablation patterns become more dependent on the computer software program, which is easily adjusted and controlled. The ideal ablation pattern, which provides the smoothest peripheral transitions, the best central optics, and the least chance of regression, remains to be determined. LaserSight investigations and software modifications are now under way to optimize visual results and long-term stability of PRK.

Future Improvements

All excimer lasers have some inherent limitations, such as energy variability over time and degradation of optics that make pretreatment PRK calibration mandatory. The preoperative ablation of PMMA is the calibration technique recommended by most manufacturers to check the intended dioptric power on the lensometer. However, the lensometer does not assess homogeneity of the ablation and higher dioptric corrections become increasingly difficult to read. Multizone treatment regimens cannot be "dissected," and they may further complicate the determination of the end point. The Ex-Calibur PRK laser system, using corneal topography and PMMA corneas, is another method of preoperative calibration now under investigation at Laser-Sight.

The Ex-Calibur system utilizes proprietary artificial corneas that provide high-quality images for placido-disc videokeratoscopes and for a rastophotogrammetric topography machine (PAR Technologies, New Hartford, NY). Difference topography maps are then used to calculate the net effects of the ablation. With the rastophotogrammetric unit, elevation maps can be analyzed with a sensitivity of 5 microns. With this degree of sensitivity, the PAR system could provide an accuracy of one-third D for a 6.0-mm ablation zone, including the critical, central 1- to 2-mm of the ablation.

LaserSight is making a genuine effort to become the first excimer laser manufacturer with a real-time topography system that is directly integrated into the laser's computer-controlled galvanometric delivery system. LaserSight plans to incorporate the rastophotogrammetric topography machine developed by PAR to provide real-time corneal elevation feedback to the LaserSight delivery system. In effect, this information, even on highly irregular corneas, will allow the laser to deliver excimer laser energy in whatever pattern is necessary to achieve a spherical result.

References

1. Gailitis RP, et al. Solid-state ultraviolet laser (213nm) ablation of the cornea and synthetic collagen lenticules. *Lasers Surg Med* 11:556–562, 1991.
2. Ren Q, Simon G, Parel JM. Ultraviolet solid-state laser (213-nm) photorefractive keratectomy (in vitro study). *Ophthalmology* 100: 1828–1834, 1993.
3. Ren Q, et al. Ultraviolet solid-state laser (213nm) photorefractive keratectomy (in vivo study). *Ophthalmology* 101:883–889, 1994.
4. Asbell PA, et al. The mini-excimer laser: Second-generation 193-nm photorefractive keratectomy for myopia. *Ophthalmology* 101(9A):102, 1994.
5. Lin JT, et al. Advantages of LaserSight Mini-Excimer PRK laser using low-energy scanning method. Presented at the 15th Congress of the Asia-Pacific Academy of Ophthalmology, Hong Kong, March 9, 1995.
6. Gordon R, et al. Ablation surface characteristics of mini-excimer second generation 193 nm photorefractive keratectomy (PRK) for myopia. *Invest Ophthalmol Vis Sci* 36(4)(Suppl.):S706, 1995.
7. Lin DT, et al. Corneal topographic differences between a scanning laser and broad beam lasers. Presented at the American Society for Cataract and Refractive Surgery, San Diego, CA, April 2, 1995.

17 Autonomous T-PRK

Marguerite McDonald and Larry C. Van Horn

History

Autonomous Technologies Corporation (ATC, Orlando, FL), founded in 1985, has been involved in military- and NASA-sponsored coherent laser radar research applied to strategic target tracking, weapons fire control and rendezvous/docking of space vehicles. ATC developed many state-of-the-art system architectures and signal processing innovations. The application of this technology to tracking eye motion was ATC's first commercial venture. Once the prototype eye tracker was developed and had been demonstrated, it became obvious that the appropriate business decision was for ATC to apply its laser system engineering discipline to developing a PRK system. The tracker-assisted photorefractive keratectomy (T-PRK) system is the result of a 2-year engineering development effort. The first T-PRK system was used for primate trials in mid-1994, and the first humans were treated in Crete, Greece, in January 1995.

Unique Aspects of the Hardware

The Laser System

The ATC T-PRK system is a self-contained excimer laser refractive surgery system. It incorporates a high-performance eye tracker, LADARVision, to provide automatic centration of the eye and line-of-sight stabilization of the treatment beam to negate the effects of saccadic eye motion during surgery. The small (~1-mm) beam is controlled by a high-precision scanning system to provide optimal postoperative shape and surface smoothness of the cornea.

The patient's bed and head rest are integral parts of the system. The patient is positioned supine with his or her head directly under the output window, looking directly up at the output window. The surgeon sits at the viewing microscope during the procedure and controls the excimer laser using the foot switch. The control panel and system control computer video monitor may be positioned so that the surgeon or an assistant (or both) have access to them during the procedure.

In the T-PRK system (Fig. 17-1), the excimer laser enclosure, system control computer, and all other electronics are mounted under the patient bed.

The laser is a small argon-fluoride excimer laser with an output wavelength of 193 nm. It is capable of a pulse repetition frequency of 100 Hz and has a nominal energy per pulse of 5 mJ. The cavity length is approximately 30 cm. The 500-milliwatt average output power of the laser is very favorable with respect to cooling (air cooling is sufficient), reliability, gas lifetime, size, and power requirements.

The entire excimer laser subsystem (which includes the laser, electrical control interface, argon-fluorine-neon premix gas supply bottle, exhaust gas filters, cooling fans, gas regulator, and associated plumbing) is contained in an enclosure. The excimer laser enclosure is designed to provide a failsafe container for the fluorine gas when the lid is closed; filters will absorb essentially all of the fluorine in the event of a gas leak inside the enclosure. The excimer laser enclosure

Fig. 17-1. Photograph of T-PRK system with locations of subsystems identified.

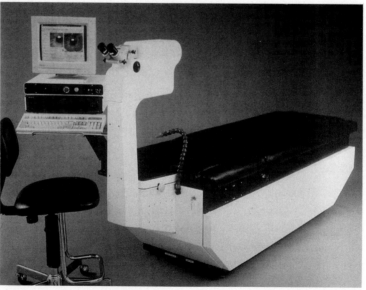

is an integral part of the optics module, which provides an optically rigid structure for the excimer beam control and eye-tracker optics.

The premix gas bottle is approximately 40 cm long and 10 cm in diameter. It contains about 25 laser gas changes. The effective laser gas life is several days, with about 5% power degradation each day. The T-PRK system can tolerate significant power degradation because the effective treatment energy delivered to the surface of the eye is the sum of several thousand pulses integrated over the treatment zone with very precise spatial relationships between each pulse. As the output energy decreases over time for a given gas fill, the calibration procedure that is executed prior to each surgery defines the number and spatial distribution of the pulses required for the treatment as a specific function of the characteristics of the laser energy distribution at that time.

The system may be installed in a room with a minimum 30-inch door opening. The recommended floor area requirement is 11×13 feet, which allows space for the surgeon and assistant as well as access to all four sides of the system. System dimensions are $231 \times 160 \times 130$ cm ($91 \times 63 \times 51$ inches), and it weighs approximately 273 kg (600 lb). It operates from a standard 15-ampere, single-phase, 120-volt circuit. The maximum current draw occurs when the effluent vacuum pump is turned on. The continuous current requirement is less than 5 amperes. An uninterruptable power supply protects the system from power transients and ensures the completion of a surgery in case of a power failure.

The control panel and system computer video monitor are mounted on a swing arm so that they may be positioned for access by either the surgeon or assistant.

The Delivery System

A fundamental characteristic of the T-PRK system is the ability to place each pulse on the surface of the cornea with extremely high position accuracy (< 50-micron peak error). There are two independent, two-axis pointing systems. The one mounted near the laser at the bottom of the column scans the laser in the precise pattern that has been determined for the surgery based on both the refractive correction parameters entered by the surgeon and the calibration of the energy distribution of the laser beam. This scanning system provides less than 10-micron root mean square (RMS) position error in each axis at the cornea. The eye-tracker system, LADARVision, controls the two-axis tracking mirrors that provide a stabilized line of sight to the eye for the excimer beam. The eye tracker responds with enough speed and accuracy that the measured peak position error is 37 microns when a target moving at 100 degrees per second reverses direction. This peak error is reduced by 50% within 3.8 ms. The tracker jitter was measured at less than 15 microns RMS. The target used for these tests provided a smaller signal-to-noise ratio than the eye does, therefore the tracker jitter for a human eye would be less than 15 microns.

The extreme accuracy with which each laser pulse is placed on the cornea allows the use of sophisticated shot-pattern algorithms. These algorithms were developed using a high-resolution computer simulation of the laser-tissue interaction and were optimized for surface shape and smoothness using polymethylmethacrylate (PMMA) and then bovine and porcine eyes prior to human blind eye studies.

The optical system transmits approximately 30% of the laser output to the surface of the cornea. There are three transmissive elements and ten reflective elements in the excimer beam path. The overall optical transmission of the system is 50–100% more efficient than other systems that must use beam homogenizers. The energy distribution of the output laser beam is of sufficient quality that no optical filtering or homogenization is required. The T-PRK system is not very sensitive to beam quality due to the fact that the effective treatment energy is delivered over the ablation zone as the integrated sum of several thousand pulses.

The system includes a stereo viewing microscope with zoom magnification and variable illumination. The viewing microscope is focused by adjusting the elevation of the patient's head. When the patient is in the proper position and looking straight up (i.e., aligned with the fixation light), the view of the corneal surface through the microscope is exactly the same as that "seen" by the laser. When the patient's gaze is not aligned with the fixation light, however, the eye tracker maintains the laser alignment with respect to center of the pupil, but the view through the microscope shows the offset of the patient's eye from proper fixation.

LADARVision provides automatic centration about the center of the undilated pupil. The center of the undilated pupil is marked by the surgeon before dilation. The surgeon aligns the eye tracker to the mark before starting the laser ablation. The surgeon should have the patient look at the fixation light during the initial positioning and center the eye in the viewing microscope before aligning the eye tracker.

The system automatically turns on a vacuum pump to operate the suction hose for effluent removal during a procedure. The flow is sufficient to remove the ablation effluent but is intended to effect the hydration state of the corneal surface only minimally.

There is a 20-cm working distance between the output window and the corneal surface. This provides sufficient room for a microkeratome

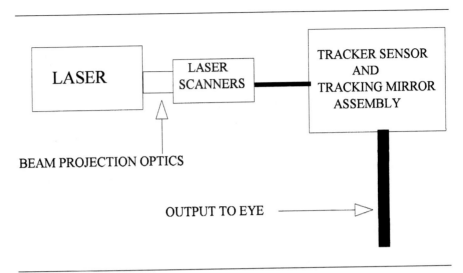

Fig. 17-2. Conceptual schematic of excimer beam path for T-PRK system.

to be used for the laser in-situ keratomileusis (LASIK) procedure while the patient is properly positioned on the bed.

Figure 17-2 shows a schematic representation of the beam delivery system. The laser beam is focused to a 1-mm diameter at 8 inches (20 cm) below the output window by the beam projection optics and a mechanical shutter. The corneal surface is properly placed by adjusting the elevation of the patient's head while using the maximum zoom magnification of the viewing microscope. The excimer beam scanners, which are located near the excimer laser at the bottom of the column, provide two-dimensional translation of the beam to produce the scan pattern on the cornea. The beam is directed up the column to the optics head, where it is combined with the eye tracker. The eye tracker sensor controls the dual-axis tracker mirror assembly, which provides a stabilized line of sight to the eye for both the tracker beam and the scanned excimer beam.

Maintenance Considerations

System reliability is an integral part of the T-PRK system. One of the motivations for using a small beam in combination with an eye tracker was to allow a low-average-power laser to be utilized. Operation at low power levels lengthens the lifetime of both the laser gas and the critical laser components, including the cavity end mirrors and discharge electrodes. Additionally, the laser is relatively simple, with no cryogenic gas purifiers or mechanical gas circulators.

Optical coating and substrate damage is another significant reliability issue for excimer laser systems. The T-PRK system excimer beam is expanded in the delivery system by the beam projection optics near the output of the laser. The last optical element, the output window, is about 20 cm from the beam focus at the position of the eye. This greatly reduces the energy density to which the remaining optics are exposed, thereby significantly increasing the lifetime of the optical coatings and substrates.

The T-PRK system uses one high-pressure gas cylinder, which is contained in the laser enclosure, to supply the premixed argon-fluorine-neon gas. The bottle holds approximately 25 gas fills. Typically, a gas fill may be used for several consecutive days. The gas should be changed at least once weekly.

The effective ablation characteristics of the laser are determined during a calibration procedure prior to each surgery. The energy per pulse may vary from 0.9–1.6 mJ at the eye and still produce the desired clinical results. The test-ablation material enables the evaluation of the two critical ablation characteristics: (1) the volume of material ablated per pulse (which is directly related to both the energy per pulse and the spatial energy distribution of the beam) and (2) the uniformity of the ablated surface resulting from a pattern of about 100 pulses (which verifies the quality of the beam delivery optics over the area of the ablation zone as well as the proper spatial distribution of the laser pulses by the shot-pattern algorithm). If the spatial energy distribution of the beam is not acceptable, the volume of material ablated per shot is either too small or too large, which would indicate a problem with either the laser or the beam projection optics. If the ablated surface is not sufficiently uniform, optical component damage is indicated.

As in any excimer laser, the laser cavity end mirrors have a finite lifetime due to the high photon energy associated with the wavelength of the laser radiation. The windows in the T-PRK system laser eventually need to be replaced. All maintenance and service activities, such as replacing halogen filters, testing the fluorine detector, or optical component replacement must be done by a qualified technician trained by ATC.

Safety Features

The T-PRK system complies with the pertinent FDA regulations relating to medical laser systems (e.g., foot switch control of the laser, laser shutter, keyed switch power control, and safety interlocks for access panels).

LADARVision ensures that the proper position of the ablation zone is maintained throughout the procedure. The tracker is composed of two critical subsystems: (1) the laser radar to measure the position of the eye and (2) the two-axis tracking-mirror assembly, which responds to the position errors generated by the laser radar. The laser radar measures the position of the eye several thousand times per second. The open loop gain crossover frequency (which is the figure of merit used by servomechanism designers to characterize the ability of an electromechanical system to respond to external inputs) of the tracker-mirror assembly combined with the laser radar is greater than 600 radians per second, or about 100 Hz. This exceptionally high performance allows even the highest-speed saccadic eye motions to be tracked with peak position errors of about 30 microns.

The argon-fluoride-neon gas mixture that is used in the laser is contained in a single high-pressure gas bottle. The concentration of fluorine is much less than 1%, but this small amount of fluorine, which does present a hazard, is controlled by the laser enclosure. The gas bottle and all related plumbing is in the laser enclosure. The laser enclosure is designed so that during operation, all of the gas escaping the enclosure must go through one of two filters that absorbs the fluorine. The high-pressure gas bottle is fitted with a small-aperture Cedoux valve to limit the rate at which gas may flow from the bottle in the event of a valve or regulator failure. There is no requirement for external ventilation or gas scrubbing equipment.

A suction hose is placed near the surface of the eye during the ablation procedure to ensure that the effluent is captured. The vacuum system is connected to a filter that traps all the particles in the effluent as the air is pulled through. This filter is changed during normal maintenance and servicing.

The T-PRK system has an uninterruptable power supply (UPS) to ensure that a procedure is not interrupted in the event of facility power surges or outages. This UPS also supports an independent safety system, which is operational even when the system power is switched off. The safety system consists of a single board computer and several sensors. The computer continuously monitors the following conditions: fluorine gas inside the laser enclosure (2 ppm and 5 ppm), gas pressure in the laser, temperature in the laser enclosure, and airflow in the enclosure. The safety system provides visual and audible warnings whether the system is switched on or not and also provides warning messages to the operator if an unsafe condition occurs during surgery. There is also an emergency stop button, which properly sequences the system down automatically in the event of an emergency.

Software-User Interface

An IBM-compatible PC with Windows-based software is used in this system. The user interface consists of a minimal control panel for physical switches and status indicators. These include the (1) shot counter, (2) floppy disk drive, (3) emergency stop button, (4) video recorder, (5) illumination control, (6) gas leak indicator LED, (7) safety status indicator LED, (8) power-on LED, (9) mouse, (10) keyed power switch (on, off, reset), and (11) the laser emission indicator LED. Except for the laser control foot switch, the remainder of interface with the user occurs via the computer-generated graphical user interface (GUI), which is controlled by a mouse.

Figure 17-3 shows the GUI, or operator's interface, for the T-PRK system. The main screen is shown at the top. The power button controls power distribution to the subsystems when the keyed power switch is on. The status of the tracker, laser, shutter, and excimer scanner subsystems is displayed on the lower left side along with the status of the calibration and alignment procedure. The graphic button bar along the top provides access to all the user functions. A direct

Fig. 17-3. Graphical user interface (GUI). This Windows-based software screen displays the status of the tracker, laser, shutter, scanner, calibration, and alignment subsystems. The untracked and tracked images show the respective alignment of the eye as seen through the microscope and as tracked by the laser during ablation. When the patient maintains fixation on the fixation light source, the untracked and tracked images are the same.

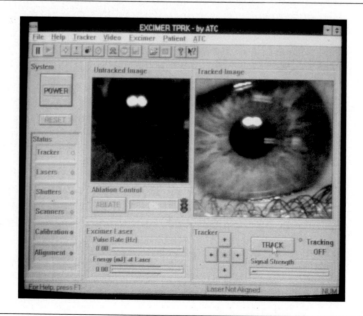

video view (the same as the viewing microscope) of the eye is displayed in the untracked image area, and the tracked image area shows the video view of the eye through the tracker-mirror assembly. When the tracker is engaged, eye motion is apparent in the untracked image, and the tracked image presents a stationary eye.

The steps for setting up the system for a surgical procedure are controlled by the software. Various procedural steps must be performed and the results accepted before the software allows the next step to be executed. Also, all hardware subsystems' status must be acceptable to proceed. A summary of the process (in sequential order) for setting up the system and performing a procedure is outlined in Table 17-1.

In setting up the system, the excimer energy measurement is performed by referring to the dialogue box on the lower right, which appears in the "untracked image" area. Next, the geometry adjust procedure is accomplished by noting the four sets of cross-hairs that appear in the "tracked image" area (Fig. 17-4A). A target material is ablated by the laser in the four quadrants (A, B, C, and D), after which the cross-hairs are centered on each ablation to tell the computer where the ablation occurred. This allows the computer to compensate for any subtle, temperature-dependent optical or mechanical misalignments that may be present. The last step in preparing the system for a surgery is to calibrate the ablation rate (Fig. 17-4B). This is done by executing a known shot pattern on the calibration material and verifying that the result is accurate within an appropriate tolerance. If the result is not within the tolerance, the measured result is entered into the computer, which adjusts the ablation calibration factor. The accuracy of the adjusted calibration factor is then verified by a second ablation and the result accepted before the surgery may proceed. These steps must be completed before all surgical procedures. The system setup is designed to be easy to perform in a short period with minimal mistakes.

Table 17-1. T-PRK system setup and treatment

1. Turn on the system power.
2. Enter patient and surgery data.
3. Enable automated excimer energy measurement.
4. Enable and verify automated geometry adjustment.
5. Perform the ablation volume calibration test.
6. Enable automated shot pattern generation.
7. Align the ablation zone.
8. Ablate the patient's eye.
9. Exit and power system down.

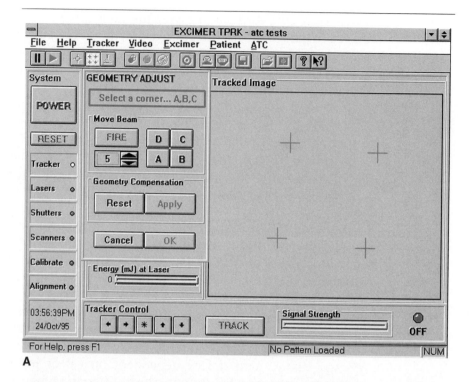

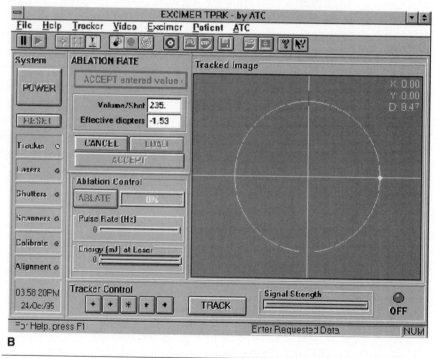

Fig. 17-4. **A.** Geometry adjust screen, which allows the computer to realign the tracker based on the four-quadrant geometry of a test ablation. **B.** The ablation rate screen, which allows the computer to adjust the ablation calibration factor according to the results of a test ablation.

The patient and surgery database allows the operator to enter patient data and the surgical parameters. After the system setup procedures are complete and the required patient data and surgical parameters have been entered, the computer generates the specific shot pattern and shot sequence that is appropriate for the ablation to be carried out and the spatial energy distribution for the laser at that time. The patient data and surgical parameters are stored, along with the pertinent physical parameters for the system (such as laser energy, ablation calibration factor, geometry calibration factors), after the surgery is complete.

Ablation Parameters and Capabilities

The ability to provide myopic, hyperopic, astigmatic corrections with advanced blend zones is designed into the T-PRK system. The small scanned spot allows the system to ablate nonsymmetric patterns. This feature supports the correction of irregular astigmatism.

The excimer scanners support ablation zones up to 10 mm in diameter to accommodate hyperopic blend zones, for example. The spot diameter is approximately 1 mm, although a uniform ablation with a very smooth surface can be generated up to the maximum ablation zone. The laser is capable of 100 pulses per second, and the average energy density is about 180 mJ/cm^2. The scan rate provides a rate of 20 seconds per diopter for myopic corrections with a 6-mm ablation zone. The shot pattern and shot sequence are defined to provide graceful degradation if a procedure were interrupted (the ablation is executed in several layers per diopter, each of which is an independent correction). The shot sequences are designed to minimize the effects of effluent from previous pulses. The general nature of the shot pattern is a nonsequential spiral for ablations that have central symmetry. The system is capable of utilizing multizone algorithms (with a large number of zones) to provide large refractive corrections while minimizing the ablation depth.

The physical configuration of the system also supports LASIK procedures.

Advantages and Disadvantages

Preliminary Results

The T-PRK system was first tested on a series of animal and human cadaver eyes; encouraging results led to a two-part series of procedures in nonhuman primates at the Delta Primate Center in Covington, Louisiana. Although it became clear that the original volume-per-shot calculations were overestimated, the animals did experience a dioptric shift, as measured by topography, retinoscopy, and keratometry. More important, all animals healed quickly, and no infections or recurrent erosions or other sight-threatening complications occurred. The monkeys had only mild corneal haze, which cleared quickly. Timed histologic samples showed extraordinarily smooth ablations without steps, and no subepithelial scar formation. At this juncture, Ioannis Pallikaris of Crete, Greece, commenced the first clinical trials of the T-PRK system in human subjects. The ATC protocol is shown in Table 17-2.

After the volume-per-shot calibration was adjusted, based on a blind eye protocol (5 patients), a sighted eye study was undertaken in two phases. In the first phase a total of 50 sighted patients were treated for myopia between −1 to −6 D with 6 mm ablations [1]. Follow-up data were available for 49 patients at 1, 3, and 6 months, and for 43 patients at 9 months. Overall, there was some refractive undercorrection evident postoperatively that was reduced by a stepwise adjustment in calibration. However, the mean refractive error showed excellent stability between 3 and 9 months. Despite the undercorrection, there was excellent retention of best spectacle-corrected visual acuity with 20/20 or better achieved in 98% (41/42) of eyes at 9 months. Corneal haze was trace or less in all eyes at 9 months (Fig. 17-5). Patient satisfaction with the procedure at 6 months was quite good, with improvement of preoperative symptoms (e.g., glare, halos, grittiness, redness, burning, and photophobia) noted more frequently than worsening. Eighty-two percent of patients noted a marked or extreme improvement of vision following surgery, and 97% would undergo the procedure again.

To date, 96 eyes have been treated in the second phase of the study. Follow-up data is available on 48 eyes at 1 month, 38 eyes at 3 months, and 15 eyes at 6 months. Early refractive data show consid-

Table 17-2. Autonomous Technologies protocol for patient treatment

1. Mark the center of the normal pupil.
2. Dilate the eye to optimize tracker performance.
3. Run system setup and calibration procedures and surgery setup.
4. Position patient; patient fixates on the fixation light.
5. Give topical anesthetic and remove epithelium rapidly.
6. Wait 2 minutes to reduce the variation of corneal tissue hydration from patient to patient.
7. Track the eye, and adjust the ablation center to the mark.
8. Perform the ablation until the program is completed. Apply bandage contact lens and appropriate drops.

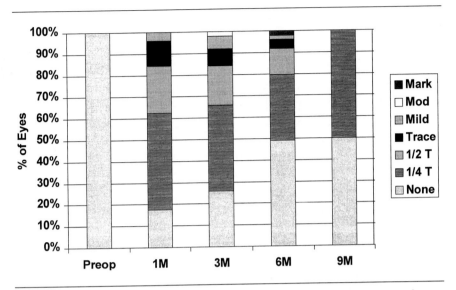

Fig. 17-5. Percentile distribution of corneal haze grading at 1 month, 3 months, 6 months, and 9 months following treatment with T-PRK for myopia of −1.0 to −6.0 D. Only 1 patient had grade 2 (moderate) haze at the 3-month visit.

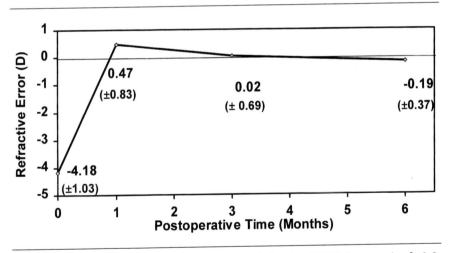

Fig. 17-6. Mean spherical equivalent refraction following T-PRK for myopia of −1.0 to −6.0 D with follow-up in 48 eyes (1 month), 37 eyes (3 months), and 15 eyes (6 months). At 3 months, 84% (31/37) are within 0.5 D of intended correction.

erable improvements in accuracy of refraction (Fig. 17-6). Uncorrected visual acuity was 20/20 or better in 80% (12/15) at 6 months. Early return of best spectacle-corrected visual acuity was noted, with 94% (45/48) at 20/20 or better by 1 month. The 3-month data show that no eyes have lost 2 or more lines of best spectacle-corrected visual acuity, and 84% (31/37) are within 0.5 D of intended correction.

Comparison to Other Systems

ATC's T-PRK instrument combines very sophisticated eye tracking with precisely scanned narrow beam shaping. ATC believes that narrow beam shaping—made legitimate and effective only through sophisticated high-speed tracking such as that found in the LADAR-Vision eye tracker—is the technology platform of the future. The active tracker is able to compensate for saccadic eye movement during surgery, allowing the laser ablation to continue and virtually eliminating shaping error caused by eye movement. The narrow beam excimer provides a smooth ablation and allows the application of flexible algorithms to correct complex visual disorders such as astigmatism and hyperopia.

Future Developments

The research and development plan leverages the T-PRK platform to address a wider range of indications including astigmatism, hyperopia, and the many combinations of hyperopic and myopic sphere and cylinder through the implementation of proprietary shaping algorithms with precise blend zones. T-LASIK is under development to incorporate the eye-tracking capability of T-PRK in the LASIK procedure. ATC is developing CustomCornea, a technology designed to further extend the precision and flexibility of T-PRK by incorporating advanced eye measurement technology to determine the more subtle errors of the human visual system and generate custom ablation patterns ideally suited for each patient.

References

1. Pallikaris I, et al. Tracker-assisted photorefractive keratectomy for myopia of −1.00 to −6.00 diopters. *J. Refract Surg* 12:240–247, 1996.

18 Novatec LightBlade

Casimir A. Swinger, Shui T. Lai, and Ernest W. Kornmehl

History

In 1990, while the phase II investigational trials of excimer photo-refractive keratectomy (PRK) were beginning, one of the authors, Shui T. Lai, a laser physicist, was developing patentable new PRK technology based on a solid-state laser. An active eye tracker was also developed to enhance the reproducibility and accuracy of the procedure. Early excimer PRK results had demonstrated marginal predictability, regression, and haze. Lai and Swinger, an aerospace engineer who with coworkers introduced refractive surgery in the United States in 1977, decided that in order to eliminate the many intrinsic disadvantages and limitations of the excimer laser, drastic changes were needed. In the fall of 1990, Lai and Swinger jointly founded the corporation, Novatec Laser Systems, Inc (Carlsbad, CA).

The Novatec laser was designed to be versatile: not only does it perform superbly in surface PRK, it also offers the best in accuracy and gentleness for intrastromal and intraocular applications. A host of new applications, including intrastromal radial keratotomy (RK), arcuate keratotomy (AK), and PRK, were demonstrated, with fine control in location and dimension of cavity created in the stroma. Laser trephination (for corneal grafts), laser microkeratome, laser phacoemulsification, and laser capsulorhexis and iridotomy were also demonstrated by mid-1992.

The first solid-state PRKs on rabbits and primates were performed in early 1993. These first test results, based on a double-blind study, were shown to be indistinguishable from those of a VISX 20/20. Rigorous refinement of nomograms and continued technological development ensued. After repeated trials performed on more than 100 rabbits, the U.S. trial of blind humans was initiated in the spring of

1994. The ensuing success of the phase I results led to a rapid approval of phase IIa trials by the U.S. Food and Drug Administration (FDA) in November 1994.

The first sighted eye procedure using the Novatec laser was performed before the 1994 American Academy of Ophthalmology meeting in San Francisco by Casimir A. Swinger. The patient was a 62-year-old female with −3.50 D preoperatively. She was +0.25 D at the third day postoperatively, with uncorrected visual acuity (UCVA) of 20/30. She was plano at 6 months, and her UVCA was 20/20. Although not all phase IIa patients treated with the Novatec system achieved the same level of accuracy, the majority of them (60% at 1 month) are within 0.5 D of emmetropia. These sighted eye results clearly demonstrate that the Novatec solid-state laser has the potential to become a leader in PRK technology.

Unique Aspects of the Hardware

The Laser System

The Novatec LightBlade laser was specifically designed for PRK surgery (Fig. 18-1). Its hardware features are unique among ultraviolet (UV) ablating sources in that the laser light is stimulated through a solid-state laser crystal rather than a complex halogen gas. Consequently, no excimer gas cylinders, refill, or disposal is necessary. The

Fig. 18-1. The Novatec LightBlade solid-state PRK laser workstation; LightBlade Model 200.

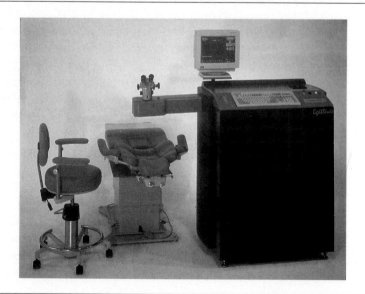

laser beam profile has a gaussian spatial energy distribution because it operates in the fundamental mode. The formation of hot spots, or fluctuations in the laser beam, seen with multimode excimer lasers is not possible in the fundamental mode. The energy density or fluence is set at 100 mJ/cm^2, which is approximately half the value found in most currently used clinical excimer lasers. Together with a small beam diameter of 300–500 microns, the pulse energy is about 200 times less than that of a typical excimer laser. The smaller spot results in a more localized acoustic shock, making the laser ablation almost inaudible. Another major benefit of having a steady uniform energy distribution in the laser beam is the reduced potential for damage to the optics. The Novatec laser beam requires no beam homogenization, leaving fewer optical components that are susceptible to UV damage. Assuming that the humidity and dust are reasonably controlled in the surgery suite, the estimated lifetime of the optics are in the range of 2000–3000 procedures. With current excimer laser systems, the replacement of optical components is necessary after every 300–400 procedures.

Another advanced feature of the Novatec laser is remote diagnosis via modem. With a dedicated modem telephone line, the Novatec laser is connected to the computer of a service engineer. Minor system maintenance can be performed in real time, minimizing down time and costs.

The physical dimensions of the current system are relatively compact, and further size reduction is anticipated in the near future. The dimensions (length, width, and height) of the laser system are 100 × 66 × 120 cm, and the system weighs approximately 550 kg. Its footprint is 2 × 3 ft. The LightBlade system is on four rollers and can be moved easily from room to room. The entire system, with patient's chair and instrument tray, can fit into a 12 × 12-ft room, although a room of 15 × 15 sq ft or larger is recommended. Because it uses no toxic gases, there is no requirement for special ventilation, liquid nitrogen, or a large window in the room in case of emergency. The laser is water cooled, and closed-loop recirculation is preferable when available. The electrical requirements of the system are 208 V in 3 phase and approximately 50 amps, drawing a total power of 15 kW.

The Delivery System

The Novatec delivery system can be divided into three areas: patient alignment, automated eye tracking, and the scanning beam.

Patient Alignment

The patient's chair can be equipped with either a swivel feature, centered at the base of the chair, or with rollers, so that the entire chair is movable. The swivel feature allows the patient to be seated clear of the delivery arm and then swung underneath it, and the rollers allow the chair to be used in surgical procedures at other locations.

Once the patient's head is in rough alignment, the computerized motion control can be used for fine positioning of the cornea within 0.1-mm increments. This fine alignment occurs along three orthogonal axes and may be performed rapidly if needed. The range of movement permits positioning of the patient's fellow eye for bilateral procedures. The vertical alignment of the cornea is achieved by two crossing helium-neon (HeNe) beams overlapping at the corneal apex. The horizontal position of the cornea is achieved by centering the entrance pupil. Because of the small size of the laser beam, one can achieve perfect coaxiality of the surgical beam, the patient's visual axis, and the physician's line of sight by adding a small mirror under the surgical microscope. The coaxial beam enhances the proper centration of ablation, which has important bearing on visual outcome.

Automated Eye Tracking

Current PRK procedures require patient fixation, which is believed to work well with short procedures in the range of 15–20 seconds. With longer procedures, however, patient anxiety and distraction from the ablation noise can lead to eye jittering and drift. The Novatec system is equipped with an automated eye tracker that locks onto the position of the cornea. Its tracking range covers an area 10 mm in diameter, within which the surgical beam follows eye movement freely and with high speed. The beam position is updated every 2 milliseconds, which is among the fastest response times offered on the market. Both patient and surgeon are able to be more relaxed with the eye tracker, and centration is maintained during the entire procedure. For longer and more complex PRK procedures, such as those for hyperopia and irregular astigmatism, the eye-tracking function is mandatory.

Scanning Beam

With the advancement of PRK technology, delivery systems have evolved from large stationary beams with a motorized diaphragm to beam wobbling, sweeping, or scanning with or without a diaphragm or rotating mask. The goal has been to reduce the pulse energy on the cornea, to expand the capacity for larger-zone ablations, and to minimize the optics necessary to homogenize a less than perfect excimer laser beam profile. The Novatec surgical beam covers a small area of about 0.3–0.5 mm in diameter and is capable of addressing any localized corneal irregularity with sufficient spatial resolution. Computerized scanning places no limit on the ablation zone size. Single collimated fundamental mode pulses maintain a consistent gaussian

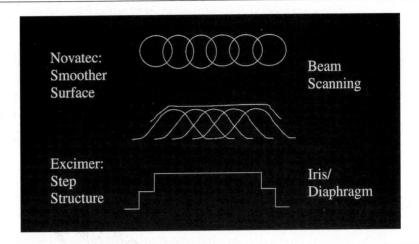

Fig. 18-2. The corneal surface smoothing effect of a Novatec computerized scanning laser beam versus the step structure resulting from diaphragmatic control.

profile that is independent of vertical focusing. By overlapping the gaussian etch profile within the pattern of the scanning beam, a smooth cornea surface is achieved without the etching steps of an iris diaphragm (Fig. 18-2). Central islands were not observed in any of the Novatec-treated patients, which may be due to the fact that the ablation pattern with each pulse is identical irrespective of the laser beam location on the cornea.

Maintenance Considerations

Much of the Novatec laser system's hardware is proprietary, making the exact maintenance requirements and need for laser servicing unknown. Because the Novatec LightBlade is generated with a solid-state crystal, no excimer gas is used in the system, thus obviating the need for gas cylinder replacement, gas evacuation, and frequent replacement of optics and components in the cavity, which otherwise would be exposed to the highly reactive fluorine gas. Closed-loop water cooling is recommended; it requires replacement of an in-line water filter when the color of the filter turns from white to grey.

The laser itself has internal diagnostics that monitor various aspects of the laser, the eye tracker, and the laser power. Automatic adjustments are made by computer when necessary. Routine maintenance is recommended every 6 months so that optical alignment is not required of the system operator. Optical element damage is infrequent, and the lifetime of optics are expected to be 1–2 years, depending on frequency of use. Other factors that may affect the optics' lifetime, alignment, and laser operation are the maintenance of room temperature and control of humidity and dust in the surgical suite.

Other maintenance issues (system shutdown and need for repair) are easily resolved via modem. The computer software program offers a modem maintenance file on the main menu, which has a direct telephone connection to Novatec headquarters. In addition to uploading and downloading files via modem, a remote system diagnostic is easily implemented through a telephone line, making laser servicing simple and particularly useful for users outside the United States.

Safety Features

Special ventilation and toxic gas containment are not required with the solid-state system. The Novatec system has several features to ensure the safety and efficacy of the PRK surgery.

Eye Tracker Warning

When the signal level is insufficient for the eye tracker to function properly, the HeNe alignment beams blink to warn the operator. The laser cannot be activated until the situation is remedied.

Scanner Fault Detection

When the scanner fails to follow the computer instruction to direct the laser beam in a prescribed manner, a warning flag is raised, and the laser beam is disabled. No surgery can be performed until the fault condition is resolved. The scanner fault detection function is activated continuously whenever the scanner is instructed to direct the laser beam.

Surgical Procedure Interrupt

If the procedure is interrupted for any reason, the computer keeps track of the break-off point. The surgeon may reposition the patient and continue the procedure without any compromise. With a new PRK ablation module, if the procedure has to be terminated, the ablation profile on the cornea is a fraction of the intended correction over the entire optic zone rather than a small zone with the full intended correction. In this way, the Novatec ablation algorithm minimizes symptoms of glare and halos seen with small ablation zone size. Without the new algorithm, recentering of the eye to complete the procedure from the point of interruption in a later session is typically difficult; however, with the Novatec ablation algorithm, critical alignment is not crucial because the additional correction will be similar to any new ablation.

Calibration

Once a day, before treatment, calibration testing is required to ensure that adequate energy delivery and ablation depth are achieved. A screen for the calibration procedure, when requested, guides the user through the procedure. The operator is asked to place a factory-supplied polymethylmethacrylate (PMMA) plate in the surgical field and initiate the ablation process. A uniform, flat (plano) layer of the PMMA material is removed, and the depth is measured by the operator. If the measured depth differs by more than 5% from the intended depth, the actual measured depth is entered into a query, and the computer adjusts the internal calibration. The procedure is repeated to ensure that the computer has implemented the modified value. The second calibration measurement usually produces an accuracy within 2% of the intended value.

Software-User Interface

Table 18-1 reviews the steps for setting up the Novatec system before treatment. When the system is turned on, there is a 20-minute

Table 18-1. List of steps to set up the Novatec LightBlade laser system for treatment

1. Turn on the power switch. The system needs 20 minutes to warm up, during which time the computer performs all system initialization procedures. The monitor displays a clock for the time countdown.
2. When the information screen appears, select the desired function from the following menu:
   Calibration procedure
   Surgical procedure (myopia or other PRK)
   Patient file (updates or enters new patient information)
   Modem maintenance (accesses a direct connection through a telephone line to Novatec headquarters where system maintenance, diagnostics, and uploading or downloading of files can easily be performed)
3. Select Calibration, and follow the required steps before treating the patients each day.
4. Select Patient File to enter the patient information required for the treatment to be performed.
5. Select from Myopic PRK, Hyperopic PRK, Astigmatic PRK, and other procedures. The operating parameters for the PRK procedure can then be entered. The computer displays the operative parameters again for confirmation and informs the surgeon of the tissue ablation depth and the ablation time for the procedure.
6. Once the surgeon accepts the operative parameters with an affirmative answer, the laser is ready for the ablation. The eye tracker is automatically engaged when the cornea is aligned and the foot pedal depressed.

warmup period, in which the computer performs all system initialization procedures. The monitor displays a clock for the time countdown.
When the system is warmed up, a patient information screen appears,
requesting information about the patient. A menu then offers a choice
of four functions: (1) calibration procedure, (2) surgical procedure
(myopia, astigmatism, hyperopia, or other procedures), (3) patient
file, to update or enter new patient information, and (4) modem
maintenance. "Modem maintenance" accesses a modem that links the
user with Novatec headquarters for system maintenance, diagnostics,
and file loading over a telephone line.

After calibration, the patient identification and other pertinent
information, such as date and time of the procedure, laser parameters,
and procedural treatment plan, are recorded in a patient file in the
system's computer. This file can be printed out if a printer is available,
or transferred to a floppy disk to generate a hard copy at any PC
workstation.

After the operating parameters for the PRK procedure are entered, the computer displays these parameters again for confirmation and informs the surgeon about the tissue ablation depth and
the ablation time for the procedure (Fig. 18-3). Once the surgeon
accepts the operative parameters with an affirmative answer, the
laser is ready for the ablation. After the patient's cornea is aligned,
the eye tracker is automatically engaged when the laser beam activation foot pedal is depressed. Seeing a faint blue fluorescence on
the cornea in a darkened room confirms that the ablation process is
taking place.

Fig. 18-3. Screen showing operative parameters for confirmation of a surgical
procedure.

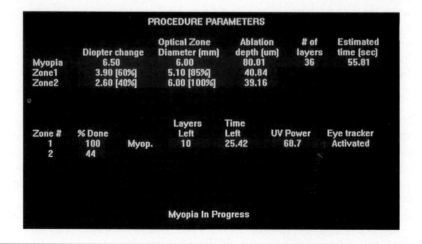

	Diopter change	Optical Zone Diameter (mm)	Ablation depth (um)	# of layers	Estimated time (sec)
Myopia	6.50	6.00	80.01	36	55.81
Zone1	3.90 [60%]	5.10 [85%]	40.84		
Zone2	2.60 [40%]	6.00 [100%]	39.16		

Zone #	% Done		Layers Left	Time Left	UV Power	Eye tracker
1	100	Myop.	10	25.42	68.7	Activated
2	44					

PROCEDURE PARAMETERS

Myopia In Progress

Ablation Parameters and Capabilities

Before any PRK procedure, three principal parameters are required: (1) the preoperative keratometry, (2) the desired dioptric change, and (3) the ablation zone size. The corresponding diopter power at the spectacle plane is converted to the power at the corneal apex, which is used for the ablation profile. A 6-mm, single-zone, circular scanning pattern was used in the early U.S. clinical trials. When patient treatments are not restricted by protocol requirements, multiple zones of variable diameter can be chosen from a menu. For hyperopia, an annular scanning pattern with an ablation zone of 9.5-mm diameter has been used with good results. For astigmatism, both a linear scanning pattern for a purely cylindrical correction and an elliptical scanning pattern for combined myopia and astigmatism are offered. The usual abrupt edge of a purely cylindrical ablation on the cornea can be smoothed out with an extended taper zone to avoid epithelial hyperplasia, and hence regression. Overall, the flexibility of the Novatec software offers surgeons the ability to modify and tailor the nomogram to suit their personal experience in conjunction with differences in postoperative regimen.

The Novatec scanning approach also permits a detailed modification of a corneal surface, going beyond the current simple lens correction approach. Based on the difference map of preoperative corneal topography and an ideal base curvature of the cornea, a detailed elevation map of the tissue to be removed can be generated, including any localized irregularity and astigmatism. This information is then fed into the computer to guide the laser beam during ablation of tissue elevated beyond the ideal intended base curvature. Two major attributes of the Novatec beam delivery make this possible: (1) the small size of the scanning laser beam, which provides good spatial resolution, and (2) the consistent ablation depth of each laser pulse.

Advantages and Disadvantages

Preliminary Results

At the time of this writing, the required number of patients for the U.S. FDA phase IIa low-myopia protocol have been successfully treated and followed for at least 6 months. The study required 50 normally sighted eyes with preoperative best corrected visual acuity of 20/40 or better and 1–6 D of myopia with less than 1.5 D of astigmatism. The intraoperative protocol involved epithelial removal and a single 6-mm optical zone. Following the ablation, tobramycin-dexamethasone ointment (TobraDex) was applied with a pressure patch. Topical nonsteroidal anti-inflammatory medication and a bandage contact lens were not administered. Postoperatively, fluorometholone 0.1% (FML) was applied 4 times per day for 1 month and tapered over the next 8–16 weeks, depending on response.

All 50 eyes have undergone surgery, with 50 eyes having 6-month follow-up. Intraoperatively, there were no complications, and surface quality was excellent during the procedure, with no significant wetness or dryness at the surface. Additionally, no sound was heard during the ablation procedure. The postoperative findings are summarized below.

Epithelialization

Twenty-three eyes re-epithelialized in 2 days, 24 eyes in 3 days, and 3 eyes in 4 days, for a mean of 2.6 days.

Refractive Correction

The preoperative spherical equivalent was -3.32 ± 1.27 D with a range of -1.13 D to -5.75 D. At 1 month postoperatively in all 50 eyes, the mean spherical equivalent refraction was -0.01 ± 0.69 D with a range of -1.13 D to $+3.38$ D, for a mean change of -3.31 D (Fig. 18-4). The mean spherical equivalent at 3 and 6 months was -0.37 and -0.37, respectively.

Fig. 18-4. Mean spherical equivalent refraction of Novatec phase IIa results over a 6-month period.

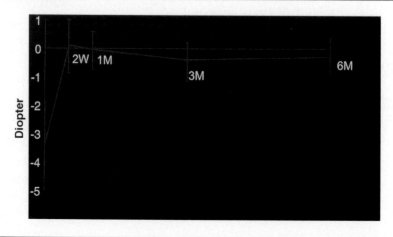

Haze

Haze was graded from 0 (clear) to 4 (opaque). At 1 month, there was a mean haze of 0.5 (trace) and maximum haze of 1.0 (mild); at 3 months, the mean haze was 0.4 and the maximum was 2.0 (moderate); and at 6 months, the mean haze was 0.3 and the maximum, 2.0.

Accuracy

At 1 month, 98% of the eyes were within 1.00 D of the intended correction, with 64% within 0.5 D of emmetropia (Fig. 18-5). At 3 months, 88% were within 1.00 D, and at 6 months, 84% were within 1.00 D (Table 18-2).

Uncorrected Visual Acuity

At 1 month, 76% had uncorrected visual acuity of 20/25 or better and 48% were 20/20 or better; at 3 months, 78% were 20/25 or better and 48% were 20/20 or better; and at 6 months, 96% were 20/40 or better, 80% were 20/25 or better, and 56% were 20/20 or better (Table 18-3).

Best Spectacle-Corrected Visual Acuity

At 1 month, 100% were 20/30 or better and 80% were 20/20 or better; at 3 months, 100% were 20/25 or better and 92% were 20/20 or better; and at 6 months, 100% were 20/32 or better and 94% were 20/20 or better.

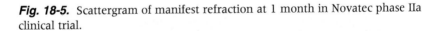

Fig. 18-5. Scattergram of manifest refraction at 1 month in Novatec phase IIa clinical trial.

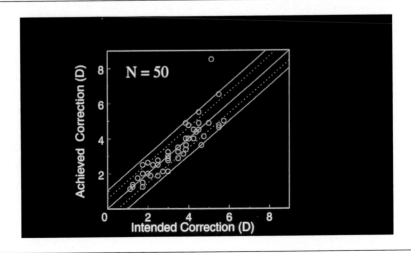

Table 18-2. Novatec PRK accuracy in phase IIa trials (n = 50)

Deviation from intended outcome	1 month	3 months	6 months
± 0.50 D	64%	60%	64% (50%)*
± 1.00 D	98%	88%	84% (75%)*
± 2.00 D	98%	98%	98%

*Numbers in parentheses are the US FDA recommended panel standards used for approval of the Summit excimer laser.

Table 18-3. Six-month follow-up of Novatec LightBlade phase IIa trials (50 eyes)

Uncorrected visual acuity	Percent of eyes
20/12.5 (1.6) or better	6%
20/16 (1.2)	18%
20/20 (1.0)	56%
20/25 (0.8)	80%
20/40 (0.5)	96%

Note: Numbers in parentheses indicate European standard of visual acuity management.

Topography

There were no abnormalities or central islands in any eyes.

Complications

At 3 months, there was one case of steroid-induced ocular hypertension, one steroid-induced cataract, and one retinal depigmentation, possibly from the fiberoptic illumination source of the microscope. The patient with retinal depigmentation now has a normal vision field, and the visual acuity is not affected.

Hyperopia Trial Results

Nine sighted eyes with previous corneal surgery underwent hyperopic PRK using a 6.0- to 6.5-mm optic zone and a 9.0- to 9.5-mm ablation diameter. Four of the eyes had failed holmium:yttrium-aluminum-garnet laser thermokeratoplasty, 1 eye was an overcorrected RK, and 4 eyes were overcorrected PRK patients. The mean preoperative spherical equivalent was + 3.95 D (range 1.00–6.63 D) and the mean postoperative spherical equivalent was −0.08 D, for a change of + 4.03 D.

III Economic Considerations

19 Medical Economics of Photorefractive Corneal Surgery

Robert E. Fenzl, Michael A. Romansky, Richard Saver,
Nils Bonde-Henriksen, and Stephen M. Blinn

As changes in the practice of ophthalmology alarm many American practitioners, a large number are looking to photorefractive keratectomy (PRK) to provide some easy solutions to reduced incomes resulting from managed care contracting. The most significant impact of PRK may lie not in the financial benefit it brings to individual ophthalmologists but in the financial dilemmas it could pose for them.

Like any product manufacturer, excimer laser manufacturers expect to recover their development costs and receive a reasonable return on their investment. When those costs include 10 years of independent research and development and significant regulatory review in various countries, the investment that the manufacturer must recover is significant. Given the time and money expended to bring excimer lasers to market, it should come as no surprise that they are priced at approximately $500,000 and that, as of June 1996, a royalty per procedure of $250 is imposed by the laser manufacturers.

The appeal of excimer lasers is that they will simplify refractive surgery to the point that many ophthalmologists will be encouraged to participate in the perceived PRK windfall. When performed by an experienced surgeon, radial keratotomy (RK) can produce results similar to PRK for low myopia. The development of excimer lasers makes it possible for a much larger group of ophthalmologists to participate in refractive surgery and produce uniform results. More important, a computer-controlled laser system that produces predictable results has far greater marketing potential than the hands of the steadiest and most gifted surgeon using a "knife" to operate on a patient's eye. However, too many high-cost excimer lasers competing in the same market are a recipe for financial disaster. Ophthalmolo-

Table 19-1. Comparison of cataract and PRK patients

Variable	Cataract	PRK
Age	Old	Young
Visual needs	Essential to maintain independence	Functional, nonessential
Financing	Third-party payer, universally covered	Out-of-pocket
Cost of entry for M.D.	Low	High
End economic result	Highly reimbursed initially (1970s–1980s); dramatic drop in compensation recently	Competition will drop fees more rapidly; high cost of doing business squeezes profits

gists need to give careful consideration to their particular situation when deciding if, when, and how to participate in PRK.

The era of laser refractive surgery will introduce a new economic paradigm to the field of ophthalmology. The biggest mistake that ophthalmologists can make while attempting to evaluate the potential for excimer PRK in their practices is to assume that the growth of excimer PRK will parallel prior successful economic experiences with the practice of cataract surgery in the 1970s and 1980s.

To illustrate this important distinction, one needs to carefully compare and contrast the attributes of cataract and PRK patients (Table 19-1).

Cash Flow Considerations

Participation in PRK can be a costly proposition. Before you commit to buying an excimer laser or utilizing the services of a particular excimer laser management company, careful thought should be given to what your financial commitments will be and what you can realistically expect as a return on your investment. With PRK, the cost of obtaining patients will likely shock you.

If you decide to buy an excimer laser system, the $500,000 price of the laser is just the beginning and does not include the other "incidental" costs of sales tax, shipping, and liability insurance (Table 19-2). Having made this enormous investment, you must now expend additional resources to maximize the likelihood that you can generate sufficient patient flow to pay for your investment. The excimer and the broad appeal of PRK lead many to believe that a new era of "retail" medicine is emerging.

The expenditure of $500,000 probably will require you to focus substantially on PRK. Be prepared to absorb a variety of additional

Table 19-2. Startup cost of laser refractive surgery practice

Excimer laser*	$500,000
Laser suite preparation	$50,000–100,000
Legal costs	$20,000–50,000
Total	$570,000–650,000

*Includes laser purchase.

costs. Changing the focus of your practice may require physical changes to your existing office space and infrastructure. This may mean changing or adding personnel and office hours to accommodate your new patients, adding telemarketing and fulfillment capabilities, and changing the way you interact with other eye-care professionals.

Because PRK is a new procedure, considerable marketing will be required to introduce it to the public and begin to create a demand for the service. Perhaps the greatest misconception regarding PRK is the cost of marketing. Many experts talk of a "per-patient" marketing cost. What they fail to mention is that to be involved at any level you must absorb certain minimum marketing costs, regardless of how many patients you generate. Once you have an established PRK practice, it may be possible to calculate a "per-patient" cost, but in the early stages you should think instead of a minimum marketing cost required to establish your PRK practice.

The cost of establishing a PRK practice varies from market to market, but in a typical mid-sized city, expect to spend at least $250,000 a year to generate interest. Much of this money is often spent long before the first patient is treated, and there are no guarantees that this, or any other level of spending, will generate the desired return.

Other costs related to the laser can add up. Upgrades in technology can cost as much as $30,000 a year. Gases will cost laser owners another $10,000 or more each year, and maintenance agreements will cost as much as $50,000 per year after the first year (Table 19-3). In addition, the laser manufacturers will require payment of a per-procedure fee of as much as $250 (Pillar Point Royalty).

Many ophthalmologists will eventually ask themselves the difficult question, Should I purchase an excimer laser? For the vast majority the answer is no.

Purchasing a costly excimer laser system will, by necessity, force you to focus heavily on providing PRK services. In many ways, the investment in an excimer laser is similar to the investment in creating an ambulatory surgery center for cataract surgery. The costs of equipment and physical improvements merely allow you to enter the field,

Table 19-3. Annual fixed expenses of laser refractive surgery practice

Amortized startup cost (includes laser purchase)*	$145,000/year
Maintenance of laser	$ 50,000/year
Laser upgrades	$ 30,000/year
Gas for operating laser	$ 10,000/year
Total	$235,000/year

*Assumes total startup costs of $570,000.

and significant additional commitments are required to make the business successful.

As you conduct your evaluation to determine whether purchasing is a viable alternative for you, consider the following information and how it applies to your particular circumstance. To make a proper evaluation, various scenarios involving surgical volume and fees must be considered. These scenarios are based on the costs that an individual ophthalmologist is likely to incur in establishing a PRK practice (see Tables 19-2 and 19-3). Additional costs specific to the development of a group PRK practice are outlined later in this section under Special Group Costs.

Startup costs are one-time costs that must be incurred to place the laser in your practice. The laser suite preparation costs are based on the assumption that your existing space is large enough to accommodate the new service and can be modified as needed. Special consideration must be given to the ventilation capabilities of the proposed space as well as the ability to tightly regulate temperature and humidity. If shared space with other surgical or diagnostic equipment is planned, the presence of certain chemical substances or the potential for substantial generation of particulate debris that might contaminate the laser's optical pathway are co-variables that must be carefully considered. If major modifications are required because of local fire and safety regulations, or OSHA regulations, your costs could increase.

Legal costs vary from state to state and will be affected by various factors. The costs shown in Tables 19-2 and 19-3 assume traditional expenses associated with establishing a new service in a state where "reasonable standards" exist. These costs can include development of documents needed to participate in PRK, including informed consent agreements and comanagement agreements. If your state requires PRK clinics to meet the same requirements as ambulatory surgery centers, you can expect your legal costs to increase significantly. If you are also required to obtain a Certificate of Need (CON), additional legal costs may be incurred.

Table 19-4. Startup cost of laser refractive surgery practice with laser leasing

	Cost
Excimer laser (sales tax, shipping, insurance, maintenance)[a]	$75,000–85,000
Laser suite preparation[b]	$50,000–100,000
Legal costs	$20,000–50,000
Total	$145,000–235,000

[a]Generally requires $250 per case variable payment as an additional variable cost (source: Excimer Vision Leasing, Walnut Creek, CA).
[b]Assumes creation of new, freestanding facility.

If you are fortunate, you may be able to amortize these one-time startup expenses over a 5-year period. This may not be possible for a number of reasons. Lenders in your area may be unwilling to use an economically unproved excimer laser as security on a loan. More important, the first-generation laser system that you purchase may be supplanted by updated technology in less than 5 years. If you were able to amortize the $570,000 startup costs (see Table 19-3) at 10% over 5 years, the resultant payments would be approximately $145,000 per year. As seen in Table 19-4, leasing a laser dramatically reduces startup costs but will increase variable costs by $250 to $300 per case if the lease operates on a pay-as-you-go basis. A leasing arrangement makes it much more affordable to enter the laser center business from the standpoint of startup capital, but profit margins are similar unless very large volumes of cases are performed. Losses are reduced at lower volumes.

Fixed Yearly Costs

Having amortized your startup costs, you must now consider other annual operating costs that you will incur with the purchase and operation of an excimer laser (see Table 19-3). Maintenance of the laser is required if you expect to protect your warranty. Refinements of the excimer laser will continue, and upgrades will be required if you intend to compete for patients. As patient volumes increase, the amount of gas used will also increase; therefore, the $10,000 projected cost may be higher if you do a high-volume business.

Variable Costs

Other costs are incurred based on the number of PRK procedures performed. These costs are included in the following broad categories:

Supplies	$50–100 per treatment
Marketing	$200–300 per treatment
Royalty	$250 per treatment
Total variable costs	$500–650/treatment

In this context, supplies include the cost of your office personnel's time related to the PRK treatment as well as the cost of disposables. At a minimum, each patient will consume some portion of the time of your technical staff and billing department. Marketing requires an initial minimum investment regardless of the number of treatments generated, but a realistic scenario from the international experience to date would assign a marketing cost of $300 per procedure.

Special Group Costs

Many ophthalmologists will consider joining with colleagues and friends to create a PRK partnership or corporation that purchases or leases and operates an excimer laser. Although this can reduce your individual financial liability, additional costs are necessarily incurred, and complex relationships must be sorted through. Participating in such an arrangement allows you to share expenses and reduce your personal level of financial risk. The group shares the fixed and variable costs described above, but it also incurs new costs, including rent, personnel, insurance, billing, equipment (office and medical), and licensing requirements (increases significantly if CON is needed). The total potential costs of a PRK partnership or corporate practice may exceed $100,000 annually.

A group partnership or corporate PRK venture will typically require a new, freestanding facility with enough room to accommodate the significant patient flow needed to meet costs and satisfy each member of the group. For a high-volume practice, that probably means 1500–2000 square feet of space. The cost of this space varies from market to market, as does the cost to staff the facility with a receptionist, laser nurse technicians, and a competent (i.e., well-paid) manager. A group practice or freestanding site will require its own general liability coverage. A freestanding facility must also have its own billing capacity and the general office equipment and supplies necessary for any business or practice. Finally, obtaining a CON would significantly increase your costs. In many states, a group could not operate a center without first obtaining a CON. If you are in a state that requires a CON for ambulatory surgery centers, you should expect that a PRK center will also require a CON.

These group expenses are likely to cost well in excess of $100,000, depending on your market. For the purposes of this evaluation, a conservative estimate of $100,000 is used to calculate additional expenses related to a group purchase and operation of an excimer laser. If a group of surgeons is able to arrange for shared use of appropriate space in an existing medical practice facility, they may dramatically decrease expenses via shared overhead not only for space but for personnel, ancillary equipment, phone lines, and billing services. Under this scenario, costs may be allocated in such a manner that the laser center pays only for those services it uses within the construct of the larger facility.

Using the cost assumptions discussed above, it is then possible to determine your return on investment based on projected patient flow levels and patient fees. Many groups have spoken of obtaining patient fees of up to $2000 per treatment. International experience and common sense, however, indicate that PRK will be a price-sensitive product and that the existence of many laser purchasers will drive prices down in order to drive patient volumes up. The global fee charged to patients is more likely to fall in the $1200–1500 range.

Surgical Fee Pricing and Profit Margins

Any ophthalmologist interested in participating in PRK will want to make a return of at least 30% on the global fee. That 30% has to cover surgical consultations, surgery, and postoperative follow-up visits. On a $1500 patient fee, that 30% return, or $450, must then be weighed against the actual time involved in providing the necessary services. Most ophthalmologists will seek an even higher return, but even at the 30% rate of return the numbers are not an overwhelming incentive for an individual to purchase a laser, as shown in Tables 19-5 and 19-6. As is obvious from the scenarios provided in these tables, it is practical to purchase a laser only if volumes in excess of 1000 cases per year are anticipated. Such a goal is much more likely to be achieved by a large group of surgeons and is another strong argument for creating a laser center as a group venture within an existing facility

Table 19-5. Individual PRK provider profits at $1500 per treatment

Number of treatments	Revenue	Fixed yearly costs	Variable costs (@$650)	30% return (@$450)	Additional profit or loss
300	$ 450,000	$235,000	$195,000	$135,000	(–$115,000)
400	$ 600,000	$235,000	$260,000	$180,000	(–$ 75,000)
500	$ 750,000	$235,000	$325,000	$225,000	(–$ 35,000)
600	$ 900,000	$235,000	$390,000	$270,000	+$ 5,000
750	$1,125,000	$235,000	$487,500	$337,500	+$ 65,000
1000	$1,500,000	$235,000	$650,000	$500,000	+$115,000

Table 19-6. Individual PRK provider profits at $1200 per treatment

Number of treatments	Revenue	Fixed yearly costs	Variable costs (@$650)	30% return (@$360)	Additional profit or loss
500	$ 600,000	$235,000	$325,000	$180,000	(−$140,000)
750	$ 900,000	$235,000	$487,500	$270,000	(−$ 92,500)
1000	$1,200,000	$235,000	$650,000	$360,000	(−$ 45,000)
1250	$1,500,000	$235,000	$812,500	$450,000	+$ 2500

utilized for other purposes (i.e., the practice of other aspects of ophthalmology) as opposed to individual ownership.

With a patient fee of $1500 per treatment, the individual excimer laser owner must perform 600 procedures before realizing the desired 30% return. When the PRK fee drops to $1200 per treatment, not only does the dollar value of the 30% return diminish (from $450 to $360 per procedure), but the ophthalmologist must now treat 1250 eyes before achieving the 30% return rate.

U.S. Food and Drug Administration (FDA) protocols may well require that every patient receive a 2- to 3-day follow-up, a 10-day follow-up, and follow-up visits at 1, 3, 6, and 12 months. The ophthalmologist's return must generate sufficient revenue to allow him or her to make a fair and reasonable fee for these services. If co-management is being considered, the return must be sufficient to cover those costs as well.

Groups of ophthalmologists who purchase and operate excimer lasers will incur some costs beyond those incurred by individual practitioners. Although these costs and others are shared by the group, they require the group to perform even more procedures than the individual must perform before reaching the desired 30% return rate (Tables 19-7 and 19-8).

If international experience with individual excimer laser operators and excimer laser management companies is any indication, few operators will generate more than a few hundred procedures in the first year of operation. If this holds true in the U.S. market, it could cause rapid price compression and result in a large resale market for excimer laser systems. Unlike most ophthalmologists, some of the excimer laser management companies can afford to take a long-term view and accept initial losses. These companies also have significant economies of scale not available to individual and small group excimer laser operators, which reduces the number of procedures necessary to break even. A few of the management companies may also be able to secure more favorable terms of purchase because of the number of machines they purchase. The financial advantage of participation through a management company for a physician is further enhanced

Table 19-7. PRK group practice profits at $1500 per treatment

Number of treatments	Revenue	Fixed yearly costs	Variable costs (@$650)	30% return (@$450)	Additional profit or loss
500	$ 750,000	$335,000	$325,000	$225,000	(–$135,000)
750	$1,125,000	$335,000	$487,500	$337,500	(–$ 35,000)
1000	$1,500,000	$335,000	$650,000	$450,000	+$ 65,000
1250	$1,875,000	$335,000	$812,500	$562,500	+$165,000

Table 19-8. PRK group practice profits at $1200 per treatment

Number of treatments	Revenue	Fixed yearly costs	Variable costs (@$650)	30% return (@$360)	Additional profit or loss
1250	$1,500,000	$335,000	$ 812,500	$450,000	(–$97,500)
1500	$1,800,000	$335,000	$ 975,000	$540,000	(–$50,000)
1750	$2,100,000	$335,000	$1,137,500	$630,000	(–$ 2,500)
2000	$2,400,000	$335,000	$1,300,000	$720,000	+$45,000

by the elimination of the risk of technological obsolescence that one assumes as an owner of an excimer laser. Laser access companies provide an opportunity to generate income regardless of the level of participation (Tables 19-9 and 19-10). Tables 19-9 and 19-10 take a conservative approach and assume that a doctor using a management company's laser will make $400 on a per-procedure patient fee of $1500. The $400 is the portion of the fee that remains once the doctor has paid the $250 per-procedure royalty, $300 per-procedure marketing cost, and a $550 per-procedure laser access fee. The costs for the group-owned laser are those fixed costs plus the variable costs and special group costs discussed earlier. One major limitation of publicly held excimer laser management companies, however, is the pressure they may receive from stockholders to drive up demand for the procedure, and hence stock prices, in the short-term. Many such entities are under significant pressure from venture capitalists, investors, and stockholders; these individuals often want a quick return on their investment and hence the company may not always act in the long-term interest of others, such as practicing physicians.

An individual ophthalmologist must perform more than 522 PRK procedures on a privately owned machine before his or her return is similar to what it would be using the laser management company excimer laser. Few doctors can expect to do 500 PRK procedures annually, unless they operate within a group. For practitioners who simply want to offer PRK to their own patient base and are not interested in doing extensive marketing, a laser management

Table 19-9. Profit comparison: Individual vs. management company ($1500 patient fee)

	With own laser	With management company laser*
200 cases	−$65,000	+$ 80,000
400 cases	+$105,000	+$160,000
522 cases	+$208,700	+$208,800
600 cases	+$275,000	+$240,000
800 cases	+$445,000	+$320,000

*Assumes management company fee of $550 per case.

Table 19-10. Profit comparison: Group vs. management company ($1500 patient fee)

	With group-owned laser	With management company laser*
400 cases	+$ 5000	+$160,000
600 cases	+$175,000	+$240,000
744 cases	+$297,400	+$297,600
800 cases	+$345,000	+$320,000
1000 cases	+$515,000	+$400,000

*Assumes management company fee of $550 per case.

company or creation of a group partnership provides a reasonable opportunity to generate income and serve their own patients while minimizing financial risk.

The numbers are somewhat more positive for a laser operated by a group of ophthalmologists. The group must do more than 744 PRK procedures on the group's machine before the return is similar to what it would be using the laser management company laser. Although the group number may seem much more attainable than the individual number, the effort and aggravation associated with establishing and maintaining any partnership are difficult to quantify and should be carefully considered before pursuing this option, regardless of the potential return. The disclaimers concerning the assumptions used in calculating the costs also apply when considering establishing and operating a group PRK center.

One additional option that has not yet been discussed, but should become more common as a surplus of serviceable lasers reaches the market, is laser leasing. This option transfers much of the debt risk from the physician to the leasing company. If appropriate clauses and financial planning are in place to arrange for equipment upgrades and replacement, such arrangements can also serve as a hedge against technological obsolescence. At the time of this writing, excimer laser leasing is only available through one company. Availability of this option should increase with time, and laser leasing may provide physicians a cost-effective entrée into the business of laser refractive surgery in the future.

Access Alternatives

Several obvious options are available to ophthalmologists who wish to participate in PRK:

1. Buy your own excimer laser system.
2. Join with a group of ophthalmologists to purchase or lease a system.
3. Work for or obtain privileges at a laser-equipped hospital.
4. Affiliate with a group of optometrists who will help to purchase and support the laser through patient referrals.
5. Affiliate with an excimer laser center management company.

Your choices will depend on the market where you practice, the level of participation that you seek, the risk you are willing to assume, and the return you desire. Clearly, purchasing your own laser exposes you to the greatest risk. Beyond the obvious up-front investment, you will have the added worries that the technology may become outdated or that competitive forces will cannibalize your market before you can recover your costs. On the positive side, if things work out favorably, your reward could be substantial.

Each of the other options listed reduce your risk and your reward in some manner. Because most ophthalmologists are familiar with the traditional options mentioned, we will focus on the less traditional laser management and leasing companies.

Laser Center Companies

Laser center management companies offer plans that vary widely, require different levels of financial participation, impose different levels of constraint, and differ in how they reward the ophthalmologist. Because of these differences it is important that you ask the right questions when considering an affiliation with an excimer laser management company. Questions you need to ask include the following:

Does the excimer laser management company have the financial resources needed to make multiple purchases of laser systems, upgrade and maintain the systems, and market its services? What is the source of its funding, and will funding be available in the future?

A laser center management company must have the funds necessary to establish the business and to see it through slow growth and aggressive competition. If it does not have these resources, you could find yourself affiliated with a center that goes out of business. Ask the company to show you its financial statements, and learn how much cash they have available to fulfill their obligations. A single center requires well over $1 million to get up and running in a competitive market.

Does the company have an existing excimer laser center business?

There is a lot to be said for experience, particularly when it comes to managing a business that is very expensive to get into and requires extensive marketing experience to reach out to prospective patients effectively. Ask to tour the company's existing facilities.

What is the company's level of understanding of the industry and emerging technologies? Who else is affiliated with the company?

Find out if the principals have a background in eye care and the use of lasers. It is important that your partner have the ability and the connections needed to understand and react to changes in the industry. You want to be affiliated with a group that sees change coming and is proactive rather than reactive. Ask to see a list of ophthalmologists or institutions who are expected to play active roles in the company. Industry leaders, both individuals and institutions, tend to look before they leap, therefore, their participation is generally a good sign.

Does the company intend to do marketing from which you can benefit? Have they had experience marketing to refractive patients?

In many instances, marketing costs will exceed the cost of the laser. A significant marketing effort will be needed just to generate the patient flow needed to cover the fixed costs of a PRK center. Successful marketing to PRK patients usually requires a process of testing various approaches. If your partner has already gone through this costly process, it could mean more cash available for effective marketing in the future.

What excimer laser systems does the company currently use or intend to use? Can the company obtain access to the additional systems needed to meet future expansion plans?

The two laser manufacturers that are the leaders in the FDA approval race will produce a total of less than 250 systems in the first year after approval. With a very limited supply of FDA-approved lasers in the United States, it is critical that you understand exactly what type of purchase plan your new partner has. The companies listed later in this chapter collectively claim to be opening more than 600 centers in the United States alone, thus far outpacing projected patient demand and equipment production capacity, even without including systems that will be purchased by individual ophthalmologists. Lasers that are still years away from securing FDA approval will not do you much good if another group establishes a center in your area with an FDA-approved laser and gets a head start in marketing and providing PRK services in your market. Ask for evidence of a commitment from the laser manufacturer. Anyone can *claim* to be able to secure lasers—*getting* them in a timely fashion may be a problem.

How many centers does the company intend to open? Where will they be located?

Remember the old adage: If it sounds to good to be true, it probably is. If the company's plans are not realistic, you should think twice about working with it.

Does the company require a financial contribution from you or require you to use its centers for a specified period of time?

If you are required to make an up-front investment beyond the cost of training and certification, tread carefully. Any investment you make should be recouped by performing a few treatments. If not, you are no longer a user, you are now a partner, and your return should reflect that. There should be no need to commit yourself to a laser center for longer than 1 year. Long-term commitments sometimes lead to complacency. The center should expect to compete in the marketplace and adjust to the changing dynamics of your particular community. If it does not, you will want to have an escape clause.

Does the company provide PRK training programs and offer assistance with difficult cases?

Although many ophthalmologists find some of these courses repetitive, a well-thought-out plan should require physicians to hone their surgical skills and follow an established protocol, at least in the early years of commercial availability. Occasional problem cases will arise, and you will need to consult with experienced PRK providers on how to best proceed with postoperative care. Training and continuing assistance helps to ensure that you do not find yourself affiliated with a center that starts to generate poor results—and poor press—because no one is staying on top of quality control issues. An investment in training protects you and your business.

How will you make money through the center? What is the usage fee for the laser? What happens if price compression occurs?

You alone can determine whether the center's plan allows you the opportunity to make a reasonable fee for providing PRK services. The talk of fees in the $1500–2000 range sounds inviting, but $1200–1500 seems much more realistic. Make sure that the center's plan provides ample room for you to make money when the inevitable price compression occurs.

The following excimer laser center management companies (listed alphabetically) plan to provide PRK services in the United States. Regardless of your choice, a careful analysis is warranted before you make any decision on how to participate in providing PRK services. This list was compiled in early 1996 and represented the best information available at that time. Providers and their terms for participating are likely to change considerably over time. Do not rely on this data when making a decision to affiliate with a particular excimer laser center management company; rather, use it as a guide to help you make your initial contacts.

Beacon Eye Institute, Inc.   This Canadian-based company has opened its initial clinic in Toronto but plans to expand to every U.S. state. The company's plans emphasize the use of referrals from optometrists and guarantees that participating optometrists will provide the postoperative care to their patients. Ownership options are available. Call (817) 332-7590.

Equivision   This group intends to place lasers in 15 high-volume practices. Group headquarters are in Georgia. Some centers will provide comanagement opportunities. Call (404) 320-6111.

Excimer Vision Leasing   This is the first company to offer true laser leasing. The capital obligations of the lease are minimal, typically comprising only the sales tax on the equipment and a maintenance contract. Arrangements to ensure timely replacement of equipment at reasonable cost as technology advances are available. Physicians must agree to use the leased laser for a period of years. The company is based in Walnut Creek, California.

Global Vision, Inc.   This Florida-based company intends to locate its first U.S. centers in Texas and Florida. They presently operate in several international sites. The company plans to provide comanagement opportunities. Limited partnership ownership of centers is available. Call (800) 217-0876.

Laser Focus, Inc.   This Ohio-based company intends to open centers primarily in Midwestern towns with populations under 1 million. Physicians must agree to use only the company's centers for 4–5 years. Call (800) 246-4296.

LaserSight Centers   This publicly owned, Florida-based company is a laser manufacturer that operates 11 centers in China and intends to open centers in the United States. The company plans to operate mobile as well as fixed-site centers. The company will collect patient fees and pay the physician $500 to provide PRK services. Its mobile laser concept may require a separate FDA approval process. The company's own laser system is not likely to complete the FDA approval process before 1998 at the earliest. Call (803) 768-3505.

LaserVision Centers   This publicly owned, Missouri-based company operates 22 centers in Canada and Europe. The company currently operates a mobile laser in Canada and intends to operate similar units throughout the United States. Its mobile laser concept will require a separate FDA approval. The company intends to open more than 54 company-owned centers and 24 franchised centers. Physicians will pay the company for the use of its equipment and services. The company also has a nationwide agreement with Columbia/ HCA Health Care. Call (314) 434-6900.

New Image Centers   This Massachusetts-based company is owned and operated by Summit Technology, a publicly owned laser manufacturer. The company operates three centers in the United Kingdom and intends to operate in various U.S. markets. Call (617) 890-1234.

Sight Resources Corporation   This publicly traded, Massachusetts-based company owns Cambridge Eye Doctors, a chain of retail optical-optometric outlets in Massachusetts, and operates centers in New England and several other U.S. markets. Physicians will be able to use these centers to treat patients for a fee of $550 or send their own patients to be treated for $850 and provide the follow-up care themselves. Physicians must participate in the company's PRK training program. Call (800) 867-3387.

Refractive Laser Centers   This California-based company intends to open 20 centers in various markets. The company provides a shared-laser partnership with 10–15 physician partners at each site, each making an initial investment of $8000. Call (909) 621-9116.

Refractive Laser Managers   This California-based company provides management services and capitalization to laser surgery centers. General partners will join with limited partners (at $20,000 per share) at each center. Call (415) 382-8297.

The Laser Center, Inc. (TLC)   This Canadian-based company operates a center in Windsor, Ontario. The company intends to open two more Canadian sites and 45–50 centers in the United States, primarily in the Midwest. Each center will set its own fees. TLC plans most centers to have a dedicated surgeon paid by the company and will allow affiliated physicians to pay a user fee to perform their own surgeries. Call (800) 852-1033.

20/20 Laser Centers   This Maryland-based company initially intends to open three centers in the Washington, DC area. The company then intends to open centers in 10–15 U.S. cities by the end of 1997. The company will maintain 80% ownership of each center and make 20% available for equity partnerships. Physicians must participate in twice-yearly continuing medical education (CME) seminars. Call (301) 961-2020.

Vision America Laser Centers   This Tennessee-based company intends to open centers at existing Health Network and Omega Health Systems managed care sites. The company intends to open 50 sites in the United States. Partners will share the costs of establishing the centers. Call (901) 683-4169.

Vision Correction, Inc.   This Minnesota-based company operates mobile RK and automated lamellar keratoplasty (ALK) units. The company intends to operate 10 mobile PRK units and service approximately 100 surgeons in smaller Midwestern cities. The mobile laser concept will require a separate FDA approval. No up-front investment is required, but surgeons must complete training and CME programs offered by the company. Call (800) 824-7444.

Vision Correction Group (VCG)   This group, based in Georgia, intends to offer consulting advice to parties interested in opening laser centers in U.S. markets. Atlanta's Emory Vision Correction Center opened in early 1995 and is owned by VCG. Call (404) 248-4605.

Vision International   This North Carolina–based company operates four international centers and intends to open centers in the United States. Ophthalmologists can own up to 20% of each center. Call (910) 485-3432.

Marketing

As many potential PRK patients are young, healthy, and not under the care of an ophthalmologist, a significant percentage of PRK patients are likely to select a PRK provider based on advertising and promotion. For many ophthalmologists, PRK will represent the first time that they are truly required to market their practice.

You cannot market successfully unless you have a well-researched strategy that identifies the target market and has the appropriate mix of marketing techniques. Your particular approach will depend on how much you wish to expend on the effort and what you hope to achieve (i.e., how many treatments you hope to perform).

The first step of any successful marketing program is to identify the market segment that you need to target. For PRK, this would appear to be a simple process. Generally speaking, the PRK market consists of patients in their late twenties to late forties who are myopic, from −1 to −6 D with less than 1.5 D of astigmatism.

To do effective marketing, you need to learn which local marketing vehicles will serve your potential PRK patients best. Developing an appropriate marketing mix may be difficult and may involve a series of stops and starts before you find the right combinations. Your mix may include traditional paid advertising through television, radio, print, and direct mail; news releases and public relations; brochures and videos for use within your practice and at selected locations in the community; and making presentations to community groups in your area. Marketing is not limited to paid advertising, although there is a cost associated with every form of marketing that you undertake. However you reach your potential PRK patient, the message must be complemented with a call to action that makes it clear what the potential patient must do next.

Whatever the blend used, you should ensure that your marketing complies with the guidelines established by the American Society of Cataract and Refractive Surgery (ASCRS) and the Federal Trade Commission (FTC). The ASCRS guidelines offer guidance on specific issues related to advertising refractive surgery services, which are readily obtained by contacting the organization's national headquarters at 4000 Legato Drive, Fairfax, Virginia.

To market effectively, you need to fine-tune your message constantly. Without the right advertising message, the best-laid marketing plans can go awry. A compelling message tells something about you, who you are, and why the patient should put faith in you. The message is delivered in everything you do, from how the phone is answered in your office to the quality of your brochures and advertising.

Marketing really consists of two forms of communicating with patients: (1) the outbound communication represented in the message you send to patients in your advertising and collateral materials and (2) the inbound communication, which occurs when patients call you seeking information and advice. A good outbound message can be destroyed by a poor internal mechanism for responding to inquiries.

Once a potential refractive surgery patient first learns of the procedure, it generally takes 6–18 months for him or her to proceed with treatment. This period provides ample opportunity for the patient to lose interest or go elsewhere. With this kind of lead time, it is critical that your staff be properly trained to deal with inquiries and maintain interest in your services. As with many other things in life, the first impression is often the most important, so hone up on telephone skills and make sure that your staff does the same. Happy patients are the most effective marketing tool available, so make sure that you and your staff keep your patients happy.

Refractive surgery patients often have different needs when compared to the traditional patients of ophthalmic practices. The refractive surgery patient is young and healthy, whereas the typical ophthalmic patient is older and is not healthy. These differences not only affect your external marketing approach, they also affect internal marketing. Many successful RK providers have found it necessary to have separate appointment days for these two distinct groups. Whereas older, retired patients can more easily accept waiting room delays, younger refractive surgery patients will demand that you are prompt with your appointments. In fact, you may need to extend your hours to make your services more convenient to refractive surgery patients.

Marketing takes many forms, some easily recognizable and others less so. A clean, comfortable, well-appointed waiting area tells something about you that the patient will not get from an ad. Freshly painted walls do the same. Shabby, older finishes may not inspire confidence in your ability to provide modern laser surgery. Similarly, handsome personalized brochures can create a positive impression. As with the interior finishes of your office, a cheaply prepared brochure does not send the message that you must send to refractive surgery patients.

Several options are available for obtaining brochures and other collateral materials, such as videos. It is possible to create many of these materials yourself. A creative staff member or a local printer who has done work for you in the past may be a logical choice and offer a way of reducing your costs. Another alternative is to use one of the many companies that produce generic pieces that can be personalized. These companies advertise regularly in the professional journals. If you decide to work with a laser center management company, the company often offers promotional materials as an enticement to use its facilities.

Before you order materials, you must decide how you intend to use them. Brochures and collateral materials are always a good thing to have displayed in your office, but they can also be used more extensively. If you arrange to speak to local groups, it is important to have handouts available that reinforce your message. Some materials should be designed to be mailed out to anyone who calls your office requesting information. You may also want to do mailings to targeted groups in your community. If you have a dispensary in your practice, mailings can be directed to everyone in your database or to everyone who appears to be a good candidate. It is also possible to buy mailing lists that target particular groups within a specific market. These lists might be as specific as "everyone between 25 and 50 who wears contact lenses," or they may be as broad as you wish.

Brochures and collateral materials should support your larger marketing effort. At this early stage of public acceptance of PRK, marketing the service requires flexibility, creativity, and perseverance. Sending the wrong message will hurt any advertising campaign, but even the right message may not work if the target group is not hearing it often enough to encourage them to respond to your call to action. A successful campaign combines a good message with the right media outlets and the appropriate frequency of message to ensure that the message is heard. The typical refractive surgery patient needs to hear a radio ad as many as eight times before acting on it (i.e., calling your office).

Your choice in constructing a marketing plan will depend on your available resources. Again, PRK center management companies are likely to have deeper pockets and more options available to them but will exact a higher price from the physician for providing such services. Ultimately, you want to spend the least amount of money necessary to get your message to the highest number of qualified candidates for treatment. To accomplish this requires careful examination of the various media options in your market and the marketing alliances available to you.

Traditionally, radio and newspaper ads have been the most effective manner of attracting refractive surgery patients. Television can also generate results but requires a much heavier investment. As with radio and newspaper, you need frequency to get your message through on television. Infomercials can also be used, but be forewarned that the quality of a potential lead from this source declines dramatically depending on the time of day that the program airs.

An advertising program should be carefully constructed to meet the specific requirements of your practice and your market: No single program will work for everyone. Whatever mix of print and broadcast media you use, make sure your message is consistent and does not confuse the prospective patient. Generally, it is a good idea to target radio stations with the formats that have the highest number of listeners in the 25–50 age bracket (e.g., news stations, adult contemporary, sports). Sunday and Wednesday (coupon day) tend to be good days to buy newspaper space. In both instances you need to advertise with sufficient frequency and duration for the message to reach your audience.

Once your initial flight of ads is complete, you can back off and evaluate the response. Any good advertising program must include a way of measuring effectiveness in real terms, such as the cost of acquiring each lead. This cost should be tracked according to the advertising medium used. A truly efficient operation tracks leads for as long as 18 months because this is the time it often takes refractive surgery patients to decide to proceed with treatment. Throughout that time the prospect should receive periodic contact from you, keeping you fresh in the prospect's mind as the obvious choice for refractive surgery.

Finally, and perhaps most important, know your competition. If you have a market to yourself, you have very different advertising needs than if you are competing against other PRK providers. This is where creativity and flexibility are critical. If you find yourself in a marketing battle against a more heavily armed competitor, it may be time to rethink your strategy.

Patient Flow

For the vast majority of ophthalmologists participating in PRK, patient flow will not disrupt their existing practice.

Industry analyst Arthur D. Little Company projects that 1,438,000 PRK treatments will occur in the United States in the third year after FDA approval. Recent polls indicate that as many as 10,000 ophthalmologists intend to get involved in PRK. If these numbers are accurate, the average ophthalmologist will perform 144 procedures that year. This level of volume is far from sufficient to support the cost of a laser. Furthermore, the average is likely to be significantly less than these projections because a relatively small number of ophthalmologists and centers run by excimer laser management companies may perform a disproportionate share of the procedures because of their aggressive and well-funded marketing programs.

Many ophthalmologists will only participate in PRK to protect their existing patient base. For these participants, securing access to a laser through one of the laser center management companies or local hospital or surgicenter makes a great deal of sense.

For the small percentage of ophthalmologists who become high-volume PRK providers, access to an excimer laser and a good marketing campaign are only the beginning elements of a successful PRK practice. If patient volume indicates you may become a high-volume PRK provider, your office should be designed to allow you to realize that goal while providing the highest quality of care. You are now marketing to an enormous group of potential patients who have very little in common with your typical patient, who comes to you with some pathology.

Refractive surgery patients are younger and more likely to shop around. When prospective patients contact your office, you must be prepared. If you are not equipped to handle them in a professional manner, you run the risk of offending them or jeopardizing their faith in you as a provider. With the high cost of generating patients, you cannot afford to let this happen.

Your first major decision is formulating a "call to action" in your marketing campaign. Do you intend to have interested individuals call or show up at your office? If so, get ready to deal with peaks and lulls in activity that can frustrate both you and your staff. If your media campaign involves radio or television, you must be prepared to handle a large volume of calls whenever ads are run. This type of calling pattern can thoroughly disrupt your normal practice. Before purchasing ad space, think about the impact on your practice and the phone skills of your staff. Are your existing phone system and staffing sufficient to handle peak-time calling? The phone skills needed to deal with "retail" medicine may be quite different from the phone skills needed in your everyday practice.

Busy phone lines and frustrated staff not only cost you expensive PRK leads, they can also drive away traditional patients who are calling to schedule an appointment or secure prescriptions and other medical advice. This can be a real disaster for your existing practice. One alternative is to use telemarketing to ease the burden. Telemarketing can be provided by private companies who specialize in this. Because they charge you by the call and are not necessarily concerned with whether the call becomes a patient, this process can be expensive. On the other hand, this arrangement lets you test the effectiveness of your advertising without incurring the additional staff and systems required to establish your own in-house telemarketing operation. Your local marketing outlets should be able to give you a sense of typical response rates to different products. Once you get a sense of the response level, you can determine whether you are ready to bring the telemarketing service in-house. Whatever your choice, it is a cost you must absorb and cover with increased patient flow.

Understandably, few patients are ready to undergo PRK without first having the opportunity to ask questions or learn more about the procedure. For every 100 calls you receive seeking information on PRK, less than 30 people are likely to be sufficiently motivated to do anything more than receive your promotional literature. The remaining group may be interested in attending a seminar on PRK. Group seminars are obviously more efficient than individual sessions, but they also pose a greater risk because it only takes one unfortunate comment to turn off the entire group. Individual seminars give more of a traditional medical feel to the procedure, but these are time consuming. With either choice, you must factor in the time spent in these meetings when calculating your return on investment.

Professional "closers" can get a higher rate of seminar attendees to go forward with the procedure than most physicians may be able to accomplish. You should expect your rate to be significantly lower than that of salespeople, particularly in the first year or more when you are becoming familiar with the procedure and the questions that prospective patients are likely to ask. After the pent-up demand for PRK is addressed, the procedure will be marketed to an even broader group. Expect the percentage of callers who agree to attend your seminar and the percentage of attendees who move forward with the procedure to decline when this occurs.

In the end, the PRK patient you operate on represents at least 10 people who called your office seeking information. Your patient also represents a much larger group that you pay to advertise to but who, for whatever reason, do not respond to your message. For that reason, patient referrals are extremely important in keeping your marketing costs down. A happy patient will spread the word about your service and will do so at no cost to you, whereas patients driven by your marketing are extremely expensive. Physicians who send the most patients out into the community also reap the reward of having more unsolicited patients contacting their office. Because of this, high-volume refractive surgery providers actually have lower marketing costs per procedure. Word of mouth is by far the cheapest and most effective form of marketing.

Optometric Comanagement

If initial international experience with PRK and the U.S. experience with RK are any indication, optometry will not generate a large volume of PRK cases in the U.S. market.

When considering the impact that optometrists might have on patient flow, it is important to recognize how optometric practices work. The optometric business is extremely competitive, and there is generally little margin for error. In many ways, PRK represents a considerable risk to an optometrist. Because optometrists generally control the vision correction needs of entire families, it is critical that they provide service that does not put their relationship with the individual or family at risk.

If optometrists must speak to 20 patients before they generate one PRK referral and only stand to make a few hundred dollars in co-management fees on that patient, there is very little incentive for them to support PRK. With a similar expenditure of time, the optometrist could likely have generated considerably more income selling eyeglasses or contact lenses. You cannot expect to have optometrists sending you PRK patients unless you support them in their efforts. In the end, given the time and potential headaches, the financial reward from PRK may not be there for the optometrist.

In 1994, approximately 92.8 million Americans purchased eyewear. RK patients (about 150,000 people or 300,000 procedures) represented approximately 0.16% of that market. For an optometrist who sees 2500 patients per year, that translates to 4 RK patients a year. Even if PRK penetration of the market were double that of RK, the optometrist would generate 8 PRK patients per year. If you were able to put together a network of 10 optometrists (easier said than done), it would still generate only 80 patients per year. Regardless, the high cost of obtaining patients should make ophthalmologists think twice before discounting comanagement or any other direct route to patients with common refractive disorders.

Although many ophthalmologists are not interested in participating in PRK optometric comanagement networks, economic reality and time constraints may require it. The large number of relatively routine follow-up visits required by PRK are likely to make comanagement of patients a necessity. For high-volume PRK practices and center management companies, the required regimen of follow-up visits will make comanagement an absolute necessity. An established PRK provider who is treating 6 first eyes and 6 second eyes each week will, after 1 year, also be providing more than 50 follow-up visits each week. As the number of treatments grow, the follow-up requirements become even more overwhelming. For this reason alone, high-volume ophthalmologists and PRK centers should consider co-management arrangements that allow them to maximize time spent in more productive pursuits.

Comanagement can work for you, but you must remember its limitations. Comanagement takes another slice out of a refractive surgery pie that is already being asked to feed many different interests (e.g., laser costs, surgical fee, marketing, support staff). If optometric partners are able to generate patients, they may demand a bigger slice of the pie and they will certainly be susceptible to enticing offers from your competitors. Although a good and trustworthy comanagement partner can allow you to pursue more lucrative or stimulating work, a bad partner can increase your liability and your headaches. A well-established protocol for follow-up visits is essential, but prior thorough assessment of your prospective partner is even more critical.

Will comanagement of PRK patients work for you? That depends on your market, your history of interaction with optometrists, the time you have to support them, and the economic needs of optometrists in your area. For some individual ophthalmologists, comanagement can work, but in the majority of cases it will not work for either the ophthalmologist or the optometrist.

Medicolegal Considerations

Legal and regulatory issues will also affect your decision on if, when, and how to participate in PRK. A complicated maze of laws and regulations apply. This section highlights several potential legal issues. Of course, you should seek legal counsel and carefully scrutinize PRK investment, ownership, employment, and affiliation opportunities. Because many of the applicable laws vary from state to state, there is no uniform model of PRK participation and, after a legal review, you may have to reconsider your preferred option from among those discussed above, under Access Alternatives. *You should be wary about affiliating with an excimer laser management company that is shopping the same model to physicians in different markets.*

As a threshold issue, if you are planning to perform procedures such as LASIK, which falls outside the sphere of FDA-approval, you must be aware of the commercialization and marketing restrictions applicable to advertising off-label uses of medical devices, such as the excimer laser. You do not want to become involved in activities that will attract the attention of the FDA and the Federal Trade Commission.

Corporate Practice of Medicine

Many states adhere to a legal doctrine known as the "corporate practice of medicine." In the interest of ensuring that the physician is the party making medical decisions, application of the doctrine essentially prohibits business corporations from employing physicians or exercising undue control over their practices. The corporate practice of medicine doctrine may limit your ability to accept employment with or participate at a laser center owned and operated by non-physicians. To comply with the doctrine, the laser center company may have to turn over the "reins" of the practice to the participating physicians and recover its return on investment through fees received under a management services arrangement. If you are planning to enter into a joint venture with an excimer laser center management company to develop a laser center, the corporate practice of medicine laws could limit your ability to share the financial risk of practice operations with your venture partners. In performing "due diligence," it is incumbent on *you* to ascertain whether the company is overreaching these laws, as you may be liable for essentially delegating your responsibilities to a corporate partner.

Like the corporate practice of medicine doctrine, several state laws prohibit the corporate practice of optometry. These laws may affect how you affiliate with optometrists in providing PRK services. You may not be able to employ optometrists directly and instead may need to consider independent contractor relationships. You should also question the proposed arrangements of business corporations that promise to line up a network of optometrists, on your behalf, to provide referrals and render pre- and postoperative care. The corporate practice of optometry laws may, as a practical matter, limit how much control such corporations can actually exercise over network optometrists and hence fortify a stream of patient referrals to your practice.

Regulation of the Laser Center

You should realize that a license may be needed for use of the excimer laser at its intended location. Many states require a nonhospital facility housing a laser to obtain an ambulatory surgery center license. Complying with licensure requirements can be time consuming and costly. In many states, the facility would have to be equipped with a full operating room suite and capable of administering general anesthesia, even though these requirements are inapplicable to PRK. Most states have an exception from facility licensure requirements for physician's offices. However, *the availability of the physician's office exemption may depend on whether regulators deem PRK to be surgery, an answer that still varies from state to state.* If you are trying to fit within a physician's office exemption, *your ability to share the laser with physicians from other practice locations may be limited.* To the extent that licensure requirements are not burdensome, you should consider voluntarily seeking licensure for the laser treatment clinic because this may essentially provide you with "grandfathered" protection from future changes in state law and, on a current basis, with something akin to a franchise in your area.

Securing a license is a matter of perseverance and money. Related to the question of licensure is whether a CON will be required for use of the excimer laser at its intended location; obtaining a CON can be costly and time consuming, and certain states have implemented CON moratoriums for surgical centers in "oversupplied markets." Like the licensure laws, most states exempt physician's offices from CON requirements. If you intend to avail yourself of such an exemption, however, you must be careful to stay within the regulatory parameters. *For example, sharing the laser with physicians from other offices who are not members of your group practice, charging other physicians a user's fee to have access to the laser, or billing patients a facility fee could lead to loss of the office exemption and trigger CON review.* In addition, a CON is often required for the purchase of major medical equipment. In most states, the purchase price of the laser would likely fall below the expenditure thresholds for CON review, but you should be familiar with your state's requirements before making a commitment to proceed with developing a laser center.

Organizational Structure

If you plan on participating in PRK in some type of joint venture because of issues of cost control or the possibility of ultimately selling what might be an appreciating asset, a choice will have to be made as to the appropriate organizational structure. You should consider whether the joint venture will be organized as a business corporation, professional corporation, limited liability company, or other type of entity. If you are seeking other physicians to make an investment stake in the joint venture, you will also need to check whether offerings need to comply with state or federal securities registration requirements; typically, involving more than 25–35 investors places you in the position of possibly having to register an offering in the entity as a security.

Billing

Another critical issue is whether your proposed billing arrangements and allocation of PRK revenues comply with state fee-splitting laws. Certain states have fee-splitting statutes that are intended to prohibit agreements to divide fees in exchange for patient referrals. Such laws were not passed with modern health care delivery arrangements in mind, and they can present significant obstacles to your business plans. For example, your state's fee-splitting statute may prohibit charging the PRK patient a flat global fee covering your services and the services of optometrists for pre- and postoperative care. Moreover, fee-splitting laws may limit your ability to share PRK revenue with corporate partners or other joint ventures on a percentage basis. *As a general rule, whoever provides the service should collect payment directly from the patient for the services provided.*

Referrals and Comanagement

Antikickback issues are likely to arise because, in an increasingly competitive environment, ophthalmologists feel pressured to secure referrals of PRK patients from optometrists. Because PRK will not initially be covered by Medicare or Medicaid, *the federal antikickback statute will likely not apply* so long as you are not involved in an arrangement that involves the bundling of PRK with other Medicare- or Medicaid-covered services. However, state antikickback laws may still apply. You should be cautious about entering into any arrangements, express or covert, with an optometrist (or referring ophthalmologist) whereby patients are referred to your practice for PRK in return for your promise to send the patients back to the referring provider for the economic benefit of providing postoperative care. While you may plan and expect to send a patient back to a referring provider for a substantial component of the postoperative care after PRK, this decision must be a medical one and should remain the choice of the operating surgeon and the patient. Where an optometrist or a referring ophthalmologist is providing pre- or postoperative services (e.g., from the United States to a Canadian surgeon), the portion of the global fee that he or she receives should be commensurate with the fair market vaiue of the services delivered; any excess payment above fair market value or amount billed to the patient can be inferred to be in exchange for the referral of the patient.

Comanagement arrangements with optometrists should also be carefully considered from a legal standpoint. Although a few state medical boards take the position that only physicians may provide postsurgical care for PRK, in most states there are no express prohibitions on physicians and optometrists coordinating care of the PRK patient before and after surgery. Nevertheless, comanagement agreements should be structured so that they are not perceived as simply referral and fee-splitting schemes. *Coordination of services for providing quality of care should be the prime consideration in such arrangements; you must trust that increased revenues will naturally follow.* Protocols should be developed to cover postoperative care, including details as to how complications are identified and reported and if or when the patient should be referred back to the physician.

Malpractice

You should give some consideration to the increased malpractice liability exposure in performing PRK. Because the procedure is elective (unlike cataract surgery) and the patient pays for it out of his or her own pocket, the patient's expectations will be higher, and because the patient is likely younger and employed, any bad result could mean that the patient will suffer higher economic damages. As such, physicians performing PRK are at increased risk for malpractice liability and higher awards to the patient for economic loss. This liability risk may be compounded if you are entering into comanagement arrangements with optometrists or referring physicians because you may be held jointly liable for the malpractice of your comanagement partners. Securing informed consent is imperative, and this means a comprehensive and meticulously documented discussion of the risks associated with the procedure, including plain and simple disappointing results in terms of improved visual activity. You should consult with your insurance carrier to ensure that you have appropriate coverage. Moreover, as the FDA requires that credentialling standards for physicians performing PRK, you should complete appropriate training courses.

Refractive Surgery in a Changing Health Care Delivery System

Comprehensive health care reform in the United States met its demise when the Republicans took over Congress in the 1994 elections. However, Congressman Newt Gingrich and the Republican leadership remain committed to a number of health system reforms, which, if enacted, could affect the ophthalmologist's decision whether to move forward with practicing PRK.

1. Under all legislative plans, Medicare as a fee-for-service program will be preserved, *but* with gargantuan cutbacks in provider and physician payment rates. As such, you may be able to maintain a fee-for-service practice because many ophthalmologists primarily treat the elderly. On the other hand, looking at gradually phasing into some non–government-payable services would appear to make sense.
2. Managed care is an increasingly common part of the health care system, and any type of health care reform will only promote it. Just as ophthalmologists are competing, so are the myriad of HMOs and other managed care plans struggling to distinguish their products and attract patients. Just as basic vision (and dental) care has become a virtual "standard benefit" in many managed care plans, it is not inconceivable that the offering of refractive surgery, or more specifically, PRK, may represent such a distinguishing benefit, at least as part of a supplemental plan.
3. Congress will ultimately mandate that insurance programs offer a "standard benefits package." To the extent that supplemental in-

surance plans with separate premiums (like vision plans) are also regulated, this could affect, favorably or adversely, the offering of refractive surgery services to managed care patients.

4. There are few places in which to find revenues to pay for any element of health care reform. Taxing high-option health care plans, which might provide services beyond the standard benefits package, including refractive surgery, may be a revenue-raising option. Changes in tax law affect your patient's willingness to undergo these procedures but, at present, it is still allowable to use funds from medical savings accounts to pay for refractive surgery.

5. Malpractice reform will occur. Will Congress bite the bullet and impose limits on noneconomic damages? If so, the malpractice risks of refractive surgery discussed above could be significantly ameliorated.

Summary

Continued technological advances, coupled with the public's preference for laser technology procedures, may make PRK the preferred refractive surgery choice for many but not all patients. It is up to ophthalmologists to ensure that their individual circumstances, including the economic incentives surrounding the use of the various refractive surgery practices, do not take precedence over the best interests of their patients.

PRK has been touted as having a potentially huge market, with positive ramifications for patients and ophthalmologists throughout the United States. As with the introduction of any new procedure, there is a risk that fighting within the profession or misleading advertising by the industry could destroy the market before it has the opportunity to flourish. It will be difficult, if not impossible, in the absence of careful and comprehensive outcomes and analysis, for the government, media, and consumer to differentiate between one procedure (PRK) and another (RK), and good surgeons from less qualified doctors.

It is critically important that mechanisms be established to provide ophthalmologists with easy access to excimer lasers as well as training programs that will ensure that patients receive only the highest quality refractive surgical care. There are opportunities for ophthalmologists to participate in PRK at every level, from employee to independent contractor to investor to sponsor. This flexibility should be good news for all ophthalmologists and their patients.

Bibliography

Arons JJ: PRK: There's gold at the end of the rainbow. *Ocular Surg News* 13:42–43, 1995.

Filiano G: PRK Centers on Rise. *Vision Monday* 9(1):1, January 9, 1995.

Fourteen firms gearing up to market PRK. *AOA News* 33:14, 1994.

Hawks TF, Moretti M: Laser surgery. *Optom Manage* 30:24–33, 1995.

Kezirian GM: A rational way to plan for PRK. *Rev Ophthalmol* 2:42–45, 1995.

Lee J: Excimer lasers: How to access one. *Rev Ophthalmol* 2:47–50, 1995.

Moretti M: PRK center companies court optometrists. *Ocular Surgery News* 13:39–40, 1995.

Murphy R: How to evaluate PRK referral centers. *Rev Optom* 131:41–46, 1994.

Appendixes

A Comparison Tables of Available Photorefractive Laser Systems

Wide-field lasers

Advantages
Shorter operating time (< 30 sec)
Eye tracking and scanning not needed (optional)
Easy myopia and astigmatism correction
Further along in U.S. Regulatory Process (Summit = VISX > Technolas)

Disadvantages
High-output pulse energy needed
Good beam uniformity needed
Hyperopia correction more difficult
Higher incidence of steep central islands

Manufacturer model/ name	Summit Apex and Apex Plus	VISX Star [20/20B]	Technolas Keracor 116	Coherent-Schwind Keratom
Distributor	Summit Technologies, Inc. (Waltham, MA)	VISX Inc. (Santa Clara, CA)	Chiron Vision Corp. (Irvine, CA)	Coherent Medical, Inc. (Palo Alto, CA)
Installation considerations				
Dimension (cm) $L \times W \times H$	$165 \times 69 \times 186$	$204 \times 110 \times 150$ [$271 \times 84 \times 141$]	$220 \times 130 \times 200$	$202 \times 145 \times 153$
Weight (kg)	660	726 [955]	600	700
Electrical requirements	110 V, 15 amp, 60 Hz; or 220 V, 10 amp, 50 Hz	220 V, 1 phase, 30 amp	220 V, 1 phase, 16 amp	230 V, 1 phase, 16 amp, 3.5 kW (max)
Gas cylinder requirements	2 cylinders ArF premix, N_2	2 cylinders ArF premix, He [ArF, He, liquid N_2]	1 cylinder ArF premix	1 cylinder ArN_2, (self-contained halogen generator)
Instrumentation				
Laser cooling system	Internal water-cooled	Internal water-cooled [air-cooled]	Internal water and air-cooled	Air-cooled
Computer system	Fixed microchip	IBM PC: embedded [external]	IBM PC: external	IBM PC
Delivery system microscope	Zeiss operating microscope	Leica Wild operating microscope [Moller]	Zeiss operating microscope	Moller-Wedel operating microscope
Delivery system optics	7 (4 lenses, 3 mirrors)	9 (3 mirrors, 6 lenses/ prisms), [6 mirrors, 3 lenses]	7 (3 mirrors, 4 lenses)	8 (3 mirrors, 4 lenses, 1 integrator)

Continued

Wide-field lasers (*continued*)

Manufacturer model/ name	Summit Apex and Apex Plus	VISX Star (20/20B)	Technolas Keracor 116	Coherent-Schwind Keratom
Instrumentation (*cont.*)				
Laser beam homogenization	None	Rotating prism plus spatial integrator	Optical integrator, beam wobble (oscillation)	Prismatic integrator, telescopic zoom
Beam shaping	Iris and ablatable mask, "emphasis laser disc"	Iris and slit	Iris with beam scanning	Band with patterned or "fractal mask" apertures
Evacuation system	None	Vacuum nozzle aspirator	Suction ring (optional)	Circumferential laminar flow vacuum
Patient fixation system	Coaxial LED within illuminated ring	Single coaxial LED	Single coaxial red laser diode	Blinking coaxial laser diode
Tracking system	None	Under development (none)	Active-infrared tracking on pupil	"Passive" eye tracking
Pulse width	10 nsec	20 nsec	12 nsec	23 nsec
Working distance	17 cm	13.3 cm [9 cm]	13 cm	28 cm
Preparation				
Gas fill	Every day or after 15–20 patients	Every 3–4 days [1–2 days]	Every 10–20 patients	Every 2 weeks
Energy calibration	Internal feedback loop optional gelatin film ablation	Internal joulemeter plus ablation depth	Fluence test plate of foil overlying red plastic (65 pulses = 130 mJ/cm^2)	Internal energy monitor with feedback, fluence sensor with film ablation
Homogeneity check	PMMA profilometry	Calibration card quality plus BIP	Fluence test plate	Film (Wratten filter) ablation
Refractive check	None	Lensometry of calibration card ablation	None	PMMA platelet ablation (periodically sent to company)
Operator adjustment	None	Auto adjustment based on lens ablation reading	Keyboard adjustment of voltage alternator on number of pulses through foil	Reprogramming based on pulses for perforation of film

Procedure				
Eye fixation	Patient self-fixation	Patient fixation	Patient self-fixation	Patient self-fixation
Surgeon alignment	2 HeNe laser spots on either side of pupil	Virtual image reticle [optical reticle]	Red coaxial laser diode and angled green HeNe laser on cornea	2 HeNe laser spot alignment on cornea
Ablation time (−5 D correction)	25 seconds	25 seconds [40 seconds]	19–26 seconds	25 seconds
Treatment parameters				
Spot size (maximum)	6.5 mm (9.5 mm hyperopia)	6.5 mm [6.0 mm]	7.0 mm	8.0 mm
Pulse energy	60 mJ/pulse	53 mJ/pulse [45 mJ/pulse]	50 mJ/pulse	75 mJ/pulse
Energy density ("fluence")	180 mJ/cm^2	160 mJ/cm^2	130 mJ/cm^2	150 to 220 mJ/cm^2 (variable)
Ablation pulse rate	10–20 Hz	10 Hz [6 Hz]	10 Hz	10 Hz (1–30 Hz programmable)
Transition zone	Within 6.5 mm	Up to 8 mm [none]	Aspheric up to 7.0 mm	9.0 mm
Cost				
System purchase	$500,000–$533,000	$525,000 in U.S.	$450,000	$390,000–$520,000
Annual service contract	$40,000–$50,000	$52,500 (including optics)	$40,000	$30,000
Treatment capability (U.S. trial status)				
Myopic PRK	Expanding iris or ablatable mask	Expanding iris	Expanding iris	Band with a series of circular masks or fractal mask
Astigmatic PRK	Ablatable mask	Expanding iris and slit	Expanding iris with meridianal scanning beam	Band with a series of elliptic mask or fractal mask
Hyperopic PRK	Axicon and ablatable mask	Variable rotating slit with eccentric lens	Expanding iris with annular scanning beam	Band with a series of alternating half annular mask or fractal mask
PTK	Open iris, 1.0- to 6.5-mm circle for smoothing	Open iris and/or slit, 0.6- to 6.0-mm circle or slit for smoothing	Open iris, 0.8- to 7.0-mm circle with joystick for smoothing	Large 11.0-mm diameter mask, 0.6- to 8.0-mm circle for smoothing

Scanning-slit lasers

Advantages
Moderate pulse energy output
Excellent beam uniformity
Low incidence of steep central islands

Disadvantages
Moderately longer operating time
Eye tracking or fixation more important
Eye-based mask cumbersome (Meditec)

Manufacturer model/name	Nidek EC-5000	Meditec MEL 60
Distributor	Nidek, Inc. (Freemont, CA)	Aesculap-Meditec (Heroldsberg, Germany)
Installation considerations		
Dimension (cm) L × W × H	$137 \times 75 \times 152$	$270 \times 142 \times 150$ ($172 \times 58 \times 150$, laser only)
Weight (kg)	650	607 (450, laser only)
Electrical requirements	208 V, 1 phase, 15 amp, 50/60 Hz	230 V, 1 phase, 20 amp, 50 Hz
Gas cylinder requirements	3 cylinders ArF premix, N_2, He	1 cylinder ArF premix, N_2
Instrumentation		
Laser cooling system	Air-cooled	Air-cooled
Computer system	IBM PC	Microcomputer (Z 80-180)
Delivery system microscope	Zeiss operating microscope	Moller-Wedel operating microscope
Delivery system optics	11 (9 mirrors, 2 lenses)	7 (4 mirrors, 3 lenses/prisms)
Laser beam homogenization	Scanning and rotating broad band	Scanning slit
Beam shaping	Iris and slit	Rotating mask
Evacuation system	Aspiratory within optional suction cup	Vacuum aspiration in mask
Patient fixation system	Single coaxial LED	Single coaxial filament
Tracking system	Active eye tracking (optional)	None
Pulse width	17 nsec	15 nsec
Working distance	17.5 cm	10 cm
Preparation		
Gas fill	Once each week	Every day (6–8 patients)
Energy calibration	Internal joulemeter	Internal joulemeter with test foil ablation
Homogeneity check	None	Aluminum test foil with red base

Refractive check	Ablation PMMA lens (−3.0 D)	None
Operator adjustment	Reprogramming based on lens ablation reading	Adjustment of fluence till red is apparent on ninth pass of slit
Procedure		
Eye fixation	Patient or mechanical	Mechanical fixation
Surgeon alignment	2 slit and 1 diode laser spot alignment on cornea	Hand piece and mask alignment
Ablation time (−5 D correction)	27.2 seconds (4 scans/sec)	90 seconds
Treatment parameters		
Spot size (maximum)	9.0 mm achieved by 9 × 2-mm band	7.0–9.0 mm achieved by 9 × 1.5-mm slit
Pulse energy	25 mJ/pulse	33 mJ/pulse
Energy density ("fluence")	140 mJ/cm^2	250 mJ/cm^2
Ablation pulse rate	0.5–5 scans/sec (5–50 Hz)	1/2 scan/sec (20 Hz)
Transition zone	9.0 mm	9.0 mm
Cost		
System purchase	$440,000	$400,000 (US: $450,000 includes gas and maintenance for clinical trials)
Annual service contract	$40,000 ($17,000 limited service)	$35,000
Treatment capability		
Myopic PRK	Expanding iris with scanning and rotating beam	Rotating hourglass mask aperture
Astigmatic PRK	Expanding iris and slit with scanning and rotating beam	Variably rotating hourglass mask aperture
Hyperopic PRK	Expanding iris with scanning and eccentric rotating beam	Rotating inverse hourglass mask aperture (none)
PTK	Large-diameter scanning, methylcellulose for smoothing	Open iris or rectangle, 0.5- to 9.0-mm spot for smoothing

Flying-spot lasers

Advantages
Small energy output
Spot placement can be custom designed
Easy myopic and hyperopic correction
Solid-state laser (Novatec) avoids using toxic gases

Disadvantages
Active tracking system required
Longest operating time
Clinical data limited to date
Maintenance of solid-state laser optics unknown (Novatec)

Manufacturer model/name	LaserSight Compak-200	Autonomous T-PRK	Novatec LightBlade
Distributor	LaserSight, Inc. (Orlando, FL)	CIBA/Autonomous Technologies Corp. (Orlando, FL)	Novatec Laser Systems, Inc. (Carlsbad, CA)
Installation considerations			
Dimension (cm) L × W × H	67 × 46 × 113 (laser only)	231 × 160 × 130	145 × 66 × 120
Weight (kg)	136	273	550
Electrical requirements	110 V, 1 phase, 10 amps, 60 Hz or 220 V, 5 amps, 50 Hz	120 V, 1 phase, 5–15 amps	208 V, 3 phase, 50 amps, 15 kW
Gas cylinder requirements	2 cylinders: ArF premix, H_2 or N_2	1 cylinder: ArF premix	None (solid state)
Instrumentation			
Laser cooling system	Air-cooled	Air-cooled	Water-cooled
Computer system	IBM PC	IBM-compatible PC	Internal IBM PC
Delivery system microscope	Topcon operating microscope	Zeiss operating microscope	Zeiss OPM-1 operating microscope
Delivery system optics	5 (1 attenuator, 1 lens, 3 mirrors)	13 (3 lenses, 9 mirrors, 9 output window)	N/A
Laser beam homogenization	Overlapping spot placement	Overlapping spot placement	Overlapping spot placement
Beam shaping	None	None	None
Evacuation system	Air blowing	Vacuum suction hose	None
Patient fixation system	Single coaxial LED	Single blinking coaxial red LED	Single red HeNe laser
Tracking system	Active eye tracking (optional)	Active eye tracking (LADAR Vision)	Active eye tracking
Pulse width	2.5 nsec	25 nsec	N/A
Working distance	10 cm (15 cm optional for LASIK)	20 cm	12.5 cm
Preparation			
Gas fill	Every day	Every few days to 1 week	None
Energy calibration	External joulemeter	Ablation of material to verify energy distribution	Internal joulemeter

Homogeneity check	None	None	None
Refractive check	Ablation PMMA test block	Ablation of a known pattern to confirm the calibration factor	PTK ablation of PMMA for depth confirmation
Operator adjustment	Manual adjustment of attenuator	Calibration factor adjustment by input to computer	Calibration adjustment for depth > 5% from intended by input to computer
Procedure			
Eye fixation	Patient self-fixation	Patient self-fixation	Patient self-fixation
Surgeon alignment	2 diode laser spots aligned on inferior limbus	Eye tracker aligned on center of pupil mark	3 crossed HeNe laser beams on cornea
Ablation time (−5 D correction 6 mm zone)	30–40 seconds	100 seconds (20 sec/D)	60 seconds
Treatment parameters			
Spot size (maximum)	3.0 to 9.0 mm achieved by 0.8- to 1.0-mm spot	10.0 mm achieved by a 1-mm spot	10.0 mm achieved by 300- to 500-μm spot
Pulse energy	0.9–1.1 mJ/pulse	0.9–1.6 mJ/pulse	0.1–0.2 mJ/pulse
Energy density ("fluence")	160–180 mJ/cm^2	180 mJ/cm^2	100 mJ/cm^2
Ablation pulse rate	5 mJ/pulse (100 Hz)	100 Hz	> 200 Hz
Transition zone	Up to 9 mm	Peripheral blend zone up to 10 mm	Up to 10 mm
Cost			
System purchase	$300,000–350,000	N/A (not yet determined)	$396,000
Annual service contract	$40,000	N/A (not yet determined)	$25,000 (after first year)
Treatment capability			
Myopic PRK	Scanning spot	Spherical: nonsequential scanning spot	Opening and closing circular scanning spot
Astigmatic PRK	Scanning spot along flattest meridian (myopic astigmatism)	Elliptical: nonsequential scanning spot	Linear meridianal scanning spot or elliptical scanning spot
Hyperopic PRK	Scanning spot in annular pattern from 5 to 9 mm	Annular: nonsequential scanning spot	Annular spiral scanning spot
PTK	Scanning spot	Uniform: nonsequential scanning spot	Symmetric or asymmetric scanning spot based on topographic difference map of actual and ideal surface

B Office Essentials

The following forms are included to guide the reader in establishing a systematic process in the office for preoperative data collection, informed consent, and surgical planning and reporting. Because excimer PRK is an elective procedure performed on healthy eyes of healthy patients, it is of the utmost importance to thoroughly screen for all risk factors that might result in a suboptimal outcome, to provide patients with full disclosure during the informed consent process, and to establish a system of meticulous surgical record-keeping to minimize the chance of clerical errors that may become surgical mistakes.

To this end, we have included samples of forms used to facilitate thorough, efficient patient evaluation and surgical planning. These documents may be used as guides and adapted or updated with the advice of your own attorney to meet your specific needs.

Phone Questionnaire

Patient name: _____

Age: _____ Patient telephone # (Home): _____ (Work): _____

Address: _____

_____

_____

Patient's glasses prescription: Right eye: _____

Left eye: _____

Primary ophthalmologist or optometrist: _____

Does patient wear contact lenses   YES/NO   If YES, what kind: HARD/
GAS PERMEABLE/SOFT

_____ For soft contact lens wear, patient must remove contacts at least 2 weeks
prior to laser surgical evaluation appointment.

_____ For hard or gas permeable contact lens wear, patient must remove
contacts at least 3 weeks prior to laser surgical evaluation appointment.

Appointment date (if made): _____ With: _____

Interviewer: _____ Information Sent: YES/NO

Follow-up Call

Date: _____ Was information received: YES/NO

Additional questions or comments: _____

_____

_____

_____

_____

Appointment made: YES/NO   When: _____ With: _____

Interviewer: _____

Name: _____

Date: _____

Referred by: _____

Preoperative Examination for Photorefractive Keratectomy

Age: **Occupation:**

Refractive history:

❏refraction has changed ≤ 0.5 diopters per year

_____

_____

_____

Contact lens history:

❏contact lenses removed 2 weeks prior to exam for soft or 3 weeks for rigid

_____

_____

_____

Past ocular history: N Y

ocular surface disease	❏ ❏	_____
HZO/HSV keratitis	❏ ❏	_____
glaucoma	❏ ❏	_____
keratoconus	❏ ❏	_____
ocular surgery	❏ ❏	_____
corneal warpage	❏ ❏	_____
uveitis	❏ ❏	_____
severe dry eye	❏ ❏	_____
diabetic retinopathy	❏ ❏	_____
retinal disease	❏ ❏	_____
lagophthalmos	❏ ❏	_____
other	❏ ❏	_____

Current Medications

❏none

_____   _____

_____   _____

Family history: N Y

keratoconus	❏ ❏	_____
glaucoma	❏ ❏	_____
cataract	❏ ❏	_____
other	❏ ❏	_____

Past medical history: N Y

allergies	❏ ❏	_____
autoimmune disease	❏ ❏	_____
diabetes mellitus	❏ ❏	_____
pregnant	❏ ❏	_____
thyroid disease	❏ ❏	_____
keloid formation	❏ ❏	_____
other	❏ ❏	_____

V$_{sc}$〈   J$_{sc}$〈   V$_{cc}$〈   J$_{cc}$〈   W———

M————   Cycloplegic ————

K ———— Mires: ❏regular & sharp
                    ❏irregular

Central pachymetry: OD ___
                              OS ___

Topography ————

❏check here if topography not performed

Ocular dominance   Pupils ____ mm in light ____mm in dark
    ❑right
    ❑left

Motility *check if normal*   Tension
    ❑OD   ❑OS   ❑OU
                                    ❑applanation
External examination   ❑normal   ❑pneumotonometery
                                                ❑air-puff

Slit lamp exam   *check if normal*

lids	❑OD	❑OS	❑OU ____
conjunctiva and sclera	❑OD	❑OS	❑OU ____
cornea	❑OD	❑OS	❑OU ____
anterior chamber	❑OD	❑OS	❑OU ____
iris	❑OD	❑OS	❑OU ____
lens	❑OD	❑OS	❑OU ____

Dilated fundus exam

      check if normal

disc	❑OD	❑OS	❑OU
macula	❑OD	❑OS	❑OU
periphery	❑OD	❑OS	❑OU
vitreous	❑OD	❑OS	❑OU

Patient Education

❑ Monovision option discussed and understood by patient

❑ Risks including overcorrection, undercorrection, need for reoperation, surface or intraocular infection, glare, haloes, fluctuating vision, long-term unpredictability, and glaucoma were discussed with patient who expresses understanding

❑Alternatives including LASIK, ALK, RK, were discussed as were the inherent safety of spectacles and contact lenses with patient who expresses understanding

❑ The patient understands that substantial post-operative discomfort is likely to persist for several days following the procedure

❑ Patient has seen video

❑ The above risks and the potential for other risks that cannot be enumerated or fully anticipated were reviewed in detail with the patient and family. Benefits and alternatives were reviewed. Elective nature of surgery was emphasized. Questions were answered in full and at length. The patient expresses understanding and wishes to proceed with refractive surgery.

❑ Patient has signed informed consent

Impression:_____

Plan: _____

INFORMED CONSENT FOR LASER VISION CORRECTION

This information is being provided to me so that I can make an informed decision about having laser vision correction (LVC) to correct my nearsightedness (myopia).

NATURE OF THE PROCEDURE: In laser vision correction (LVC), laser light is used to reshape the cornea (the clear front surface of the eye). The laser light is passed through an aperture called an iris diaphragm that opens progressively using the laser treatment, thus shaping the laser beam to correct any nearsightedness. The laser reshapes the cornea by removing a thin layer of tissue from the cornea to reduce or eliminate nearsightedness (myopia).

EXPECTED BENEFIT: The goal of LVC is to reduce the level of nearsightedness to provide much better uncorrected vision without eyeglasses or contact lenses. Excellent uncorrected vision cannot be guaranteed.

ALTERNATIVE TREATMENTS: I understand that the alternative of LVC for obtaining useful vision include eyeglasses or contact lenses. Either option can provide excellent vision. Other alternatives include radial kera-totomy (RK) or laser in-situ keratomileusis (LASIK).

Like all surgical procedures, LVC is not absolutely safe. Most complications are rare, temporary, or mild. I understand that this is an elective procedure and that PRK surgery is not reversible.

I understand that the following are **POSSIBLE COMPLICATIONS OF LVC:**

UNDERCORRECTION OR OVERCORRECTION: I understand that it is not possible to predict how my eye will respond to this procedure. As a result, I may not achieve acceptable vision without glasses. It is possible I may still need eyeglasses after this procedure to obtain good vision because of residual nearsightedness or astigmatism. In many cases, but not all, an enhancement procedure can be done. It is also possible that I might be overcorrected, resulting in farsightedness. If I am farsighted, I may need eyeglasses for close as well as far viewing.

PRESBYOPIA: I understand that presbyopia is an aging change to the internal focusing structures of the eye that causes people to need bifocals or reading glasses starting in their late 30s or early 40s. LVC does not affect the ability of the eye to change its focus. I understand that if I need bifocals or reading glasses now, I will still need them after this procedure. I understand that if I do not wear reading glasses now, I will most likely need them eventually as I age.

DECREASE OF BEST CORRECTED VISION: I understand that after LVC, some patients find that their vision, even with the best possible eyeglass correction, is not as good as it was before the procedure with eyeglasses on. This can occur as a result of irregular tissue removal or the development of corneal haze. I understand that there is a remote chance of partial or complete loss of vision in the eye that has had PRK.

LONG-TERM CHANGES: I understand that my eyes may change over time, resulting in a decline in my vision and increased dependency on eyeglasses or contact lenses.

GLARE AND STARBURSTS: I may experience bothersome light sensitivity, glare, halos, or starbursts from light sources, particularly in the first few months after this procedure. This can limit my ability to drive, particularly at night. These symptoms generally resolve in 3–6 months but can persist indefinitely.

CONTACT LENS INTOLERANCE: If I want to wear contact lenses after this procedure, in some cases I may not be able to do so because of changes to the shape of my eye. I understand that, with rare exceptions, my doctor will not want me to wear contact lenses for at least 6 months after the LVC procedure.

RARE COMPLICATIONS: Rarely, a serious complication may occur as a result of this procedure, such as an infection inside the eye, a corneal ulcer, corneal swelling, inflammation of the eye, corneal scarring, decreased vision, persistent pain, or irregular healing. While many of these complications are treatable with restoration of good vision, LVC can result in partial or complete loss of vision in the eye. Other rare problems include recurrent erosions of the corneal surface, with episodes of a sharp, gritty feeling in the eye, drooping of the upper eyelid, and double vision. I understand that the long-term risks and effects of PRK surgery beyond 3 years are unknown.

PAIN: I may experience pain for up to 3 days.

Initials: _____

DRIVING: I must be accompanied home after treatment and must not drive. After the first follow-up appointment, I will be advised of the period to refrain from driving.

WORK: I may return to work 2–3 days after the treatment.

WOMEN ONLY: I am not pregnant or nursing and am not planning to become pregnant for the next 12 months. If it is possible that I am pregnant, then I will take a home pregnancy test to ascertain that I am not pregnant because pregnancy could adversely affect my treatment result. If the results of the test are positive, I will not undergo treatment until the results are proven incorrect or I will reschedule the treatment for after the pregnancy. If I become pregnant in the 6 months following treatment, I will notify my eye doctor immediately.

OTHER ISSUES:

I acknowledge that it is not possible to cover all the associated and nonassociated risks of a surgical intervention. I am aware that in the practice of medicine, other unexpected risks or complications may occur. I also understand that there may be unknown complications of LVC.

I understand that I will be sedated and agree not to drive a car until the next day after the procedure. I understand that I must have someone accompany me home immediately after the laser procedure.

I understand that my doctor may recommend the use of a bandage contact lens to make me more comfortable during the first few days after surgery, I am also aware that this intervention increases the chance that I may develop an eye infection, although this is still quite rare.

I understand that my doctor may recommend the use of steroid eye drops for weeks or in some cases months after my LVC procedure. I understand that the use of such medication increases the risk of infection, intraocular pressure elevation (glaucoma), and cataract formation.

I understand that I may be videotaped and/or audiotaped during this procedure. It has been explained to me that these tapes will be used for teaching and/or research purposes only and that my identity will not be disclosed.

In signing this consent form for laser vision correction, I am stating that I have read this informed consent (or it has been read to me) and I fully understand it and the nature, purpose, and possible risks of LVC. Furthermore, I have had all my questions answered by my surgeon and his or her staff to my satisfaction.

I have read and understand the contents of the LVC Patient Information booklet.

I voluntarily give my authorization and consent to the performance of Laser Vision Correction on my (right) or my (left) eye [circle one] by my physician and/or his/her associates assisted by hospital personnel and other trained persons as well as the presence of observers.

My personal reason for choosing to have PRK surgery are as follows:

_____

_____

Patient's Signature: _____   Date: _____

Surgeon's Signature: _____   Date: _____

I have been offered a copy of this consent form (Please initial) _____

Doctor's Order Sheet

MEDICATIONS

1. Valium 10 mg x 1 PO

2. Pilocarpine 1%
   One drop x 2 on arrival
   OD   OS

3. Polytrim drops
   One drop x 2 on arrival
   OD   OS

DISCHARGE MEDICATIONS

1. Voltaren 0.1%
   One drop q.4 hours while awake
   OD   OS

2. Dexacidin
   Apply q.4 hours while awake
   OD   OS

3. Percocet
   One tablet PO prn q. 4–6 hours
   (#6)

PRE-OP ORDERS

<u>Diagnosis:</u>   Myopia

<u>Procedure:</u>   Excimer PRK OD   OS
                  Excimer PTK OD   OS

<u>Vitals on Arrival:</u>

Allergies:

Mark brow   OD   OS   ( )

Informed Consent Signed: ( )

Driver Present   ( )

Prescription Slips Ready   ( )

POST-OP ORDERS

Bandage contact lens   OD   OS

Follow-up Appointment(s) on: _____

with: Dr. _____

Location: _____

Signature of Physician: _____ Date: _____

Preoperative Patient Data

Patient Name: _____

D.O.B.: _____ Sex: MALE / FEMALE   Operative Eye: OD / OS

Procedure: Photorefractive Keratectomy / Phototherapeutic Keratectomy

VAsc: _____   VAcc: _____   Prior Ocular Surg.: _____

Corneal Haze: _____   Vertex Distance: _____ mm

Manifest Refraction: _____   Manifest S.E.: _____

Cyclo Refraction: _____   Cyclo S.E.: _____

Keratometry: _____   Mean Keratometry: _____

Desired Correction: –_____

Epi Removal: Mechanical   /   Etoh   /   Laser + Mechanical

Fixation Method: Self   /   Thornton   /   Suction   /   Forceps

PTK ONLY

Treatment Zone Diameter: _____ mm Stromal Depth: _____

Treatment Zone Diameter: _____ mm Stromal Depth: _____

Treatment Zone Diameter: _____ mm Stromal Depth: _____

Transition (peripheral blend) Zone Diameter: _____   Pulses: _____

(Note: Maximum allowable stromal depth treatment = 250 μm for PTK)

Surgeon's Signature: _____   Date: _____

REFRACTIVE SURGERY POST-OPERATIVE REPORT

Patient Name _____ Age _____   Affiliate Doctor _____

Patient Address _____   Date of Report _____

City _____ State _____ Zip _____

▶ **Patient Comments:** _____

   Interval History: _____

	OD	OS
▶ **Surgery(s) Performed:**	_____	_____
Date(s) of Surgery:	_____	_____

▶ **Refractive Status & Ocular Examination**   Date: _____

	OD	OS
Uncorrected Visual Acuity:	dist ___ near ___	dist ___ near ___
% of time Wearing Corrective Eyewear:	dist ___ near ___	dist ___ near ___
Manifest Refraction:	_____ / ___ VA	_____ / ___ VA
Keratometry:	_____ / _____ @ _____	_____ / _____ @ _____
IOP:	_____	_____
Slit Lamp:	_____	_____
Glasses or CL Prescribed:	_____	_____
Ocular Meds:	_____	_____

▶ **Impression/Comments:** _____

_____

_____

_____

▶ **Next Follow-Up Visit:** Date: _____   Doctor: _____

▶ **Signed:** _____

Index

Index

Note: Page numbers in *italics* refer to figures; those followed by "t" refer to tables.